9H220 0X

AF675286

Nelson Yuan-sheng Kiang

Brain Mechanisms in Mental Retardation

UCLA FORUM IN MEDICAL SCIENCES

EDITORIAL BOARD

Mary A. B. Brazier, Editor-in-Chief

Nathaniel A. Buchwald
Carmine D. Clemente
Louise M. Darling
John L. Fahey
Victor E. Hall
James V. Maloney
Carl M. Pearson
Charles H. Sawyer
Emil L. Smith
Reidar F. Sognnaes
W. Eugene Stern
Bradley R. Straatsma
Emery Zimmerman

UCLA FORUM IN MEDICAL SCIENCES
NUMBER 18

Brain Mechanisms in Mental Retardation

EDITED BY

NATHANIEL A. BUCHWALD
Mental Retardation Research Center, Brain Research Institute, and
Departments of Anatomy and Psychiatry
University of California Los Angeles
Los Angeles, California

MARY A. B. BRAZIER
Brain Research Institute
University of California Los Angeles
Los Angeles, California

Proceedings of a Conference in the Series on Mental Retardation
Sponsored by The National Institute of Child Health and Human Development
Mental Retardation Research Centers Series

ACADEMIC PRESS New York San Francisco London 1975

A Subsidiary of Harcourt Brace Jovanovich, Publishers

COPYRIGHT © 1975, BY ACADEMIC PRESS, INC.
ALL RIGHTS RESERVED.
NO PART OF THIS PUBLICATION MAY BE REPRODUCED OR TRANSMITTED IN ANY FORM OR BY ANY MEANS, ELECTRONIC OR MECHANICAL, INCLUDING PHOTOCOPY, RECORDING, OR ANY INFORMATION STORAGE AND RETRIEVAL SYSTEM, WITHOUT PERMISSION IN WRITING FROM THE PUBLISHER.

ACADEMIC PRESS, INC.
111 Fifth Avenue, New York, New York 10003

United Kingdom Edition published by
ACADEMIC PRESS, INC. (LONDON) LTD.
24/28 Oval Road, London NW1

Library of Congress Cataloging in Publication Data
Main entry under title:

Brain mechanisms in mental retardation.

(UCLA forum in medical sciences ; v. 18)
Includes bibliographies and indexes.
1. Mental deficiency–Congresses. 2. Brain–Congresses. I. Buchwald, Nathaniel A. II. Brazier, Mary Agnes Burniston, (date) III. United States. National Institute of Child Health and Human Development. IV. Series. [DNLM: 1. Mental retardation–Physiopathology–Congresses. 2. Neurophysiology–Congresses. W3 U17 no. 18 1974 / WM300 B8145 1974]
RC570.B72 616.8'588 75-3581
ISBN 0-12-139050-X

PRINTED IN THE UNITED STATES OF AMERICA

Contents

List of Contributors and Participants

Names of contributors to this volume are marked with an asterisk.

***Anthony M. Adinolfi,** Mental Retardation Research Center and Neuropsychiatric Institute, University of California Los Angeles, Los Angeles, California 90024

***Joseph Altman,** Department of Biological Sciences, Purdue University, West Lafayette, Indiana 47906

***June E. Ayling,** Mental Retardation Research Center and Department of Biological Chemistry, University of California Los Angeles, Los Angeles, California 90024

***Robert E. Barrett,** Department of Neurology, College of Physicians and Surgeons, Columbia University, New York, New York 10032

***John Blass,** Mental Retardation Research Center, University of California Los Angeles, Los Angeles, California 90024

Mary A. B. Brazier, Editor for the UCLA Forum in Medical Sciences, Brain Research Institute, University of California Los Angeles, Los Angeles, California 90024

***G. A. M. Breen,**[1] Mental Retardation Research Center and Department of Anatomy, University of California Los Angeles, Los Angeles, California 90024

***Jennifer S. Buchwald,** Mental Retardation Research Center and Department of Physiology, School of Medicine, University of California Los Angeles, Los Angeles, California 90024

***N. A. Buchwald,** Mental Retardation Research Center, Brain Research Institute, and Departments of Anatomy and Psychiatry, University of California Los Angeles, Los Angeles, California 90024

***Gerald Cohen,** Department of Neurology, College of Physicians and Surgeons, Columbia University, New York, New York 10032

***Lucien Côté,** Department of Neurology, College of Physicians and Surgeons, Columbia University, New York, New York 10032

[1] Present address; Molecular Biology Department, Roswell Park Memorial Institute, Buffalo, New York 14203.

***J. de Vellis,** Mental Retardation Research Center and Department of Anatomy, University of California Los Angeles, Los Angeles, California 90024

***Marc A. Dichter,**[2] Department of Medicine, Beth Israel Hospital, Boston, Massachusetts 02215

***John Dobbing,** Department of Child Health, University of Manchester, Manchester, England

***Albert Dorfman,** Joseph P. Kennedy, Jr., Mental Retardation Research Center, Department of Pediatrics, Pritzker School of Medicine, The University of Chicago, Chicago, Illinois 60637

***Philip E. Duffy,** Department of Neurology, College of Physicians and Surgeons, Columbia University, New York, New York 10032

***D. R. G. Fuller,** Mental Retardation Research Center, University of California Los Angeles, Los Angeles, California 90024

***John Garcia,** Department of Psychology, University of California Los Angeles, Los Angeles, California 90024

***Patricia S. Goldman,** Laboratory of Psychology and Psychopathology, National Institute of Mental Health, Bethesda, Maryland 20014

***Richard Heikkila,** Department of Neurology, College of Physicians and Surgeons, Columbia University, New York, New York 10032

***Alfred Heller,** Department of Pharmacological and Physiological Sciences, The University of Chicago, Chicago, Illinois 60637

***Philip C. Hoffmann,** Department of Pharmacological and Physiological Sciences, The University of Chicago, Chicago, Illinois 60637

***Chester D. Hull,** Mental Retardation Research Center, Brain Research Institute, and Departments of Anatomy and Psychiatry, University of California Los Angeles, Los Angeles, California 90024

***Peter R. Huttenlocher,** Department of Pediatrics, The University of Chicago, Chicago, Illinois 60637

David L. Joftes, National Institute of Child Health and Human Development, Bethesda, Maryland 20014

***Seymour Kaufman,** Laboratory of Neurochemistry, National Institute of Mental Health, Bethesda, Maryland 20014

***Hayato Kihara,** The Neuropsychiatric Institute, Pacific State Hospital, Research Group, Pomona, California

***Anne Kitsikis,** Department of Physiology, School of Medicine, Laval University, University City, Quebec, Canada

James L. Lessard, Children's Hospital Medical Center, Cincinnati, Ohio

***M. S. Levine,** Department of Psychiatry, University of California Los Angeles, Los Angeles, California 90024

***Gary Lynch,** Department of Psychobiology, University of California Irvine, Irvine, California 92664

***J. F. McGinnis,** Mental Retardation Research Center and Department of Anatomy, University of California Los Angeles, Los Angeles, California 90024

***Luis Marco,** Department of Neurology, College of Physicians and Surgeons, Columbia University, New York, New York 10032

***Robert J. Marcus,** Mental Retardation Research Center and Department of Psychiatry, University of California Los Angeles, Los Angeles, California 90024

[2] Present address: Department of Neurology, Beth Israel Hospital, Boston, Massachusetts 02215.

*__Catherine Mytilineou,__ Department of Neurology, College of Physicians and Surgeons, Columbia University, New York, New York 10032

*__James Olds,__ Division of Biology, California Institute of Technology, Pasadena, California 91109

*__George Popják,__ Mental Retardation Research Center and Department of Biochemistry, University of California Los Angeles, Los Angeles, California 90024

*__Dominick P. Purpura,__ Rose F. Kennedy Center for Research in Mental Retardation and Human Development, Albert Einstein College of Medicine, Bronx, New York 10461

*__Pasko Rakic,__ Department of Neuropathology, Harvard Medical School, and Department of Neuroscience, Children's Hospital Medical Center, Boston, Massachusetts 02115

*__Guenter Rose,__ Mental Retardation Research Center, University of California Los Angeles, Los Angeles, California 90024

Fred E. Samson, Ralph L. Smith Mental Retardation Research Center, University of Kansas, Kansas City, Kansas

Richard J. Schain, Mental Retardation Research Center, University of California Los Angeles, Los Angeles, California 90024

*__S. Stefan Soltysik,__ Mental Retardation Research Center, University of California Los Angeles, Los Angeles, California 90024

*__John F. Tallman,__ Developmental and Metabolic Neurology Branch, National Institutes of Health, Bethesda, Maryland 20014

George Tarjan, Director of Mental Retardation and Child Psychiatry Program, Neuropsychiatric Institute, University of California Los Angeles, Los Angeles, California 90024

*__Thomas A. Tedesco,__[3] Department of Human Genetics, University of Pennsylvania School of Medicine, Philadelphia, Pennsylvania 19104

*__Virginia M. Tennyson,__ Department of Pathology, Division of Neuropathology, and Department of Neurology, College of Physicians and Surgeons, Columbia University, New York, New York 10032

*__Jaime R. Villablanca,__ Mental Retardation Research Center and Department of Psychiatry, University of California Los Angeles, Los Angeles, California 90024

Lesnick E. Westrum, Child Development and Mental Retardation Center, University of Washington, Seattle, Washington

*__Charles D. Woody,__ Mental Retardation Research Center, University of California Los Angeles, Los Angeles, California 90024

Stephen Zamenhof, Department of Microbiology and Immunology, University of California Los Angeles, Los Angeles, California 90024

[3] Present address: Department of Pediatrics, University of South Florida, College of Medicine, Tampa, Florida 33620.

Foreword

This volume has been sponsored jointly by the Mental Retardation Program of the National Institute of Child Health and Human Development and by the University of California Los Angeles Forum in Medical Sciences. For the N.I.C.H.D. Mental Retardation Program, it is the fourth book based on conferences organized by one of the twelve Mental Retardation Research Centers. The staff of the Mental Retardation Program has enthusiastically supported the Centers' Research Series volumes. In particular, Dr. Theodore Tjossem, Director of the Mental Retardation Program, Dr. Michael J. Begab, Head, Mental Retardation Research Centers, and Dr. David Joftes, Biomedical Sciences Administrator, provided encouragement and support for this volume. Dr. Joftes, in addition, devoted much hard work prior to and during the conference which provided the material for our book.

The Mental Retardation Research Centers have been set up at major universities throughout the United States. They were designed to conduct research directed toward an understanding of mental retardation and related aspects of human development. The Mental Retardation Research Center at UCLA is a multidisciplinary organization whose interests extend from anthropological and sociological investigations of cross-cultural aspects of mental retardation to molecular chemical studies of membrane phenomena related to metabolic deficiencies which underlie the most severe cognitive abnormalities. The UCLA Center is housed in a four-story addition to the preexisting UCLA Neuropsychiatric Institute. It has an important adjunct research group at Pacific State Hospital in Pomona, California, where epidemiological studies of mental retardation and biochemical and neurophysiological research, requiring the presence of a population of retarded patients, are carried out. The Research Center is closely aligned with a sister unit devoted to clinical aspects of mental retardation and to interdisciplinary training of professionals in the field. The Clinical Unit and the Research Center comprise a broadly based Mental Retardation Program at UCLA. This program, founded and organized under the leadership of Dr. George Tarjan, represents UCLA's approach to the understanding, prevention, and treatment of the cognitive deficiencies which afflict several millions of American citizens.

This volume is the outgrowth of a conference held at Oxnard, California, in January, 1974. The purpose of this conference was to present and to discuss neurobiological findings which might lead to an understanding of basic processes underlying the phenomena of mental deficiency. Most of the data reported at Oxnard were derived from laboratory researches. However, several of the speakers, all with long histories of accomplishment in the laboratory, concentrated their presentations on research on human beings or examination of human pathological material.

The cosponsor of this volume, the UCLA Forum in Medical Sciences, was set up by Dr. Sherman Mellinkoff, Dean of the School of Medicine, to enable publication of research material reflective of the variety of investigative efforts at the UCLA Center for the Health Sciences. This is the eighteenth volume in the Forum Series. We are grateful to Dean Mellinkoff and to the Editorial Board of the Forum for their part in the production of this book. Most especially, thanks go to Doctor Mary A. B. Brazier, the efficient and understanding Editor-in-Chief of the UCLA forum, for her encouragement and expertise during the planning and carrying out of the entire project.

NATHANIEL A. BUCHWALD

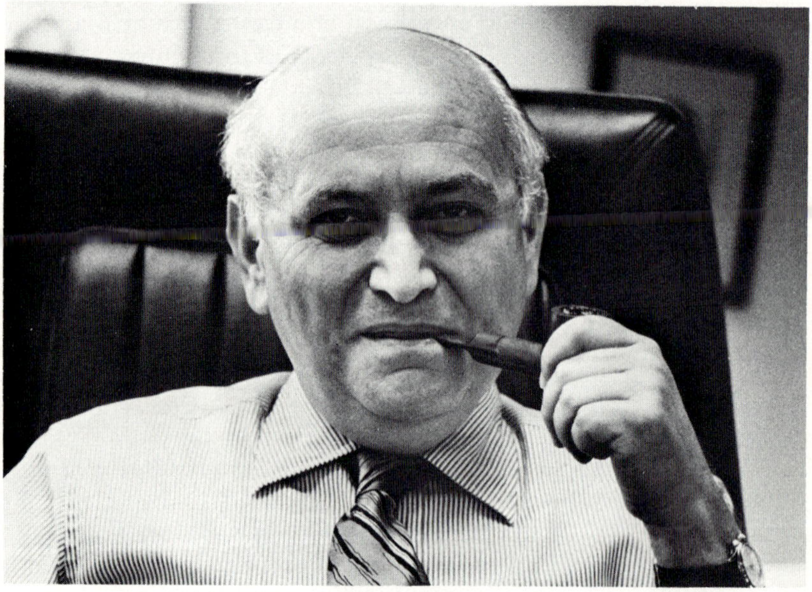

GEORGE TARJAN

Professor of Psychiatry and Director of Mental Retardation and Child Psychiatry Program, Neuropsychiatric Institute University of California Los Angeles Los Angeles, California

Welcoming Remarks

This conference seeks to examine what we know, at present, about the brain mechanisms underlying mental retardation. Progress in the study of mental retardation and human development has, of course, accelerated markedly since Congress legislated the establishment of the Mental Retardation Research Centers. These Centers and the availability of research support in developmental biology and chemistry for scientists not affiliated with the Centers have brought a whole new population of researchers and a whole new set of approaches to studies impinging on problems of mental retardation. The excellent quality of the workers attracted to this field is attested to by the people represented at this conference and by the difficulty in choosing them from the large pool of dedicated researchers in the field.

There is an old idea about scientists being uninterested in the real problems of the world, the idea that science is good for its own sake, and that if it is useful, so much the better, but that utility is not a requirement. I don't think most good scientists accept this view anymore. The fact that so many of you are devoting your efforts to problems of significance to human beings negates this idea. Even more important, I think, is the fact that you have been able to do so without sacrificing the level of your scientific efforts. Low grade scientific research, even if specifically aimed at a target such as mental retardation, has little value. It is heartening, indeed, that fine scientists have become interested in problems of mental retardation and related aspects of development. I look forward to your conference and to the time when the results of your efforts will impact upon the problems of the mentally retarded.

George Tarjan

Development of Neuronal Functions

1

Timing of Major Ontogenetic Events in the Visual Cortex of the Rhesus Monkey

PASKO RAKIC

Department of Neuropathology, Harvard Medical School, and Department of Neuroscience, Children's Hospital Medical Center, Boston, Massachusetts

A. INTRODUCTION

The neocortex in man has reached an enormous size and complexity which are approached only in some of the subhuman primates. The determination of the sequence and timing of the cellular events that occur during the development of this huge structure is essential for the understanding of the cortical abnormalities that might lead to mental retardation. Although many facts and basic concepts about neocortical development were initially obtained from the studies of the human embryos (23,31,76), the primary source of our knowledge in recent years has been experimental work in rodents. Laboratory animals were used in these studies because autoradiography and electron microscopy, two informative experimental procedures, cannot be applied to human embryos. These methods have provided important new information and confirmed some old hypotheses with more reliable data. Thus, a few basic concepts and developmental events illustrated schematically in Figure 1 are now rather well established: (a) cortical neurons are generated in proliferative zones close to the ventricular surface rather than in the cortex itself, (b) after their last division young neurons assume a bipolar shape and migrate radially to the cortical plate, (c) neurons generated first are ultimately situated in the deepest cortical layers as neurons generated later bypass earlier generated ones and assume more superficial positions, (d) the deeper neurons differentiate earlier than those situated more superficially, and (e) in rodents all cor-

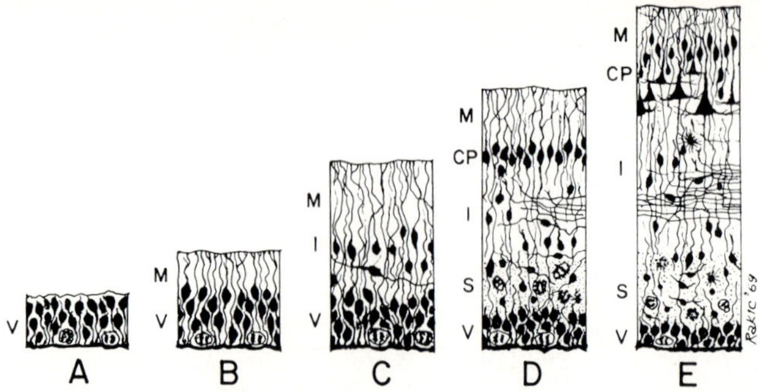

FIGURE 1. Schematic drawing of the major cellular events during the development of the mammalian cortical plate (CP). The basic principles of cell behavior during proliferation migration and differentiation stages apply, with some modifications, also to the development of other regions of the vertebrate central nervous system; this figure was used by the Boulder Committee (8) to illustrate recommended neuroembryonic terminology for ventricular (V), subventricular (S), intermediate (I), and marginal (M) zones. Further explanation in text.

tical neurons are generated during the last several days of gestation and in some species a short period after birth.

Most of these principles have been derived from the study of small lissencephalic brains. It is important to establish whether the neocortex in a large gyrencephalic brain like that of the man develops according to the same principles. At what time do cortical neurons originate during the protracted development of primate brain? Where is such an enormous number of neurons generated and what is the rate of their migration in such a large brain? What is the relationship between the time of origin and the position of neurons in the cortical laminae in the sharply layered primate neocortex? How is genesis of neurons related to the formation of fissures and gyri? The present study, which deals with these basic issues in the rhesus monkey, represents the first step in an ongoing, more detailed analysis of neocortical genesis in primates.

Several properties make the primary visual cortex of rhesus monkey a very suitable model for the study of corticogenesis. The horizontal stratification of neurons into separate layers in this species is very sharp (Figure 2B) and area 17 of Brodmann (9) can be distinguished from adjacent cortical areas at relatively early embryonic stages. Recent morphological (15,26,27,33,75) and physiological studies (e.g., 25,81) of the visual cortex in monkey have focused attention to this region. The protracted span of development increases the resolution of temporal sequences in neurogenesis (51,52) and the large size of the monkey fetus allows adequate fixation for electron microscopy (49,50).

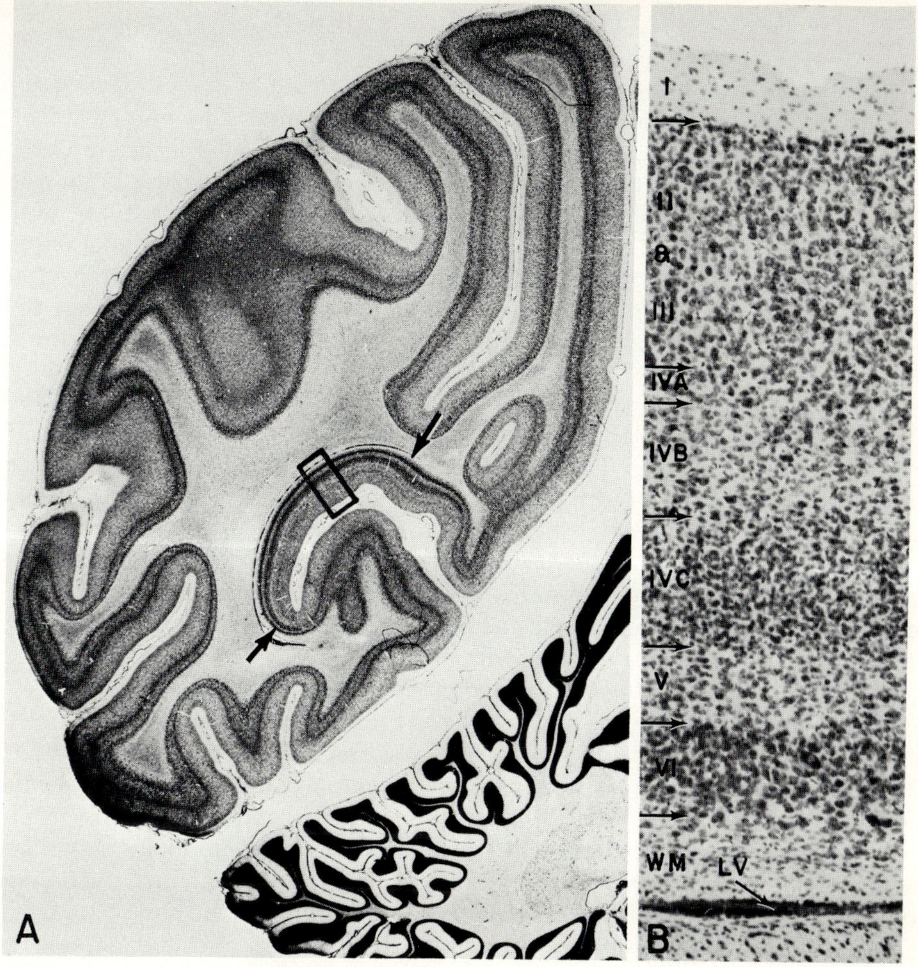

FIGURE 2. A. Coronal section through the occipital lobe and cerebellum of a 3-month-old monkey. The two arrows indicate a strip of visual cortex about 10 mm long in the depth of the calcarine fissure, where the time of neuron origin was analyzed in the present study. The area in the rectangle is enlarged in Figure 2B and on the left side of Figure 8. Thirty-micrometer section stained with cresyl violet. B. Cytoarchitectonics of the monkey visual cortex (area 17) in the depth of calcarine fissure indicated by rectangle in Figure 2A. Roman numerals indicate cortical layers according to the Brodmann's (9) classification adopted in this study. The photograph demonstrates the sharp delineation of the cortical layers in monkey with three clearly indicated horizontal fiber-rich strata (layers I, IVB, and V) dividing the cortex into three cell-dense zones. In this region white matter (WM) situated between cortex and an almost obliterated lateral ventricle (LV) is very thin.

B. TIME OF NEURON ORIGIN

The time of origin of a neuron cannot be determined by direct examination of histological preparations of the developing brain. The only available method which can provide reliable data on the time of neuron origin is ^{3}H-thymidine autoradiography (66). The procedure involves exposing brain cells to ^{3}H-thymidine at different developmental stages. Following an intravenous injection this nucleotide circulates in the bloodstream of the monkey for only a short time, that is, as a pulse, and becomes incorporated into the DNA of all dividing cells (41). Animals are killed at maturity and all "heavily labeled" neurons in the autoradiograms are those which were in the last cell division at the time of the injection. The minimum number of grains for classification of neurons as "heavily labeled" for primate specimens was arbitrarily determined for each specimen as half of the maximum grain count found in neurons of that specimen (51,52). Cells which have divided only once or twice after the injection are lightly labeled, whereas cells which had their last division before injection as well as all cells which have diluted their radioactivity through many subsequent divisions are unlabeled. By injecting a series of pregnant animals, the time of origin of cortical neurons has been determined in several rodent species (2,6,18,65). The present autoradiographic study in the monkey brain represents the first analysis of the time of neuron origin of the neocortex in any non-rodent species.

Pregnant monkeys were injected once each with ^{3}H-thymidine at the fortieth embryonic day (E40) and at E45, E50, E54, E62, E70, E80, E90, E102, E120, and E140. Gestation age was based on the assumption that ovulation and conception occurred on the twelfth day of the menstrual cycle. Pregnancy in the rhesus monkey lasts 165 days. All fetuses were delivered normally and killed at 2 to 5 months of age. Most cortical cells have already attained their final position and can be classified as neurons or glia in these "juvenile" monkeys (52). Two additional monkeys were injected at the second and eighteenth postnatal days, respectively, and sacrificed in the third month. [For more details about primate autoradiography, see Rakic (51) and Nowakowski and Rakic (41).]

No heavily labeled neurons are present in the autoradiograms of the visual cortex in animals injected at E40* or after E102. However, all animals injected at intervening ages contained heavily labeled neurons in some layer of the

* No heavily labeled neurons were seen in the visual cortex of the "juvenile" monkey that had been exposed to ^{3}H-thymidine on E40 but a few lightly labeled neurons, located exclusively in the deepest part of the cortex, were found in this specimen (52). Since heavily labeled cells were found elsewhere in the same brain, these lightly labeled cortical neurons are probably the products of several cell divisions subsequent to the time of injection. Thus it is unlikely that any visual cortical neurons were born at E40. The first neuron of the visual cortex, therefore, may actually be generated somewhere between E40 and E45.

visual cortex. Only a few neurons are labeled by injection at E45 or E102; the rate of production of neurons for the visual cortex is at maximum in terms of number of labeled neurons per unit area of the cortex at E70. On the basis of this analysis it was concluded that the entire population of cortical neurons in the monkey's visual cortex is generated during the 2-month period from around E45 to E102 (52). It is of note that preliminary examination has shown that the neurons of other neocortical areas in the neocortex of rhesus monkey are generated during approximately the same period with only a slight shifting in the time from area to area (P. Rakic, unpublished). Although no neurons are labeled in animals injected during the last 2 months of gestation or after birth, numerous astrocytes were labeled throughout the cortex (see Section F).

In the course of the study it became apparent that histogenesis of primate neocortex differs in some quantitative and qualitative aspects from that of the previously studied rodent species. Some differences are purely numerical and relate to the larger size of the monkey cortex and to the longer time necessary for its development. This point is vividly illustrated in Figure 3 which demonstrates the dramatic growth of the monkey brain. When ^{3}H-thymidine is injected into the pregnant monkey at E48, the fetal brain is less than 1% of the volume to be attained by P90. Furthermore the fetal visual cortex is represented by a relatively smaller fraction of the total hemispheric surface than at P90: it actually enlarges several hundred times during the intervening months (P. Rakic, unpublished). Since neurons in the last cell division at E48 are later to be sought as heavily labeled cells at P90 in enormously expanded cortex, light microscopic analysis is literally "a search for a needle in the haystack." In mice, where the brain grows only 3–4 times in volume during the comparable developmental period (e.g., between E14 and P30), many more labeled neurons are encountered per section. The total time period of cortical neuron production in the monkey is 10 times longer than in rodents, 60 days in monkey (52) versus only 6 days in mice (2). Since *S* phase and the cell generation cycle last approximately the same time in all mammals examined so far (5,29,66), the percentage of cortical neurons expected to be labeled in adults after a single injection of ^{3}H-thymidine at embryonic ages should be 10 times smaller in monkeys than in mice. In practice, however, the percentage of labeled neurons is even smaller because of the briefer period during which ^{3}H-thymidine is available in the circulating blood of the pregnant monkeys compared to that in rodents (41) and, in addition, the effect of DNA turnover may be enhanced by the long survival time. The practical outcome is that a larger number of autoradiograms must be prepared and analyzed in the case of the monkey.

Other differences in the histogenesis of primate and rodent neocortex appear to be biologically more significant. For example, the fact that no new neurons are generated in the last two fetal months or after birth is surprising

tions of heavily labeled neurons (Figures 4–7) were recorded with the aid of a Zeiss microscope equipped with a calibrated drawing tube. To obtain semiquantitative data all heavily labeled neurons encountered with a strip of visual cortex 2.5 mm long selected randomly in the area of the calcarine fissure (Figure 2A) were recorded (52). The location of the cortical layers and the dis-

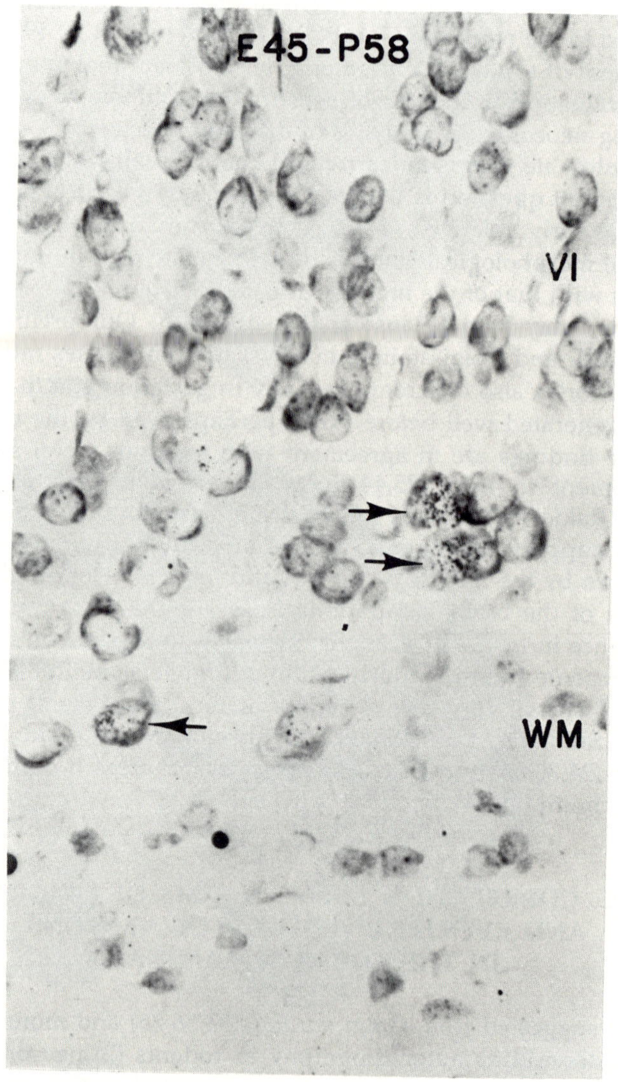

FIGURE 4. Photomicrograph of an autoradiogram of the visual cortex in a 58-day-old "juvenile" monkey that had been injected with ^{3}H-thymidine at forty-fifth embryonic day (E45–P58). Field shows deep portion of future cortical layer (VI) and underlying white matter (WM). Arrows point to the three heavily labeled neurons.

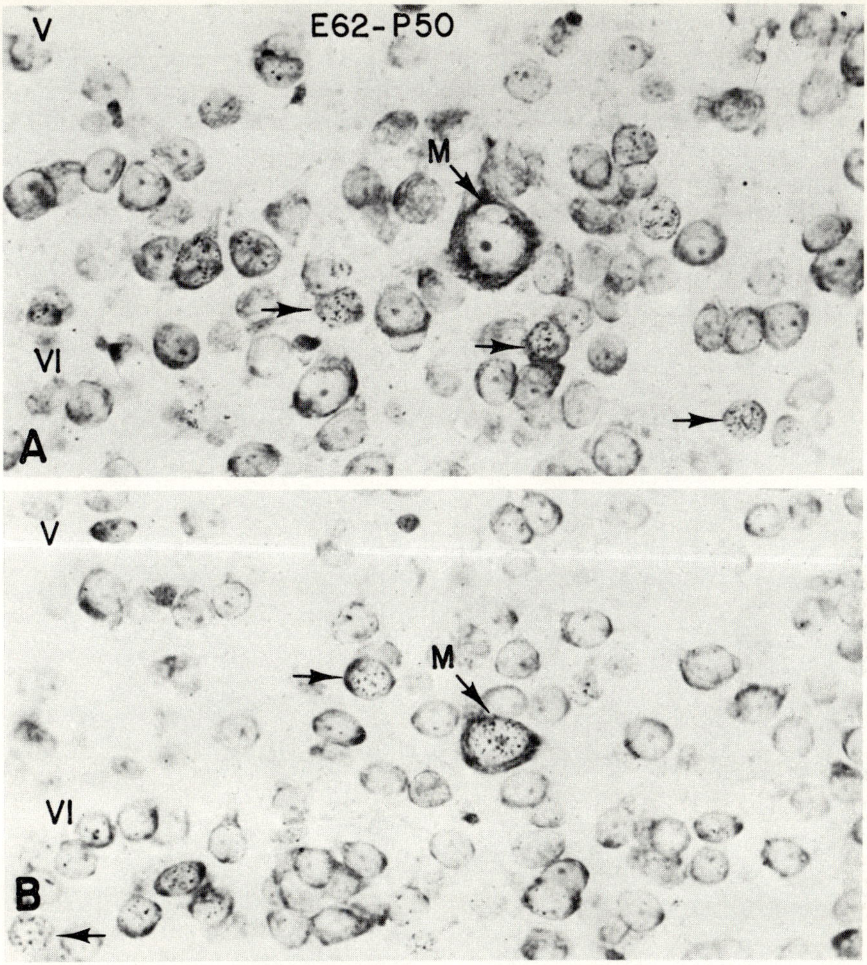

FIGURE 5. Autoradiograms of the monkey visual cortex in a 50-day-old "juvenile" animal that had been injected with ^{3}H-thymidine at sixty-second embryonic day (E62–P50). Roman numerals V and VI indicate cortical layers according to Brodmann's (9) classification as illustrated in Figure 1. Toluidine blue-stained autoradiograms are not suitable in general for further classification of neurons but so-called giant solitary pyramids of Meynert (36) are easily distinguishable (M). Some of these cells were labeled by injection at E62, as illustrated in B.

tance from the pial surface were precisely determined for each labeled cell and its position plotted along a radial vector perpendicularly traversing the cortical plate (Figure 8). The heavily labeled neurons in the brain of a "juvenile" monkey that had been injected at E45 (the earliest injection which labels heavily some neurons in the visual cortex) were localized in a narrow zone in the deeper portion of layer VI (Figure 4). Scattered neurons situated in the white matter, below layer VI, are also labeled in this specimen. In most fields a number of lightly labeled cells were detected *superficially* to the heavily labeled ones, an indication that the later generated cells take up more external positions. This was confirmed by the finding that heavily labeled neurons in the animal injected at E54 are located somewhat more *superficially*, although still within layer VI (Figure 8). The majority of neurons generated at E62 come to be situated in the upper two-thirds of layer VI, while some are localized in layer V (Figures 5 and 8). Cells with long efferent axons passing from area 17 to the midbrain (11), the so-called giant solitary pyramidal neurons of Meynert (36), situated in the rhesus monkey in layers V and VI were also labeled by an injection at E62 (Figure 5B).

An injection at E70 predominantly labels neurons that later take up resi-

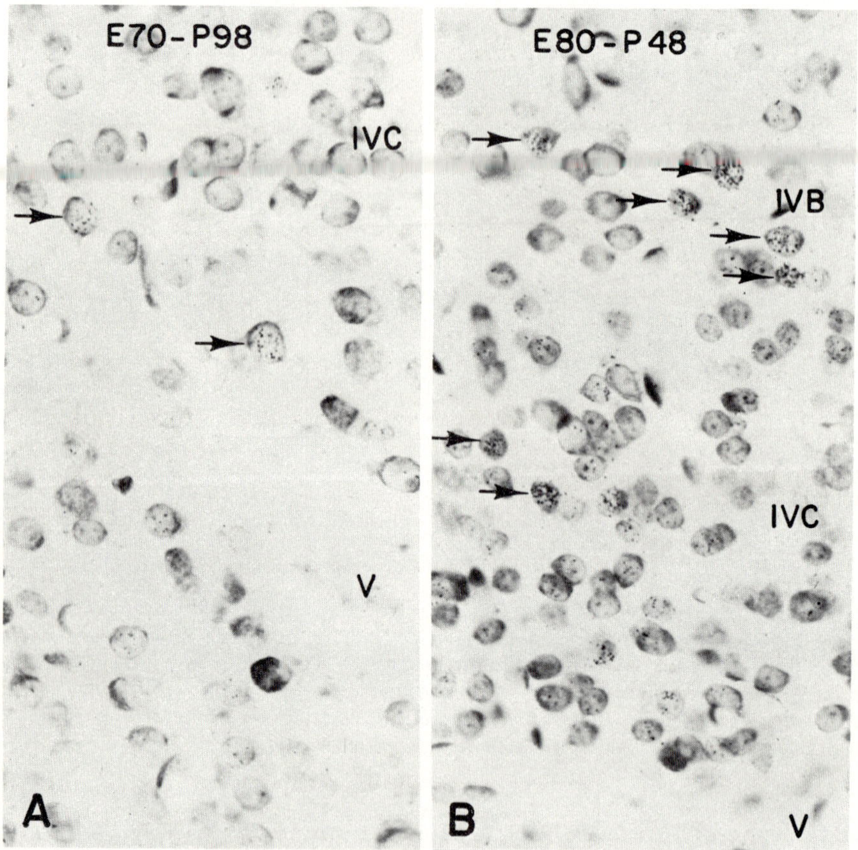

FIGURE 6. Photographs of autoradiograms of the visual cortex in two "juvenile" monkeys exposed to ^{3}H-thymidine at slightly different gestational ages. Animal illustrated in A had been injected at E70 and killed at P98; animal in B received ^{3}H-thymidine at E80 and was killed at P48. The overall distribution of labeled neurons within layers V, IVB, and IVC is different as graphically represented in Figure 8. Arrows point to heavily labeled neurons.

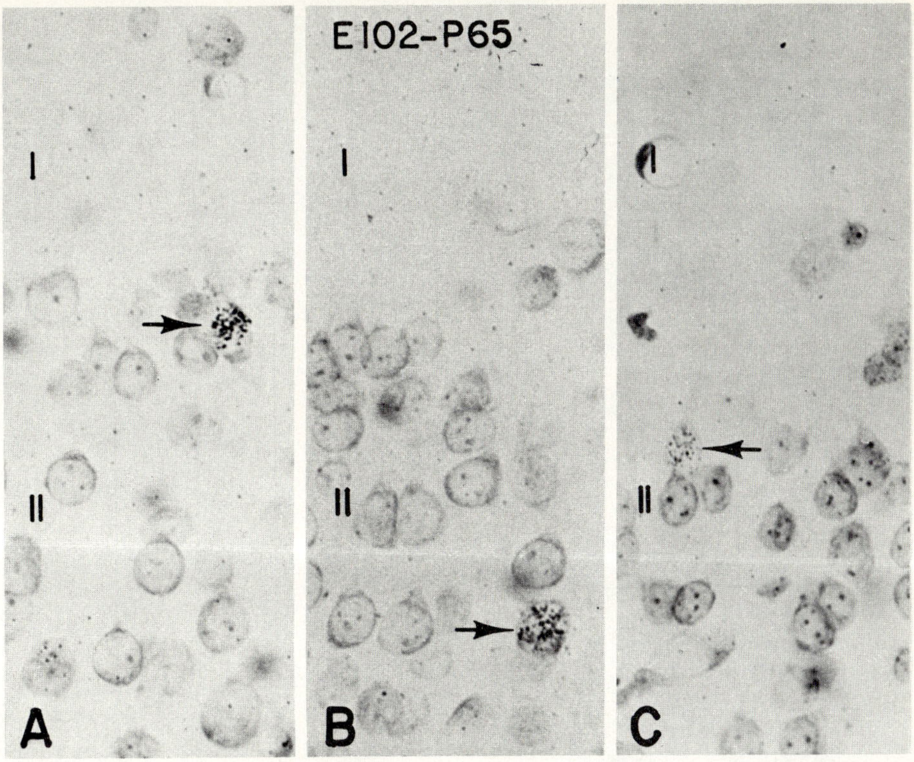

FIGURE 7. Autoradiograms of visual cortex in a 65-day-old "juvenile" monkey whose mother had been injected with ^{3}H-thymidine at E102. Photographs A to C depict the border zone between layers I and II. Only three heavily labeled cells (arrows) in more than 50 slides examined in this case were classified as neurons.*

dence in layer V but also many cells in layer IVC (Figures 5A and 8D). Neurons generated at E80 become distributed over the entire width of layer IV, with the highest concentration in layer IVB (Figures 5B and 8E); a few radioactive cells are situated in layer III. Injection at E90 labels neurons in both layers III and II (Figure 8F).

By E102 almost all neurons in the visual cortex have been born, since only a very few neurons* located at the very border between layers II and the cell-sparse layer I are labeled in the 3-month-old monkey that had been injected on this day (Figures 7 and 8G). However, in this specimen some small nuclei sit-

* Only three labeled neurons were found in 80 2.5-mm long strips of the visual cortex situated in the depth of calcarine fissure examined in 40 sections of a specimen injected with ^{3}H-thymidine at E102 and killed at P65. It was calculated that less than 1 in 10^{6} neurons was labeled in this specimen (52).

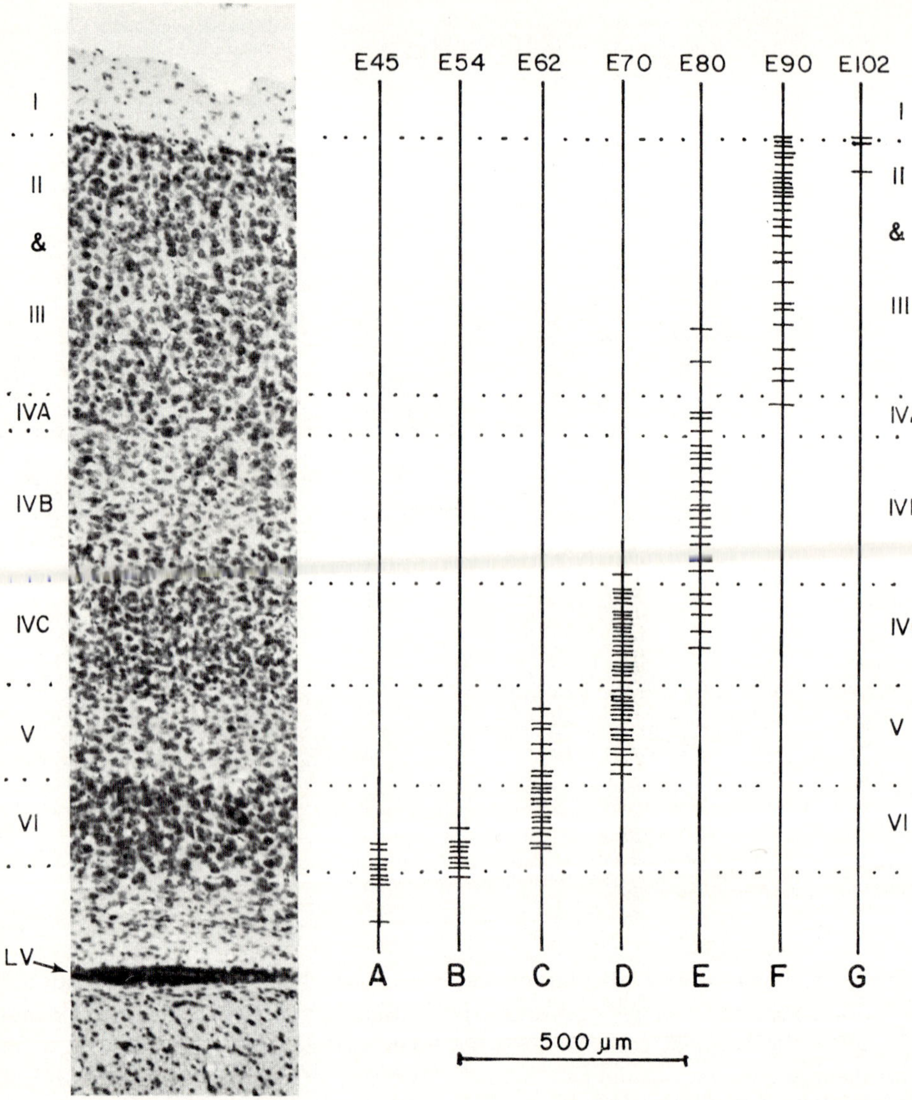

FIGURE 8. Diagrammatic representation of the positions of heavily labeled neurons in the visual cortex of juvenile animals which had been injected with ^{3}H-thymidine at various embryonic days (E) indicated at the top of each vertical line. [From Rakic (52) with permission of *Science*. Copyright 1974 by the American Association for the Advancement of Science.] On the left, for orientation, is a photomicrograph of a 30-μm cresyl violet-stained section photographed at the same magnification used for plotting of the labeled neurons with the drawing tube. Division into cortical layers, indicated by Roman numerals, are according to Brodmann (9). Horizontal markers on each vertical vector except G indicate positions of all heavily labeled neurons encountered in a randomly selected 2.5-mm long strip of the calcarine cortex. The three labeled neurons whose positions are represented in vector G were found only after examination of 80 areas of calcarine cortex each 2.5-mm wide in 40 autoradiograms from a single monkey. LV, Obliterated posterior horn of the lateral ventricle.

uated predominantly in the deeper half of the cortex are radioactive; these were classified as glial (see Section F and Figure 18).

The neurons in the plexiform layer I were not labeled in any of the specimens in this series (52). These neurons either are generated before E40, or they arise in some relatively short time interval between the ages sampled in the present series of animals.

As represented graphically in Figure 8, the position of heavily labeled neurons in the juvenile monkey's visual cortex correlates with the time of cell origin in the fetus; cells destined for deep cortical positions are generated first, and more superficial ones progressively later. Thus, most of the neurons of layer VI are born between E45 and E60, layer V between E60 and E70, layer IV between E70 and E80, and layers III and II between E80 and E100. As discussed in Section E, these data pertain only to the time of cell origin and do not reveal when the cells actually attained their permanent positions.

Autoradiographic results in this primate brain corroborate the "inside-out" pattern of cell disposition described previously in rodents (2,6,18,65). Comparison of the data in Figure 8 with those of a study in mice (10) shows that most of the simultaneously generated neurons in the monkey, particularly those generated early become eventually confined to relatively narrow strata of the cortex, i.e., the "inside-out" principle is more rigidly followed in the monkey. This may be the developmental basis for the sharper boundaries of cortical layers in the visual cortex of adult primates (52).

D. PLACE OF NEURON ORIGIN

The place where cortical neurons originate was studied in another series of experimental animals prepared for autoradiographic study. Pregnant monkeys were injected with ^{3}H-thymidine once each at E41, E45, E50, E58, E69, E87, E90, E120, and E140 and 1 hour later their fetuses were taken by hysterotomy and killed by vascular perfusion. In addition one neonatal monkey was killed at P3, 1 hour after ^{3}H-thymidine injection. Toluidine blue-stained, 1-μm plastic sections across either the entire thickness or only the inner half of the cerebral wall were prepared as described previously (49).

At E41 the cerebral wall in the occipital region is only 150 μm thick and consists of ventricular,* intermediate, and marginal zones (Figure 9A). One hour after exposure to ^{3}H-thymidine, labeled nuclei are concentrated in the outer portion of the ventricular zone, whereas mitotic figures are almost exclusively located at the ventricular surface (Figure 9A). Since animals injected at this age and killed at postnatal ages contained no labeled neurons (see above) presumably all the labeled nuclei at E41 belong to a population of proliferating cells

* Nomenclature recommendations of the Boulder Committee (8) have been adopted. See also Figure 1.

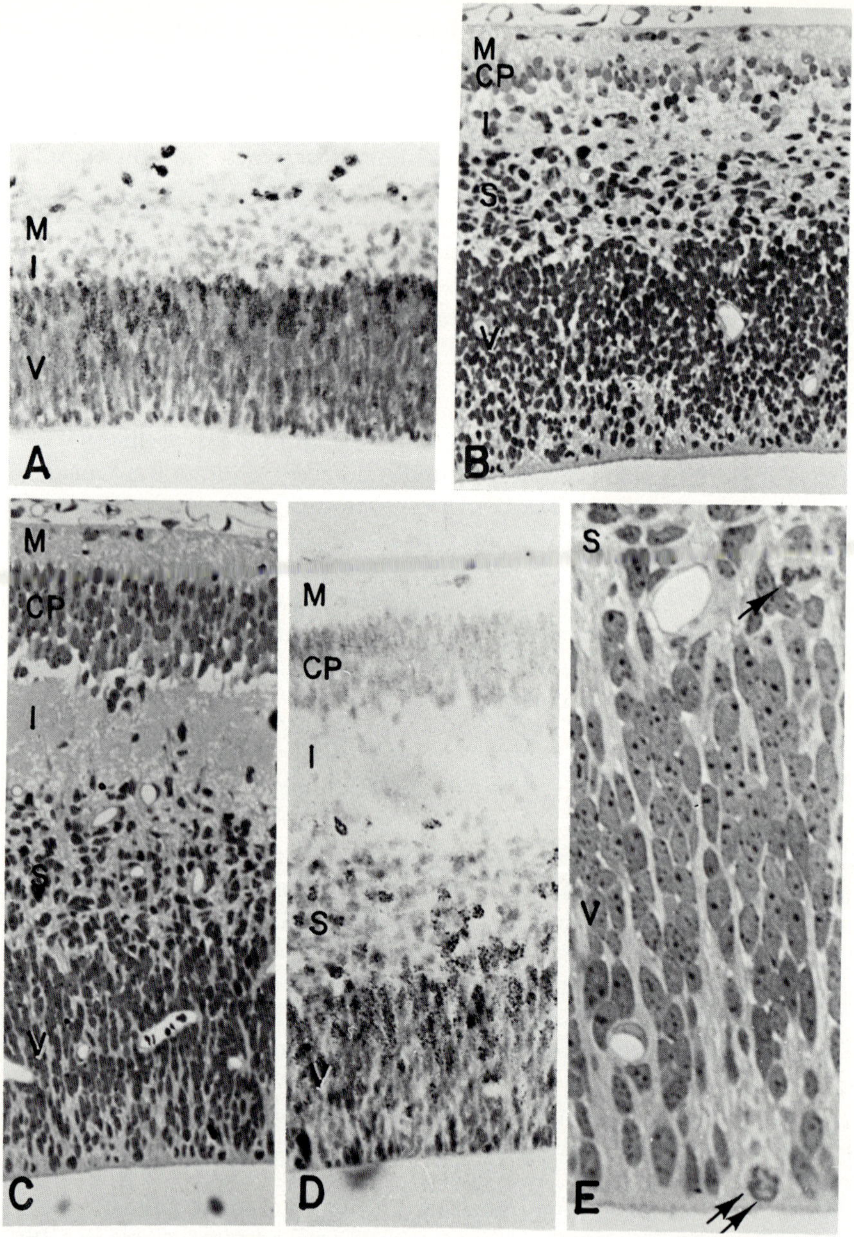

FIGURE 9. A. Autoradiograms of the cerebral wall at the posterior pole of the occipital lobe. ^{3}H-Thymidine was injected at E41, and the embryo was killed 1 hour later. Labeled cells are located in the outer third of the ventricular zone (V), very few are in the intermediate (I), marginal (M) zones or at the ventricular surface where numerous mitotic figures are present. B. Section across cerebral wall in the occipital lobe at E45. The fundamental embryonic layers are clearly delineated: ventricular (V), subventricular (S), intermediate (I), and marginal (M) zones, with incipient cor-

which are engaged in interkinetic nuclear migration, as observed in the ventricular zone of other species (61,62,67,77).

At E45 an incipient cortical plate consisting of 2–3 rows of neurons has formed in the posterior part of a cerebral vesicle (Figure 9B). This cortical plate of only a few square millimeters in surface area in the most posterior portion of the occipital lobe already contains some postmitotic neurons of the prospective visual cortex. Autoradiograms of this E45 specimen, killed 1 hour after ^{3}H-thymidine injection, reveal no labeled cells in the cortical plate itself although numerous radioactive nuclei are present in the ventricular zone. Small numbers of labeled nuclei are situated in a new cell band which develops between ventricular and intermediate zones. The presence of occasional mitotic figures in this location indicates that the proliferating cells in this band do not move to the ventricular surface for their division. This relatively inconspicuous layer of cells represent the beginning of the subventricular zone which later will become much more massive.

The only conspicuous morphological change in the cerebral wall during the next 5 to 10 days is the development of a distinctive and much thicker subventricular zone. At E53 it has approximately the same thickness as the ventricular zone and can be recognized as a layer of loosely organized cells located externally to a zone of more closely packed, vertically arranged, cells composing the ventricular zone (Figure 9C). Both ventricular and subventricular zones in the fetus injected at E53 and killed 1 hour later contain numerous labeled cells, whereas the cortical plate itself is not labeled (Figure 9D). One-micrometer plastic sections stained with toluidine blue demonstrate that mitotic figures of the cerebral wall (apart from those of endothelial cells) are confined exclusively to two well-defined locations, in the ventricular zone at the very surface of the lateral ventricle and throughout the subventricular zone (Figure 9E). These findings are in accord with established views of cell behavior in proliferative zones of the mammalian central nervous system. Ventricular cells during proliferative phases remain permanently attached to the ventricular surface to which the nucleus moves for division (21,22,61,67), whereas sub-

---

tical plate (CP) already developed. Tissue was fixed by intracardiac perfusion with a gluteraldehyde (1.25%)–paraformaldehyde (1%) mixture in phosphate buffer (pH 7.3), and by post-fixation in 2% OsO_4, embedded in Epon-Araldite, sectioned at 1 μm and stained with alkaline toluidine blue. C. Cerebral wall in the posterior region of occipital lobe at E53. Note the 2-fold increase in the thickness of the subventricular and intermediate zones and 4-fold increase in the width of the cortical plate as compared to specimen at E45 illustrated in B. Abbreviations and method of tissue preparation the same as in B. D. Autoradiogram made from a section at a comparable location in the opposite hemisphere of the specimen illustrated in C. This animal was injected with ^{3}H-thymidine at E53 1 hour before sacrifice. Labeled cells are concentrated in the outer third of the ventricular zone or scattered throughout subventricular zone—but none is present in the cortical plate. Abbreviations as in B. E. Higher magnification of the ventricular (V) and part of subventricular (S) zones. Mitotic figures in the cerebral wall are present exclusively at the ventricular surface (arrow) or throughout subventricular zone (double arrow).

ventricular cells do not contact either cerebral surface [Figure 16 and Rakic *et al.* (54)] and divide *in situ*.

Both ventricular and subventricular zones persist in parallel and produce numerous cells during the next 5 weeks as demonstrated in autoradiograms of the fetuses injected at E58, E69, E75, and E87 and killed 1 hour later. Apparently these two zones represent the only sources of cortical neurons since in these specimens the cortical plate itself contains very few labeled cells (Fig-

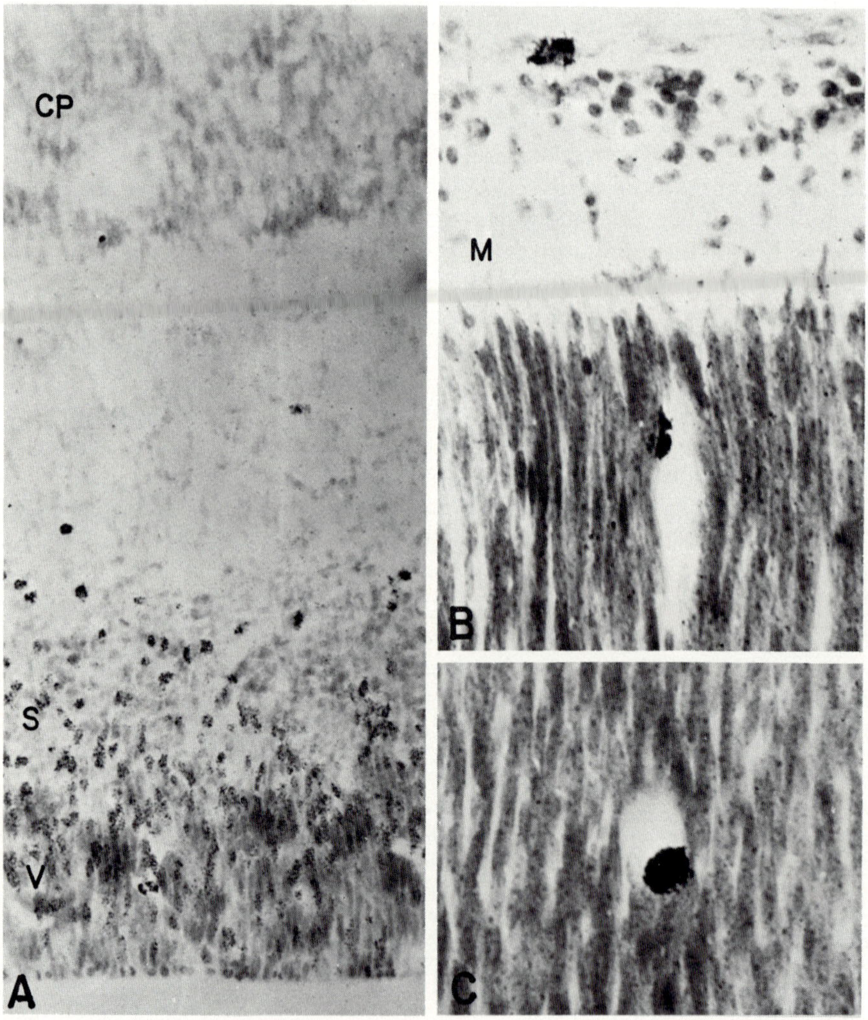

FIGURE 10. A. Autoradiogram of the cerebral wall in the region of visual cortex of a monkey fetus injected with ^{3}H-thymidine at E58 and killed 1 hour later. Labeled cells are located in the ventricular (V) and subventricular (S) zones but not in the intermediate zone or in the cortical plate (CP). Occasional radioactive nuclei which can be encountered within the cortex itself belong to endothelial cells as illustrated in B and C at higher magnification. M, Marginal zone.

ure 10A). Closer examination shows that the occasionally labeled nuclei scattered throughout the cortex in these specimens belong either to endothelial capillary cells (Figure 10B and C) or, particularly toward the end of this period, to cells of glial lineage (Figure 18). During this time period the subventricular zone gradually becomes relatively wider because the ventricular zone is narrowing. Both the number of mitotic figures (Figure 11A) and the relative number of labeled cells (Figure 11B) at later stages indicate that the subventricular zone produces a progressively larger number of cells than does the ventricular zone.

By E90, the ventricular zone becomes virtually exhausted so that thereafter the subventricular zone is the only source of additional neurons destined for the visual cortex. Indeed, in animals injected at E90 and killed 1 hour later the subventricular zone still contains many labeled cells. An apparent complication is that when injection is given at later stages, increased numbers of labeled cells are present also in the cortex itself, but these are classified as proliferating glial cells (see Section F and Figure 18). Thus, in animals injected at E120, E140, and P3 and killed 1 hour later, a few labeled cells are still present

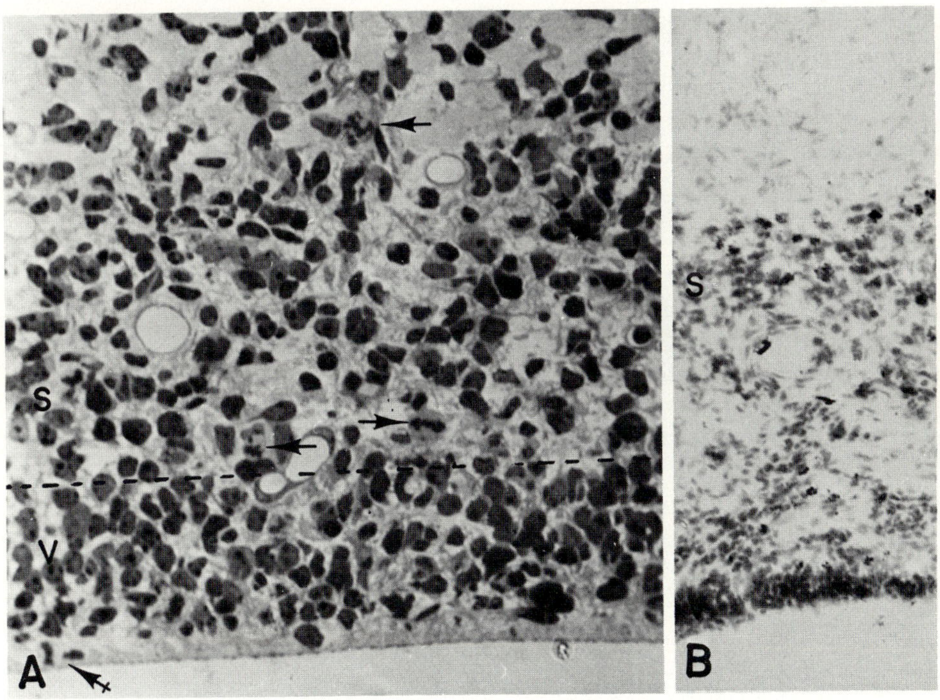

FIGURE 11. A. Photomicrograph of the inner part of the cerebral wall in the occipital lobe at E81. Ventricular zone (V) is attenuated and contains only a few mitotic figures (crossed arrow) compared to earlier stages. The subventricular zone (S) remains relatively wide and full of dividing cells (arrows). B. Autoradiogram of animal injected at E87 and killed 1 hour later. Most radioactive cells are in the subventricular zone (S).

in the vestige of the subventricular zone, and many more are found throughout the cortex. However, none of these are neuronal precursors, since in specimens injected at these ages and killed postnatally no neurons are labeled in the visual cortex (see Section B).

On the basis of these observations, it can be concluded that in the rhesus monkey, neurons of the visual cortex are generated in both the ventricular and the subventricular zones. However, the relative proportion of neurons generated in these two zones changes with time. At the earliest stages, neurons originate almost exclusively in the ventricular zone; later they are produced in both ventricular and subventricular zones, and by the end of the period of neurogenesis the subventricular zone becomes the predominant source of new cells. Further, it is not known what population of the proliferating ventricular cells is destined at any given stage to become neurons versus glia.

E. RATE AND MODE OF NEURONAL MIGRATION

Young neurons generated in the ventricular and subventricular zones eventually become displaced to the cortical plate. This process conventionally termed cell migration,* involves moving an enormous number of young neurons across increasingly longer distances from the proliferative zones to the external margin of the developing cortical plate. Disorders of neuronal migration in man may be responsible in part for cortical malformations such as microgyria, pachygyria, lissencephaly, and nodular ectopias (12), but these disorders may also cause more salient abnormalities undetectable by the usual pathological methods. Single gene mutation (10,53,68), X-ray irradiations (13,19,39), viruses (40), or drugs (32,78) may interfere with the process of production and migration of neurons in the mammalian telencephalon. Although such defects in neuronal migration to the neocortex probably contribute importantly to the etiology of mental retardation, the understanding of migration is fragmentary. A preliminary examination of the still incomplete series of autoradiograms from monkey fetuses provides some insights into this complex problem.

The migration rate of young neurons in the monkey cerebrum was studied

* In this report and in previous publications (47,48,49,53,68) the view has been adopted that until there is evidence to the contrary, "migration" is the most suitable term, whether the cell as a whole changes position [as in late stages of neocortical genesis (48,49)] or extends a cytoplasmic process outward toward and then parallel to the pia from an immediately postmitotic rounded form at the embryonic ventricular surface (21), or extends a process radially inward while holding its earlier generated axonal process in a fixed position [as in the case of the cerebellar granule cell (55)]. It would seem inappropriate, until more facts are available, to use different terms for the migration of an outward-directed process of a postmitotic ventricular cell along the surface of adjacent columnar ventricular cells (8), for the migration of a young cerebellar granule cell process and soma along a Bergmann fiber (47), or for the migration of a growing axon tip along a solid substratum *in vitro* (79).

in autoradiograms prepared from fetuses of various ages killed either 1 hour or 3, 7, or 14 days following ^{3}H-thymidine injection. In a fetus injected at E45 and killed at E48, almost all of the heavily labeled cells are found in the outermost stratum of the cortical plate. Only very few heavily labeled cells are seen at intermediate levels between ventricular zone and cortical plate. In a fetus injected at E46 and killed at E53 (Figure 12A) labeled cells form a horizontal band located in the middle of the cortical plate. External to the labeled cells lie several rows of weakly labeled or unlabeled cells which were generated following the thymidine injection. Therefore, at early stages young neurons move to the cortical plate relatively synchronously; most of them reach their destination in less than 3 days, and almost all within 7 days.

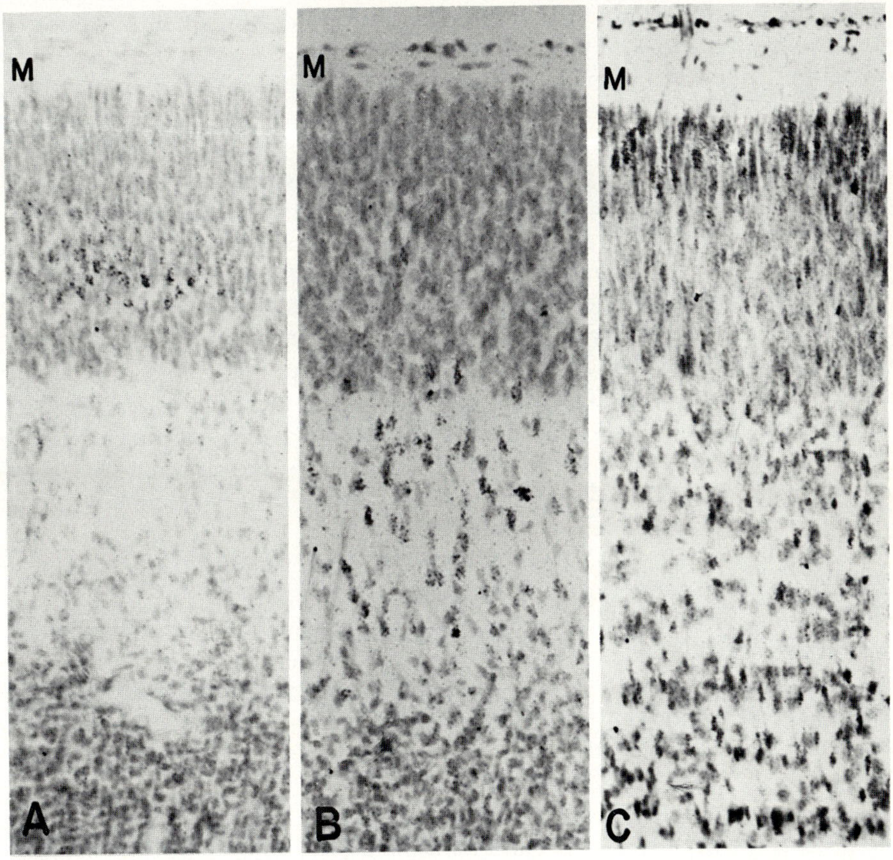

FIGURE 12. Autoradiograms of the cerebral wall in fetuses injected with ^{3}H-thymidine and killed at various times afterward. Photographs of the outer portion of the cerebral wall include molecular layer (M), cortical plate, intermediate zone, and portion of subventricular zone taken in all three fetuses at the comparable regions. Further explanation in text. A. E46–E53. B. E52–E55. C. E65–E72.

Examination of similarly prepared sections from slightly older monkey fetuses shows a considerable difference in the times when young neurons from a simultaneously generated set finally reach their permanent positions. For example, in a fetus injected at E52 and killed 3 days later at E55, only a few of the heavily labeled cells are found at their final destination in the superficial portion of the cortical plate.* Most heavily labeled cells are still located in the intermediate and subventricular zones. Apparent dissociation of cells into fast, synchronously migrating, and slow, asynchronously migrating classes is well demonstrated in a fetus injected at E65 and killed 7 days later at E72. In this specimen some labeled cells have attained their final position in the superficial stratum of the cortical plate but many are still in the intermediate zone (Figure 12C). Some neurons generated on E65 have reached their destination by E72 but the majority had not moved very far from their site of origin during the 7-day period. This difference in migratory behavior becomes even more conspicuous toward the end of corticogenesis. Thus, in the fetus injected at E92 and killed at E95 only an occasional cell has arrived at the superficial strata of the cortex (Figure 13A). Some labeled cells are passing through deep cortical layers (Figure 13B) and the majority still reside in the subventricular and intermediate zones (Figure 13C). Since in a fetus injected at E90 and killed at E97 many labeled cells are still situated in the subventricular and intermediate zones (Figure 13C), apparently at this age they take more than 7 days to arrive at their destination. The dynamics of cell movement and the exact time of arrival at the cortex will be determined when additional animals are prepared with longer intervals between injection and sacrifice.

Essentially similar changes in migration rates, but telescoped into a shorter time interval, have been observed during genesis of the rat neocortex (18). In this species at early stages (E14–E18) young neurons arrive at the cortical plate in about 2 days. However, many young neurons which originate toward the end of gestation (E19–E21) continue to migrate during the first week after birth. The first group of cells generated at E20 reach the cortex in about 3 days, the last in about 10 days. Thus the rate of arrival at the cortex among the simultaneously generated cells is variable.

If the time necessary for young neurons to reach the superficial portion of the cortical plate depends only on the length of the migration pathway, then all simultaneously generated cells should arrive synchronously at their destination. Yet at any given late stage of corticogenesis of the rhesus monkey, some cells reach their destination several times more rapidly than others. The

* The relative thickness of the lateral and medial cerebral wall is different at various fetal ages. For example at E70 the lateral cerebral wall of the occipital lobe is about two times thicker than the medial, and this difference increases to more than 4 times at E120. Since the time of the arrival of simultaneously generated neurons to the cortical plate is affected by the length of their pathway, the comparison of the autoradiograms in this study was made on roughly corresponding areas of the medioventral portion of the cerebral wall, which has an intermediate thickness.

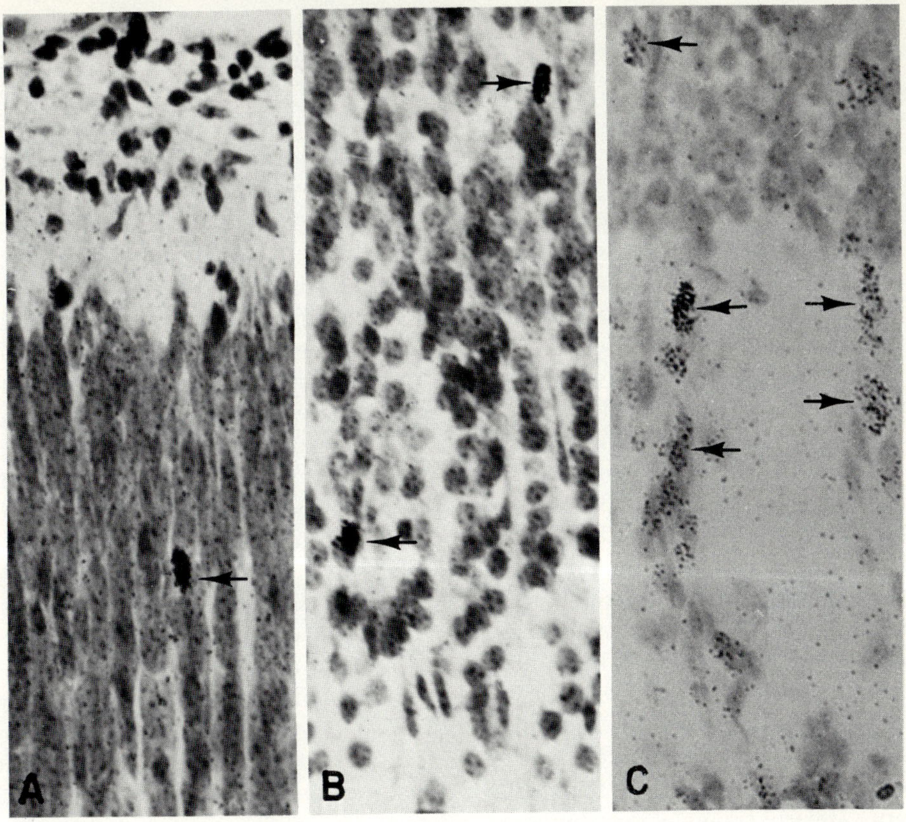

FIGURE 13. Autoradiograms of an animal injected at E92 and killed 3 days later at E95 to indicate position of heavily labeled cells (arrows). A. Molecular layer and superficial cortex. B. Deep cortex. C. Deep cortex and intermediate zone.

time of arrival might influence the final cell position in the cortical plate. Thus, neurons generated on a given day early in development come to occupy a relatively narrow zone of the mature cortex, while those generated at a given later age come to be distributed over a somewhat wider zone; also, neurons born 8 to 10 days apart may overlap somewhat in position along the radial axis [Rakic (52) and Figure 8].

One explanation for the wide distribution of cells generated simultaneously is that more slowly moving neurons reach the superficial portion of the cortex when it has already increased several hundred micrometers in thickness by the addition of many neurons, some of which were actually generated later but had migrated more rapidly (52). As a consequence the more slowly moving young neurons attain in the mature brain more superficial positions than the rapidly moving neurons generated simultaneously. At later developmental stages the difference in the rate of cell migration among simultaneously generated cell increases, as does the span of their distribution along the radial vectors across the cortex (Figure 8). A possible lengthening of the cell generation cycle at later ages (29) might also influence the time interval between injection and arrival of young neurons in the cortex. However, this effect is probably small because heavily labeled cells were located at various levels of the intermediate zones in fetuses killed 3 and 7 days after injection, thus indicating that cells already had divided. The times sampled in the present material are not suitable for distinguishing whether the difference in rate of cell arrival in the cortex is due to a differential migration rate or to the differential lags in initiation of migration. Why the difference in time of arrival to the cortex among simultaneously generated cells becomes apparent only at the middle and late stages of corticogenesis and is it in some way related to the mechanism of cell movement? These questions are considered below in the light of some studies on the mode of neuron migration.

One of the several mechanisms proposed to explain cell displacements within the central nervous system stems from the idea that the tissue is organized as a pseudostratified epithelium (61). Since the early neuroepithelium is composed of columnar epithelial cells which, at least in some phases of their intermitotic cycle, stretch from the ventricular to the external surface, it was suggested that the same arrangement might continue to exist at later developmental stages and that only the cell nucleus actually moves within the elongated but fixed cytoplasmic cylinder (7,38). Since during mitosis ventricular cells lose their external process (21,22,72), they would have to regrow and withdraw it alternatively during the cell generation cycle until finally the external process is used for nuclear translocation. This mechanism might apply at early stages of corticogenesis when the migration paths between ventricular and pial surfaces are relatively short.

In rhesus monkey fetuses at early stages, between E40 and E55, many bipolar cells whose nuclei are situated in the ventricular zone have a smooth radial process which spans the entire cerebral wall and terminates at the external surface in one or several endfeet (64). At these early stages of development, existing morphological methods do not provide features permitting classification of these cells as glial or neuronal precursors. Some of these radially oriented cells might indeed be postmitotic young neurons in which the nucleus eventually moves to a more superficial position as proposed by Morest (38). However, at slightly later stages, cells which span the entire cerebral wall assume the typical morphology of radial glial cells (Figures 14 and 19). Their somata are situated close to the ventricular surface, and have an elongated, radially oriented glial process which spans the full thickness of the developing cerebral wall [Schmechel and Rakic (64) and Section F of this chapter].

A different mechanism of cell migration has been postulated in rhesus monkey fetuses at late stages of corticogenesis (48,49). The migrating neurons appear to be relatively simple and smooth bipolar cells with a leading process

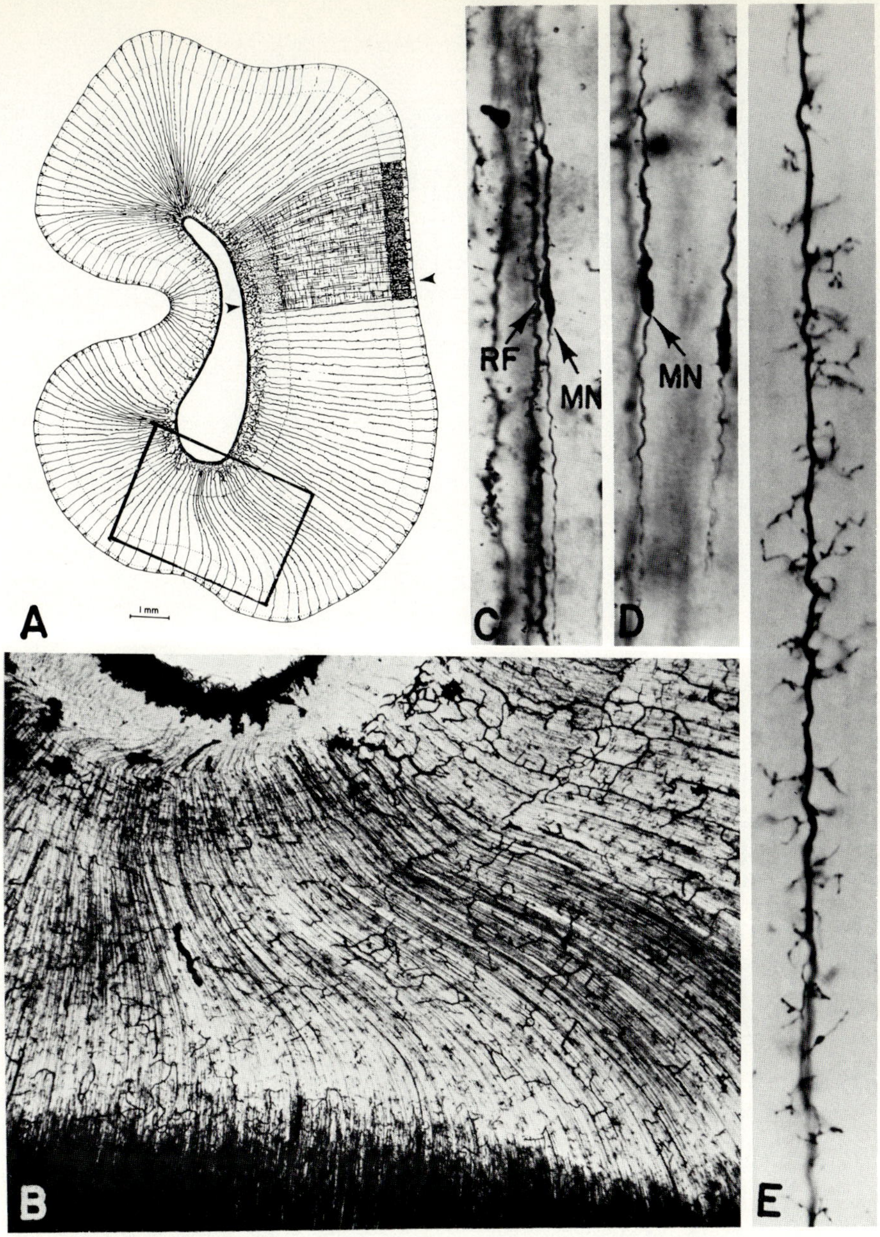

FIGURE 14. A. Camera lucida drawing of a Golgi-impregnated coronal section across the cerebral vesicles of a 97-day monkey fetus. From Rakic (49). Indentation on the left represents incipient calcarine fissure. The caliber of the radial fibers is slightly exaggerated in order to illustrate their arrangement at such a low magnification (scale equals 1 mm). Arrows indicate cerebral wall. B. Photomicrograph of the Golgi preparation used for the drawing in A taken from the area outlined by the rectangle. C and D. Photomicrographs of two migrating young neurons (MN) oriented parallel to radial glial fibers (RF) in 95-day monkey fetus. E. Photographically enlarged segment of the radial glial fiber passing through the intermediate zone. Note numerous lamellate expansions present at E95.

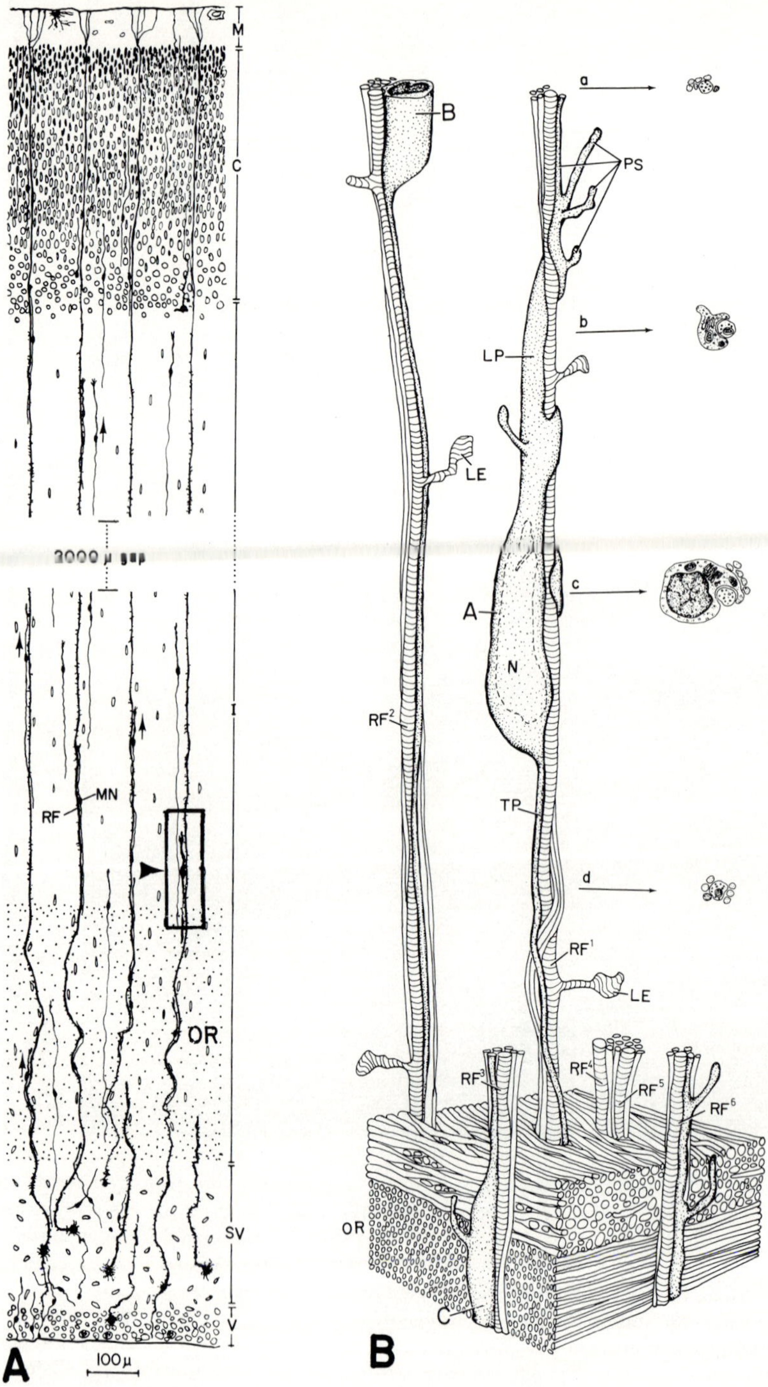
M
C
2000 μ gap
I
RF
MN
OR
SV
V
A
100μ
B
a
b
c
d
PS
LP
LE
A
N
RF2
TP
RF1
RF3
RF4
RF5
RF6
OR
C
B

whose length is only a fraction of the total migratory pathway of the expanded cerebral wall at these ages (Figure 14B). Electron microscopic examination of migrating cells suggests they find their way to the cortex by using radially oriented glial fibers as guides (48,49). Three-dimensional reconstruction of electron microscopic serial sections of 58-day fetal monkey cerebrum shows that both the trailing and the leading processes of some migrating cells are confined to the intermediate zone and do not approach either cerebral surface (54). Radial elements of the fetal cerebral wall are commonly organized in fascicles (Figure 15) consisting of one or two radial glial processes, the leading and trailing processes of several migrating neurons, and possibly afferent or efferent axons (49). The leading process of the migrating cell frequently branches and extends along more than one radial fascicle (Figure 16E). Such a process is probably capable of being retracted because, if its form and number were fixed, the cell would be unable to advance beyond fiber bundles lying transversely between its branches (Figure 16G).

Multiple neuronal processes are seen at a given level of the intermediate zone or the cortical plate since several neurons move in succession along a single radial path (Figure 15). Where they overlap, the later arriving neurons may be moving along the surfaces of their predecessors rather than along the glial fiber specifically (Figure 15B). As they enter the cortical plate the neurons that follow a given radial path become aligned in a single vertical column, an arrangement which is a prominent morphological feature of the fetal neocortex (Figure 17). The alignment of the migrating neuron along the radial glial fiber

---

FIGURE 15. A. Camera lucida drawing of the part of cerebral wall indicated by arrows in Figure 14A. Modified from Rakic (49). Composite illustration is combined from Golgi section (black profiles of cell images) and on adjacent section counterstained with toluidine blue (outlined profiles of cell nuclei). The middle 2000 μm of the intermediate zone, similar in structure to the sectors drawn, are omitted. The rectangle marked with an arrowhead shows the approximate position of the three-dimensional reconstruction in Figure 14B. Abbreviations: C, cortical plate; I, intermediate zone; M, molecular layer; MN, migrating neuron; OR, optic radiation; RF, radial fiber; SV, subventricular zone; V, ventricular zone. B. Three-dimensional reconstruction of migrating neurons, based on electron micrographs of semiserial sections. From Rakic (49). The reconstruction was made at the level of the intermediate zone indicated by the rectangle and arrowhead in Figure 15A. The subventricular zone lies some distance below the reconstructed area, whereas the cortex is more than 1000 μm above it. The lower portion of the diagram contains uniform, parallel fibers of the optic radiation (OR) and the remainder is occupied by more variable and irregularly disposed fiber systems; the border between the two systems is easily recognized. Except at the lower portion of the figure, most of these fibers are deleted from the diagram to expose the radial fibers (striped vertical shafts (RF^{1-6}) and their relationships to the migrating cells (A, B, and C) and to other vertical processes. The soma of migrating cell A, with its nucleus (N) and voluminous leading process (LP), are within the reconstructed space, except for the terminal part of the attenuated trailing process (TP) and the tip of the vertical ascending pseudopodium. Cross sections of cell A in relation to the several vertical fibers in the fascicle are drawn at levels "a" to "d" at the right side of the figure. The perikaryon of cell B is cut off at the top of the reconstructed space, whereas the leading process of cell C is shown just penetrating between fibers of the optic radiation (OR) on its way across the intermediate zone.

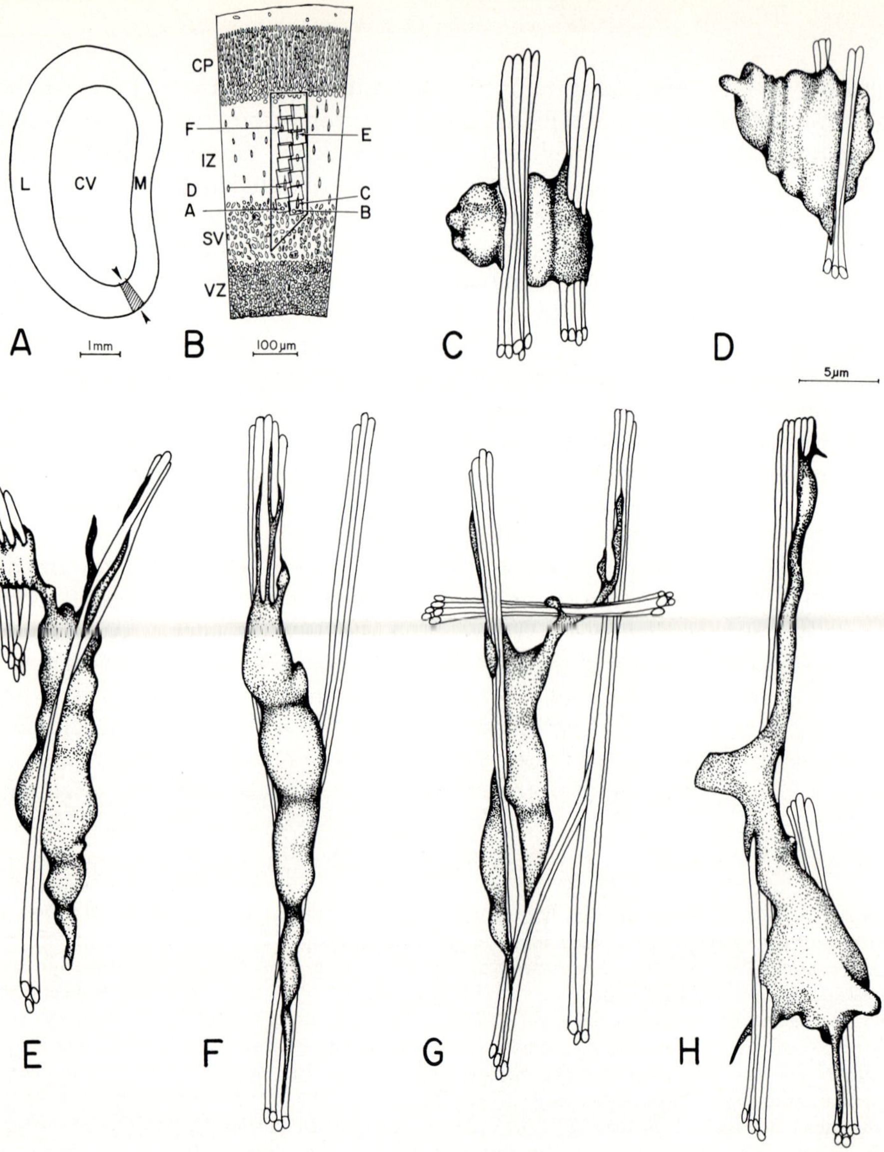

FIGURE 16. Computer-aided three-dimensional reconstruction of the cells in the occipital lobe of fetal monkey brain. Modified from Rakic *et al.* (54). A. Outline of a coronal section across the occipital lobe of a 58-day-old monkey embryo to indicate the area in which cells were reconstructed. The cerebral ventricle (CV) is relatively large at this stage and the lateral wall (L) is much thicker than the medial wall (M) on which the incipient calcarine fissure is slightly indented. The shaded area between the arrowheads indicates the position of the block of tissue that was processed for electron microscopic study. B. Drawing of a 1-μm thick, toluidine blue-stained section across the entire area shaded in Figure 16A. The cerebral wall from the ventricular surface at the bottom to the external surface at the top of the drawing consists of ventricular zone (VZ), subventricular zone (SV), intermediate zone (IZ), and cortical plate (CP). The area outlined by the rhomboid was cut serially for electron microscopic examination. The overlapping squares represent individual fields

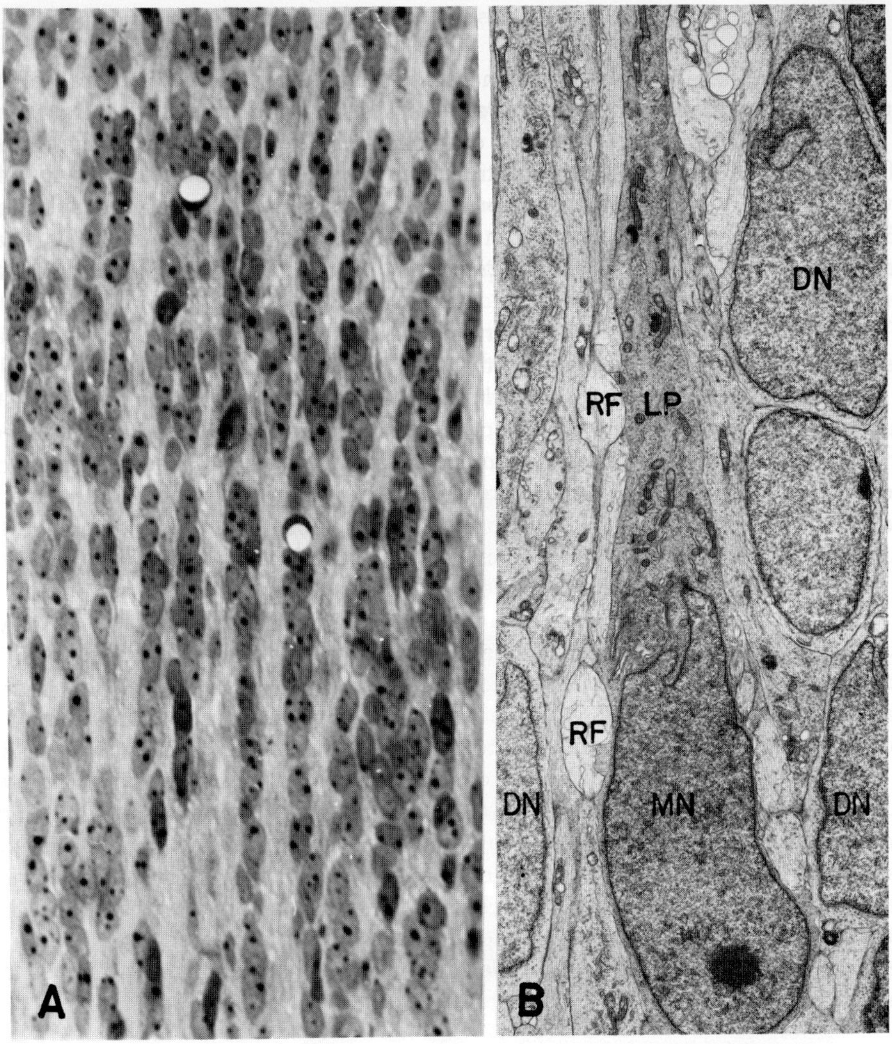

FIGURE 17. A. A portion of the cortical plate of a 97-day monkey fetus which illustrates vertical columnar organization of the cortex at this developmental stage. The top of the figure is closer to the pial surface. Photomicrograph of a 1-μm toluidine blue-stained section. B. Electron micrograph of the deep portion of the prospective visual cortex of 97-day monkey fetus. Migrating neuron (MN), its leading process (LP) aligned with a radial fiber (RF), bypasses more mature deep neurons (DN) on its way to superficial layers. The shaft of the radial fiber (RF) is only partially present within this section. It also does not have the usual amount of glycogen particles (42) because of *en bloc* staining with uranyl acetate used in preparing tissue (49).

---

photographed for the reconstruction on photomontages. Arrows A to F point to the positions of six reconstructed cells illustrated in C–H, respectively. Cells were drawn with the aid of superimposed outlines of cell profiles in serial sections at different levels traced onto transparent Mylar sheets. Some of the fibers which lie in contiguity with the migrating cells were also traced and reconstructed but most of the neighboring cells and processes were omitted. For details, see Rakic *et al.* (54).

appearance of glial cells, autoradiographic material has to be supplemented with fetal brain tissue stained with a Golgi method which adequately impregnates immature glial elements.

To analyze gliagenesis in monkey visual cortex, occipital lobes of animals aged from E48 to P1003 were processed according to Rio Hortega's rapid Golgi method (60) modified by Stensaas (70). When used on tissue fixed previously by perfusion with aldehyde mixture, this method gives good impregnations of immature glial elements in the monkey cerebellum (47) and cerebrum (49,63,64).

At early stages (E48–E70) radially oriented, bipolar cells which span the entire cerebral wall of the telencephalic vesicle have smooth somata and radial processes which terminate at the pial surface in one or several endfeet (Figure 19A). We are not able to define the lineage of any of these cells. However, already at this early age, some radial processes which end within the cerebral wall attach to blood vessels with characteristic endfeet (Figure 19A), an indication of their glial nature. This provides the first evidence for the presence of glial cells during early stages of cortical development in the rhesus monkey (64). After E70, most bipolar cells spanning the monkey cerebral wall possess lamellate expansions along the segment of radial fiber lying in the intermediate zone. Their endfeet at the pial surface stain with the periodic acid-Schiff method and their appearance in Golgi preparations (Figures 14 and 19) correlates with a class of 0.8–1.2-μm thick fibers previously shown by electron microscopy to possess many glial characteristics (49). Their morphology resembles radial glial cells described in other species (4,16,17,34,35,42,56, 57,58,71,72,76). In the rhesus monkey they become most prominent after E80 and their radial fibers are easily distinguished from the processes of migrating neurons (Figure 14B and C).

Most radial glial cells in mammalian neocortex were considered by Ramón y Cajal (56) to transform through intermediary forms into protoplasmic and fibrillary astrocytes. Transitional forms between radial glial cells and astrocytes are first observed in the monkey at E65, when the somata of some radial glial cells detach from the ventricular surface and become displaced to the intermediate zone (64). Between E75 and E120, the majority of radial glial cells acquire numerous and bushy lamellate expansions (Figure 19C). Transitional forms from radial glia to astrocytes are first seen in the deep cortical layers (at E65) then in the more superficial layers and in subpial position in layer I (E85). Thus, immature astrocytes appear in the developing cortical plate at the time when neuron production is at its peak (52). Virtually all the radial glial cells contacting blood vessels apparently transform into protoplasmic astrocytes by E120. However, many of those radial glial cells which span the cerebral wall persist longer and some continue to transform into astrocytes. After birth the number of radial glial cells continues to decrease steadily. Until P20 it is possible to verify their entire course across the cerebral wall, in the

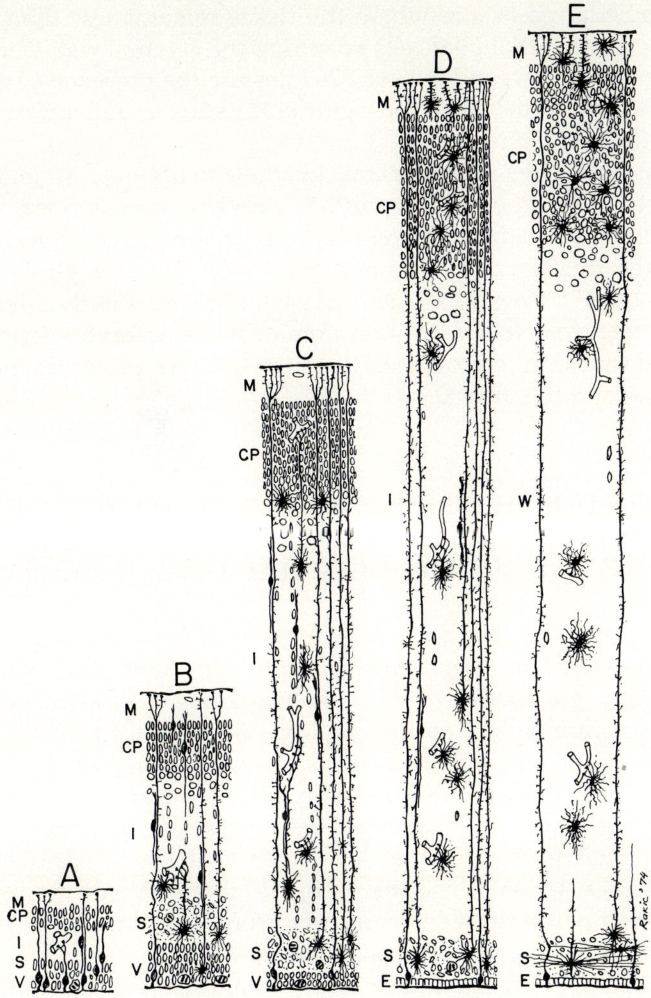

FIGURE 19. Semischematic illustration of gliagenesis in monkey telencephalon. Composite drawing is combined from impregnated cells in Golgi sections (black profiles of cell images) and cell nuclei as they appear in adjacent sections stained with toluidine blue (open profiles). In the diagrams, cell silhouettes and radial processes are represented larger than their actual size in order to illustrate their morphology at such a low magnification. Cell images in each column are typical of approximately the following age ranges A, E50–E60; B, E60–E70; C, E70–E80; D, E80–E120; E, E120–P20. Detailed description and documentation is published elsewhere (64). Abbreviations: CP, cortical plate; E, ependymal layer; M, molecular (marginal) layer; I, intermediate zone; S, subventricular zone; V, ventricular zone; W, white matter.

depth of the calcarine fissure where the tissue remains less than 2 mm thick (64). Even here, no radial glial cells spanning the cerebral wall were seen in 11 animals examined between P50 and P200 despite the presence of well-impregnated transitional forms near the ventricular surface and myriad astrocytes throughout the hemisphere.

This study indicates that certain glial elements—radial glial cells—are present much earlier in development than previously recognized. During fetal cortical development radial glial cells may serve special functions such as scaffolding for the fragile embryonic nervous tissue (56) or a guide for late migrating cells (48,49). Toward the end of gestation and shortly after birth most of the radial glial cells transform into immature astrocytes and perhaps divide again several times, thus providing the stem for both protoplasmic and fibrillary astrocytes of adult animals.

G. RELATIONSHIP BETWEEN TIME OF NEURON ORIGIN AND THE APPEARANCE OF CONVOLUTIONS IN THE OCCIPITAL LOBE

The mechanism underlying the development of fissures and gyri, which attain such prominence in the primate cerebrum and cerebellum remains a mystery. It is generally assumed without any experimental evidence that the generation of large numbers of cortical neurons in primates contributes more to an increase in cortical area than to an increase in its thickness. The expanded growth of the hemispheric surface within a limited cranial space was thought to lead to the formation of fissures and gyri. However, as reviewed elsewhere (69), it is difficult to explain the development of fissures and gyri in such simple mechanical terms. Since the occipital lobe in rhesus monkey has relatively deep sulci and prominent gyri, it is useful to correlate the time of their formation with the time of neuronal production.

Toward the end of the period of neuron genesis only a relatively shallow and widely gaping calcarine fissure exists on the medial cerebral wall (Figure 20A). The parieto-occipital notch is just recognizable on the dorsal cerebral surface (Figure 20A′). The lateral surface of the occipital lobe is still completely smooth. By E112 the brain is only slightly larger. The calcarine and parieto-occipital fissures now slightly deeper and better outlined, remain the only indentations in the occipital lobe (Figure 20B and B′). This finding is remarkable if one takes into account that virtually all cortical neurons are present by E100. It appears, therefore, that the enormous increase in surface area, which subsequently results in the deepening of primary fissures and the development of secondary fissures occurs after neurons have been generated. Therefore, the process of fissuration of the telencephalon in monkey coincides not with the genesis of neurons, but with the development of their processes and connec-

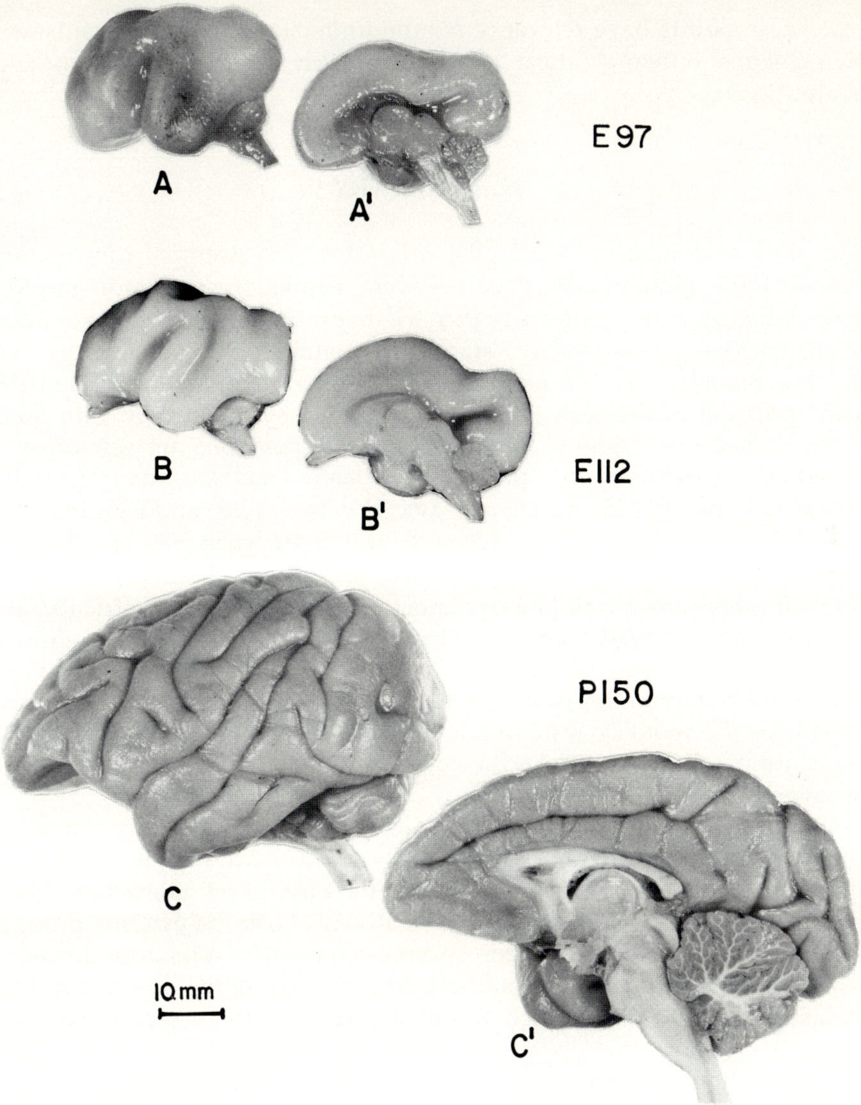

FIGURE 20. External configuration of the lateral (A–C) and medial (A′–C′) surfaces of the monkey cerebrum at E97 (A,A′), E112 (B,B′), and P150 (C,C′). All brains were fixed similarly by vascular perfusion with glutaraldehyde–formaldehyde mixture in phosphate buffer, taken from the skull 1 hour later and photographed at the same magnification.

tions as well as with the increase in glial cell numbers. However, some additional factors such as the regional differences in the migration rate of late generated neurons and the time when they attain their permanent position are still unknown and have to be worked out in relation to the formation of fissures. These points have relevance for the understanding of mechanisms underlying some human cortical dysgeneses such as microgyria and lissencephaly (12,59).

H. SUMMARY

The place and time of origin, the migration and eventual disposition of neurons of the monkey visual cortex were studied by autoradiography in animals killed at various intervals after ^{3}H-thymidine pulse labeling at embryonic (E) and early postnatal (P) stages. All neurons destined for the visual cortex are generated during about a 2-month period between E45 and E102. Neuron position in the cortical laminae correlates systematically with time of cell origin; neurons destined for deeper cortical positions are generated earlier, and more superficial ones progressively later. Thus, most neurons in layer VI are born between E45 and E60, in layer V between E60 and E70, in layer IV between E70 and E80, and in layers III and II between E80 and E102. No neurons, but numerous glia, are generated within the cortical plate itself. Initially young neurons are produced almost exclusively in the ventricular zone. Later they are probably generated in both ventricular and subventricular zones, and by the end of the proliferative period the subventricular zone becomes the predominant source of new cells. At the time when all neurons destined for the monkey visual cortex have already been produced, primary fissures are barely indicated on the cerebral surface and no secondary fissure appears as yet.

Autoradiographic analyses indicate that at early stages young neurons move to the cortical plate relatively synchronously and at a fast rate, whereas at later stages there are considerable differences in the rates of cell migration. At early stages when the migration pathway is relatively short, the external process of the ventricular cell may stretch across almost the entire migratory distance. It is possible that nuclei move without interruption within their own cylinders of cytoplasm, a mechanism which might account for the rapid, synchronous movement of cell bodies as seen in the autoradiographic material. During later stages when young neurons, mostly of subventricular origin, move across a distance which is more than 10 times the length of their leading process, migrating cells follow radial glial guides across the widened intermediate zone and through densely packed cortical plate. This type of cell displacement seems to proceed less synchronously and require more time. It is proposed that two different mechanisms of cell displacement might exist: one in operation at early stages of cortical formation when mostly ventricular cells migrate, and another utilized by subventricular cells at later stages.

The first glial elements are identifiable at E48 as bipolar radial cells which terminate with endfeet on blood vessels. Typical radial glial cells which span the entire cerebral wall are identified by E70. Transitional forms from radial glial cells to immature astrocytes in the developing visual cortex are first detected at E65, become most prominent from E80 to birth, sharply decrease postnatally, and virtually cease at 7 months of age.

Correlation of human and monkey visual cortices stained with both Nissl and Golgi methods indicates that in man the full complement of neocortical neurons is also probably generated well before birth.

ACKNOWLEDGMENT

This work was supported by Grant No. NS 11233 from the National Institutes of Health.

REFERENCES

1. Angevine, J. B. Critical cellular events in the shaping of neural centers. In: *The Neurosciences: Second Study Program.* (F. O. Schmitt, Ed.). Rockefeller Univ. Press, New York, 1970: 60–72.
2. Angevine, J. B., and Sidman, R. L. Autoradiographic study of cell migration during histogenesis of cerebral cortex in the mouse. *Nature* (*Lond.*), 1961, **192:** 766–768.
3. Artom, G. Untersuchungen ueber die Myelogenese des Nervensystems der Affen. *Arch. Psychiatr.*, 1925, **75:** 169–234.
4. Åström, K. E. On the early development of the isocortex in fetal sheep. *Prog. Brain Res.*, 1967, **26:** 1–59.
5. Atlas, M., and Bond, Y. R. The cell generation cycle of the eleven-day mouse embryo. *J. Cell Biol.*, 1965, **26:** 19–24.
6. Berry, M., and Rogers, A. W. The migration of neuroblasts in the developing cerebral cortex. *J. Anat.*, 1965, **99:** 691–709.
7. Bonin, G., and Mehler, W. R. On columnar arrangement of nerve cells in cerebral cortex. *Brain Res.*, 1971, **27:** 1–9.
8. Boulder Committee. Embryonic vertebrate central nervous system: Revised terminology. *Anat. Rec.*, 1970, **166:** 257–261.
9. Brodmann, K. Beitrage zur histologischen Lokalization der Grosshirnrinde. Dritte Mitteilung: Die Rinderfelder der neideren Affen. *J. Psychol. Neurol.*, 1905, **9:** 177–226.
10. Caviness, V. S., and Sidman, R. L. Time of origin of corresponding cell classes in the cerebral cortex of normal and reeler mutant mice: An autoradiographic analysis. *J. Comp. Neurol.*, 1973, **148:** 141–152.
11. Clark, W. E. Le Gros. The cells of Meynert in the visual cortex of the monkey. *J. Anat.*, 1942, **76:** 369–376.
12. Crome, L. and Stern, J. *Pathology of Mental Retardation.* (2nd ed.) Williams & Wilkins, Baltimore, Maryland, 1972.
13. Dekaban, A. S. Differential vulnerability to irradiation of various cerebral structures during prenatal development. In: *Radiation Biology of the Fetal and Juvenile Mammal.* Proc. 9th Annu. Hanford Biol. Symp. US At. Energy Comm., Washington, D.C., 1969: 769–777.
14. Fleischhauer, K., Petsche, H. and Wittowski, W. Vertical bundles of dendrites in the neocortex. *Z. Anat. Entwicklungsgesch.*, 1972, **127:** 213–223.

15. Garey, L. J. A light and electron microscopic study of the visual cortex of the cat and monkey. *Proc. R. Soc. Lond.* [B] 1971, **179:** 21–40.
16. Godina, G. Istogenesi e differenziazione del neuroni e degli elementi gliali della corteccia cerebrale. Z. *Zellforsch. Mikrosk. Anat.*, 1951, **36:** 401–435.
17. Golgi, C. Sulla fina anatomia degli organi centrali del sistema nervoso. *Opera Omnia* Hoepli, Milan, 1903: 397–536 (republished).
18. Hicks, S. P., and D'Amato, C. J. Cell migrations to the isocortex in the rat. *Anat. Rec.*, 1968, **160:** 619–634.
19. Hicks, S. P., D'Amato, C. J., Coy, M. A., O'Brien, E. D., Thurston, J. S., and Joftes, D. L. Migrating cells in the developing central nervous system studied by their radiosensitivity and tritiated thymidine uptake. *Brookhaven Symp. Biol.*, 1961, **14:** 246–261.
20. Hinds, J. W. Autoradiographic study of histogenesis in the mouse olfactory bulb. I. Time or origin or neurons and neuroglia. *J. Comp. Neurol.*, 1968, **134:** 287–304.
21. Hinds, J. W., and Hinds, P. L. Early ganglion cell differentiation in the mouse retina: An electron microscopic analysis utilizing serial sections. *Dev. Biol.*, 1974, **37:** 381–416.
22. Hinds, J. W., and Ruffett, T. L. Cell proliferation in the neural tube: An electron microscopic and Golgi analysis in the mouse cerebral vesicle. Z. *Zellforsch. Mikrosk. Anat.*, 1971, **115:** 226–264.
23. His, W. *Die Entwicklung des menschlichen Gehirns wahrend der ersten Monate.* Hirzel, Leipzig, 1904.
24. Flechsig, P. *Anatomie des menschichen Gehirns und Ruckenmarks auf myelogenetischer Grundlage.* Thieme, Stuttgart, 1920.
25. Hubel, D. H., and Wiesel, T. N. Receptive fields and functional architecture of monkey striate cortex. *J. Physiol. (Lond.)*, 1968, **195:** 215–243.
26. Hubel, D. H., and Wiesel, T. N. Anatomical demonstration of columns in the monkey striate cortex. *Nature (Lond.)*, 1969, **221:** 747–750.
27. Hubel, D. H., and Wiesel, T. N. Laminar and columnar distribution of geniculocortical fibers in the macaque monkey. *J. Comp. Neurol.*, 1972, **146:** 421–450.
28. Jacobson, S. Sequence of myelinization in the brain of the albino rat. A. Cerebral cortex, thalamus and related structures. *J. Comp. Neurol.*, 1963, **121:** 5–29.
29. Kauffman, S. L. Lengthening of the generation cycle during embryonic differentiation of the mouse neural tube. *Exp. Cell Res.*, 1968, **49:** 420–424.
30. Kenne, M. F. L., and Hewer, E. E. Some observations on myelination in the human central nervous system. *J. Anat.*, 1931, **66:** 1–13.
31. Koelliker, A. *Handbuch der Gewebelehre des Menschen. Nervensystem des Menschen und der Thiere.* Vol. 2. Engelmann, Leipzig, 1896.
32. Langman, J. and Shimada, M. Cerebral cortex of the mouse after prenatal chemical insult. *Am. J. Anat.*, 1971, **132:** 355–373.
33. Lund, J. Organization of neurons in the visual cortex, area 17, of the monkey (*Macaca mulatta*). *J. Comp. Neurol.*, 1973, **147:** 455–496.
34. Magnini, G. Sur la neurologie et les cellules nerveuses cérébrales chez les foetus. *Arch. Ital. Biol.*, 1888, **9:** 59–60.
35. Marin-Padilla, M. Prenatal and postnatal ontogenesis of the human motor cortex: A Golgi study. I. The sequential development of the cortical layers. *Brain Res.*, 1970, **23:** 167–183.
36. Meynert, T. Von Gehirne der Saugethiere. In: *Handbuch der Lehre, von den Geweben des Menschen und der thiere.* (S. Stricker, Ed.). Engelmann, Leipzig, 1871: 694–808.
37. Molliver, M. E., Kostovic, I., and Van der Loos, H. The development of synapses in cerebral cortex of the human fetus. *Brain Res.*, 1973, **50:** 403–407.
38. Morest, D. K. A study of neurogenesis in the forebrain of opossum pouch young. Z. *Anat. Entwicklungsgesch.*, 1970, **130:** 265–305.
39. Murakami, V., Hoshino, K., and Kameyama, Y. Mechanisms for the differential radiosensitivity of immature brain tissue: Development of hydrocephalus and allied conditions. In:

Radiation Biology of the Fetal and Juvenile Mammal. Proc. 9th Annu. Hanford Biol. Symp. US At. Energy Comm., Washington, D.C., 1969: 755–767.

40. Narayan, O., and Johnson, R. T. Effects of viral infection on nervous system development. I. Pathogenesis of Bluetongue virus infection in mice. *Am. J. Pathol.*, 1972, **68:** 1–10.
41. Nowakowski, R. S., and Rakic, P. Clearance rate of exogenous ^{3}H-thymidine from the plasma of pregnant rhesus monkeys. *Cell Tissue Kinet.*, 1974, **7:** 195–200.
42. Peters, A., and Feldman, M. The cortical plate and molecular layer of the late rat fetus. *Z. Anat. Entwicklungsgesch.*, 1973, **141:** 3–37.
43. Peters, A., and Walsh, T. M. A study of the organization of apical dendrites in the somatic sensory cortex of the rat. *J. Comp. Neurol.*, 1972, **144:** 253–268.
44. Poliakov, G. I. Progressive neuron differentiation of the human cerebral cortex in ontogenesis. In: *Development of the Central Nervous System.* (S. A. Sarkisov and S. N. Preobrazeuskaya, Eds.). Medgiz, Moscow, 1959: 11–26 (in Russian).
45. Poliakov, G. I. Some results of research into the development of the neuronal structure of the cortical ends of the analyzers in man. *J. Comp. Neurol.*, 1961, **117:** 197–212.
46. Poliakov, G. I. Development of the cerebral neocortex during first half on intrauterine life. In: *Development of the Child's Brain.* (S. A. Sarkisov, Ed.). Medicina, Leningrad, 1965: 22–52 (in Russian).
47. Rakic, P. Neuron–glia relationship during granule cell migration in developing cerebellar cortex. A Golgi and electron microscopic study in Macacus rhesus. *J. Comp. Neurol.*, 1971, **141:** 283–312.
48. Rakic, P. Guidance of neurons migrating to the fetal monkey neocortex. *Brain Res.*, 1971, **33:** 471–476.
49. Rakic, P. Mode of cell migration to the superficial layers of fetal monkey neocortex. *J. Comp. Neurol.*, 1972, **145:** 61–84.
50. Rakic, P. Extrinsic cytological determinants of basket and stellate cell dendritic pattern in the cerebellar molecular layer. *J. Comp. Neurol.*, 1972, **146:** 335–354.
51. Rakic, P. Kinetics of proliferation and latency between final division and onset of differentiation of the cerebellar stellate and basket neurons. *J. Comp. Neurol.*, 1973, **147:** 523–546.
52. Rakic, P. Neurons in rhesus monkey visual cortex: Systematic relation between time of origin and eventual disposition. *Science*, 1974, **183:** 425–427.
53. Rakic, P., and Sidman, R. L. Sequence of developmental abnormalities leading to granule cell deficit in cerebellar cortex of weaver mutant mice. *J. Comp. Neurol.*, 1973, **152:** 103–132.
54. Rakic, P., Stensaas, L. J., Sayre, E. P., and Sidman, R. L. Computer aided three-dimensional reconstruction and quantitative analysis of cells from serial electron microscopic montages of fetal monkey brain. *Nature (Lond.)*, 1974, **250:** 31–34.
55. Ramón y Cajal, S. Sur les fibres nerveuses de la couche granuleuse du cervelet et sur l'évolution des éléments cérébelleux. *Intl. Monatsch. Anat. Physiol. (Leipzig)*, 1890, **7:** 12–31.
56. Ramón y Cajal, S. *Histologie du Système Nerveux de l'Homme et des Vertébrés.* Maloine, Paris, 1911. (Reprinted by Consejo Superior de Investigacionec Cientificas, Madrid, 1977: Vol. II.)
57. Retzius, G. Studien über Ependym und Neuroglia. *Biol. Untersuch.* 1893, **5:** 9–26.
58. Retzius, G. Die Neuroglia des Gehirns beim Menschen unde bei Säugethiere. *Biol. Untersuch.*, 1894, **6:** 1–24.
59. Richman, D. P., Stewart, R. M., and Caviness, V. S. Microgyria, lissencephaly, and neuron migration to the cerebral cortex: An architectonic approach. *Neurology*, 1973, **23:** 413.
60. Rio Hortega, P. Tercera aportación al conocimiento morfólogico e interpretación functional de la oligodendroglia. *Mem. Soc. Espan. Hist. Natur.*, 1928, **14:** 5–54; republished in *Arch. Histol. (Buenos Aires)*, 1956, **6:** 132–183.
61. Sauer, F. C. The cellular structure of the neural tube. *J. Comp. Neurol.*, 1935, **63:** 13–23.
62. Sauer, M. E., and Walker, B. E. Radioautographic study of interkinetic nuclear migration in the neural tube. *Proc. Soc. Exp. Biol. Med.*, 1951, **101:** 557–560.

63. Schmechel, D. E., and Rakic, P. Evolution of fetal radial glial cells in rhesus monkey telencephalon: A Golgi study. *Anat. Rec.*, 1973, **175:** 436.
64. Schmechel, D. E., and Rakic, P. Radial glial cells in monkey telencephalon: Morphogenesis and transformation into astrocytes. *Z. Anat. Entwicklungsgesch.*, 1975, submitted for publication.
65. Shimada, M., and Langman, J. Cell proliferation, migration and differentiation in the cerebral cortex of the golden hamster. *J. Comp. Neurol.*, 1970, **139:** 227–244.
66. Sidman, R. L. Autoradiographic methods and principles for study of the nervous system with thymidine-H^3. In: *Contemporary Research Methods in Neuroanatomy.* (W. J. H. Nauta and S. O. E. Ebbesson, Eds.). Springer-Verlag, Berlin and New York, 1970: 252–274.
67. Sidman, R. L., Miale, I. L., and Feder, N. Cell proliferation in the primitive ependymal zone: An autoradiographic study of histogenesis in the nervous system. *Exp. Neurol.*, 1959, **1:** 322–333.
68. Sidman, R. L., and Rakic, P. Neuronal migration, with special reference to developing human brain: A review. *Brain Res.*, 1973, **62:** 1–35.
69. Sidman, R. L., and Rakic, P. Development of the human central nervous system. In: *Cytology and Cellular Neuropathology.* (2nd ed.) (R. D. Adams and W. Haymaker, Eds.). Thomas, Springfield, Illinois, 1975: in press.
70. Stensaas, L. J. The development of hippocampal and dorsolateral pallial regions of the cerebral hemisphere in fetal rabbits. I. Fifteen millimeter stage, spongioblast morphology. *J. Comp. Neurol.*, 1967, **129:** 59–70.
71. Stensaas, L. J. An electronmicroscope study of the organization of the cerebral cortex of the 60 mm rabbit embryo. *Z. Anat. Entwicklungsgesch.*, 1972, **137:** 335.
72. Stensaas, L. J., and Stensaas, S. S. Light microscopy of glial cells in turtles and birds. *Z. Zellforsch. Mikrosk. Anat.*, 1968, **91:** 315–340.
73. Stensaas, L. J., and Stensaas, S. S. An electronmicroscope study of cells in the matrix and intermediate laminae of the cerebral hemisphere of the 45 mm rabbit embryo. *Z. Zellforsch. Mikrosk. Anat.*, 1968, **91:** 341–365.
74. Tilney, F. Behavior in its relation to development of brain: Correlation between development of brain and behavior in albino rat embryonic states to maturity. *Bull. Neurol. Inst. NY*, 1933, **3:** 252–358.
75. Valverde, F. Short axon neuronal subsystems in the visual cortex of the monkey. *Int. J. Neurosci.*, 1971, **1:** 181–197.
76. Vignal, W. Recherches sur le développement des éléments des couches corticales du cerveau et du cervelet chez l'homme et les mammifères. *Arch. Physiol. Norm. Pathol. (Paris)*, 1888, Sect. IV, **2:** 228–254.
77. Watterson, R. L., Veneziano, P., and Bartha, A. Absence of a true germinal zone in neural tubes of young chick embryos as demonstrated by the colchicine techniques. *Anat. Rec.*, 1956, **124:** 379.
78. Webster, W., Shimada, M., and Langman, J. Effects of fluorodeoxyuridine, colcemid, and bromodeoxyuridine on developing neocortex of the mouse. *Amer. J. Anat.*, 1973, **137:** 67–86.
79. Weiss, P. *In vitro* experiments on the factors determining the course of the outgrowing nerve fiber. *J. Exp. Zool.*, 1934, **68:** 393–448.
80. Yakovlev, P. I., and Lecours, A. R. The myelogenetic cycles of regional maturation of the brain. In: *Regional Development of the Brain in Early Life.* (A. Minkowski, Ed.). Blackwell, Oxford, 1967: 3–70.
81. Zeki, S. M. The secondary visual areas of the monkey. *Brain Res.*, 1969, **13:** 197–226.

2

Effects of Interference with Cerebellar Maturation on the Development of Locomotion. An Experimental Model of Neurobehavioral Retardation

JOSEPH ALTMAN
Department of Biological Sciences, Purdue University, West Lafayette, Indiana

INTRODUCTION

The experimental analysis of the causative factors of mental retardation in man is hindered by numerous practical and moral considerations. This justifies the use of animal models, even though these models rarely, if ever, mirror adequately the complexities of human mental retardation, where biological variables are intermingled with multifarious cultural factors.

We have been engaged for several years in a multidisciplinary study of the postnatal development of the cerebellum and locomotion in rats under normal conditions and following various experimental treatments. Some of the treatments that we have used, such as undernutrition or the administration of hormones and drugs, have long been suspected among the factors that can lead to mental retardation. We recognize that experimental interference with cerebellar and motor development does not, strictly speaking, represent "mental" retardation. However, it does constitute an instance of neural and behavioral retardation, one that offers many experimental advantages over the retardation of other neural and behavioral systems. The cerebellum is an easily accessible and widely studied structure which develops in the rat to a large extent after birth when experimental manipulations can be easily applied. Moreover, the objective study of overt motor development, as opposed to many covert mental phenomena, offers many experimental advantages.

This review is restricted in scope, being essentially limited to a summary of recent work from our laboratory in which focal X-irradiation was used to interfere with the normal course of cerebellar development.

NORMATIVE STUDY OF THE POSTNATAL DEVELOPMENT OF THE RAT CEREBELLUM

The tissue of the cerebellum expands substantially from birth to 21 days, the time when rat pups are usually weaned from their mothers. A quantitative histological study showed (2) that in the sagittal plane the area of the cerebellum increases during this period over 20-fold (Figure 1) and that this increase is primarily due to the expansion of the cerebellar cortex. During the first week after birth the proliferative zone of the cerebellar cortex, the subpial external germinal layer, grows rapidly [see Altman (2, Figure 3)], while the growth of the other layers (which are essentially unformed at birth) is sluggish. This indicates that few of the cells that come into existence are differentiating at this time and that the multiplying cells are merely increasing the stem cell population of the external germinal layer. The growth of the granular and molecular layers begins at an accelerated rate toward the beginning of the second week and ends by the end of the third week (Figure 1).

The increase in cerebellar mass during this rapid growth period is due to many developmental processes. A recent study employing quantitative histology, histochemistry, autoradiography, and electron microscopy (4–6) led us to the conceptualization that postnatal cerebellar neurogenesis can be subdivided into five, largely sequential events that we shall refer to as (1) cytogenesis, (2) morphogenesis, (3) synaptogenesis, (4) gliogenesis, and (5) myelogenesis. We have studied in some detail the first three of these events.

Postnatal Cerebellar Cytogenesis

Cytogenesis refers to the first step in neurogenesis, the proliferation of precursor cells which have the potential to differentiate later into neurons. The study of cytogenesis has been greatly aided in recent years by the introduction and extensive use of ^{3}H-thymidine autoradiography which allows the visualization of newly formed cells whose DNA is tagged. Autoradiographic studies from several laboratories (32,33,46) established that whereas neurons of the deep cerebellar nuclei and the Purkinje cells of the cerebellar cortex are formed prenatally in mice and rats, the basket and stellate cells of the molecular layer and the granule cells of the granular layer are formed postnatally. Our studies have indicated (1,2,4,17) that the first contingent of differentiating cells do not migrate (see below) but settle in the lower half of the molecular layer where

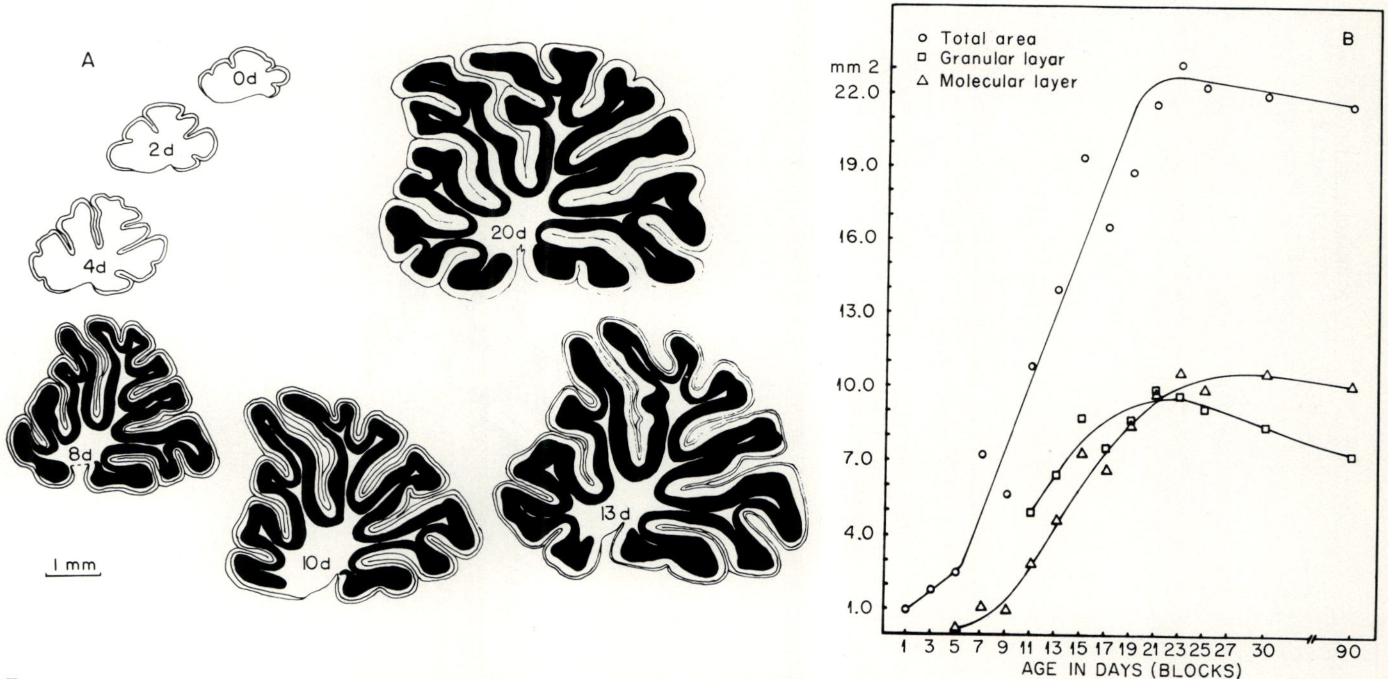

FIGURE 1. A. Tracings of sagittal, matched sections of the cerebellum from rats of different ages, as indicated (d = days). Outer band, external germinal layer; black, granular layer; white above black, molecular layer; white below black, subcortical regions, including medullary layer. B. Planimetric data of the area growth of the cerebellum in the sagittal plane shown, together with a laminar analysis. Each point represents means from several animals. Growth of external germinal layer not shown. Slightly modified from Altman (2).

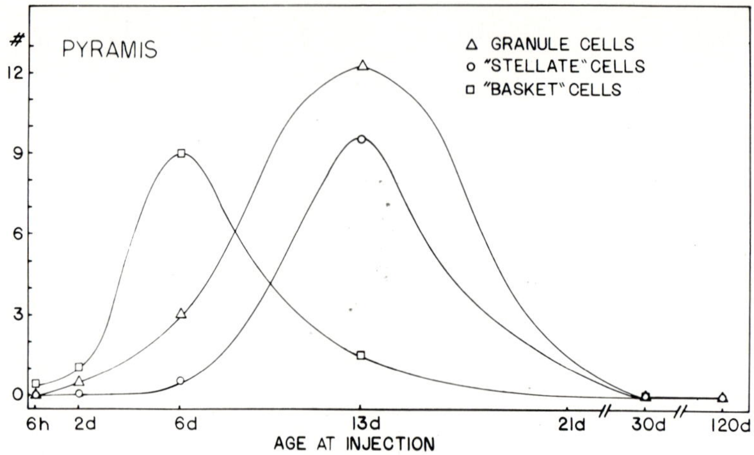

FIGURE 2. Mean number of intensely labeled cells (cells that ceased to divide soon after the day that the radiochemical was administered) in the granular and molecular layers of the pyramis in 120-day-old rats that were injected with ^{3}H-thymidine on the days indicated. Granule cells were counted in areas 130 μm^2; the much less numerous cells of the molecular layer were counted in strips 650 μm long. Intensely labeled cells in the lower half of the molecular layer were designated as basket cells; those in the upper half as stellate cells. The proportion of glia cells in the samples is unknown. Slightly modified after Altman (2).

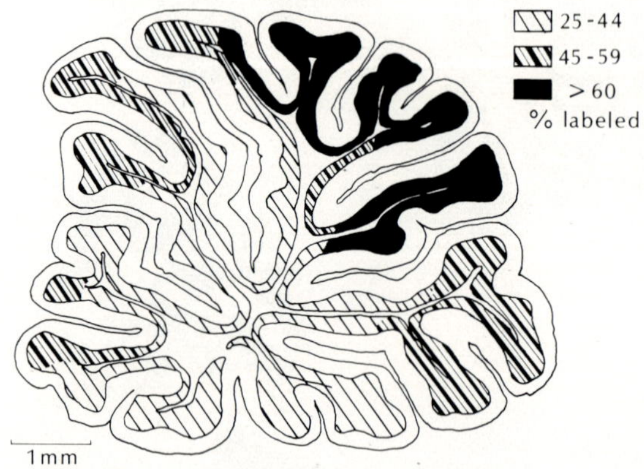

FIGURE 3. Summary of differential counts of labeled granule cells (intensely as well as lightly labeled) in the vermis of an adult rat injected with repeated doses of ^{3}H-thymidine from day 11 to 16. The obtained percentages [for details see Figure 11a, in Altman (2)] indicate regional variations in the proportion of granule cells acquired after 11 days of age. Light diagonal lines, early maturing regions; heavy diagonal lines, intermediate regions; black, late maturing regions. From Altman (2).

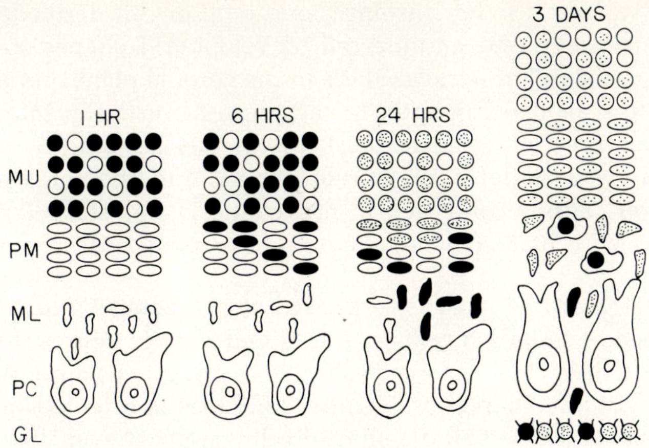

FIGURE 4. Diagrammatic representation of the pattern of cell labeling and movement in the cerebellar cortex of infant rats as revealed by autoradiography. The data relate to animals injected with ^{3}H-thymidine on postnatal day 6 [see Altman (1)] and killed at intervals thereafter, as indicated. In animals killed 1 hour after injection only the cells of the proliferative zone of the external germinal layer (MU) are labeled. In animals surviving for 6 hours, many of the premigratory cells (PM) of the germinal layer have become labeled. By this time free ^{3}H-thymidine is no longer available, indicating that the labeled cells in the premigratory zone are differentiating elements. By 24 hours after injection there is considerable label dilution in the cell population of multiplying cells and their derivatives, and some of the labeled cells are seen in the molecular layer as horizontally or vertically oriented bipolar cells. By 3 days after injection, label dilution is extensive throughout the external germinal layer. Some labeled basket cells are seen in the molecular layer (ML) and some labeled granule cells have descended through the layer of Purkinje cells (PC) and settled in the granular layer (GL). Modified after Altman (4).

they become differentiated as basket cells toward the end of the first week (Figure 2). The cells that are located in the upper half of the molecular layer, including stellate cells, come into existence during the second week. The granule cells migrate to the granular layer and differentiate during the second and third week, with 25 to 80% of them being formed between 11 and 21 days depending on systematic regional variations (Figure 3). Thus, granule cells in the depth of vermal fissures differentiate earlier than in the sulci; the ventral lobules (lingula and nodulus) mature before the anterior lobe; the last maturing vermal lobules are the tuber, declive, and culmen. The cerebellar hemispheres, with some exceptional regional variations mature later than the vermis, and the paraflocculus is the last region to mature (2). The major events in the multiplication and migration of cells in the cerebellar cortex are summarized in Figure 4.

Postnatal Cerebellar Morphogenesis

The term morphogenesis in this context refers to the initial step in neuronal differentiation, namely, the acquisition of special morphological properties by different classes of cells. For instance, one type of cell derived from the external germinal layer, the granule cell, develops a T-shaped axon. This involves the "extrusion" of parallel fibers in the coronal plane and the migration of the soma (the axon being spun in the process) vertically into the granular layer. Another type of cell, the basket cell, has its outgrowing dendrites oriented at a right angle to the parallel fibers, and the soma settles in the molecular layer. This second step in neurogenesis was studied in a series of investigations with histochemistry, autoradiography, and, in particular, electron microscopy.

The external germinal layer is composed of two zones (Figure 4). An upper zone composed of roundish cells with frequent mitotic figures that are labeled directly by ^{3}H-thymidine is the proliferative zone. The underlying zone is composed of spindle-shaped cells whose long axis is oriented horizontally in the coronal plane. These spindle-shaped cells rarely, if ever, have mitotic figures and are not labeled until several hours have elapsed after injection (by which time the injected ^{3}H-thymidine has been excreted). Observations with electron microscopy suggested that this is a premigratory differentiating zone (1). Apparently the horizontal bipolar cells "extrude" cytoplasm that becomes the horizontal branch of the future parallel fibers (Figure 5). It is presumed that when the horizontal fibers reach their final length, the cell body migrates downward through the molecular layer and eventually reaches the granular layer where its differentiation continues. As the parallel fibers are formed the undifferentiated matrix is pushed upward. Thus the horizontal branches of the parallel fibers are progressively formed on the surface of others from the bottom of the molecular layer upward by a stacking process. This building design makes possible the assembly of a matrix of very long, thin, and straight threads of horizontally oriented parallel fibers which pile up vertically according to their time of origin. The vertical branch of the parallel fiber is

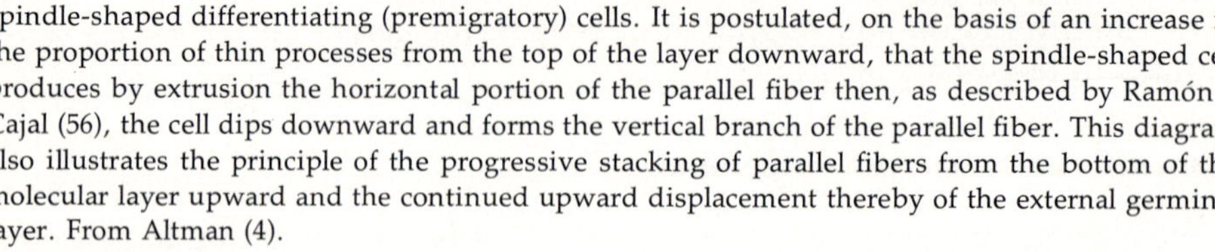

FIGURE 5. Diagrammatic illustration of the transformation of multiplying round cells into spindle-shaped differentiating (premigratory) cells. It is postulated, on the basis of an increase in the proportion of thin processes from the top of the layer downward, that the spindle-shaped cell produces by extrusion the horizontal portion of the parallel fiber then, as described by Ramón y Cajal (56), the cell dips downward and forms the vertical branch of the parallel fiber. This diagram also illustrates the principle of the progressive stacking of parallel fibers from the bottom of the molecular layer upward and the continued upward displacement thereby of the external germinal layer. From Altman (4).

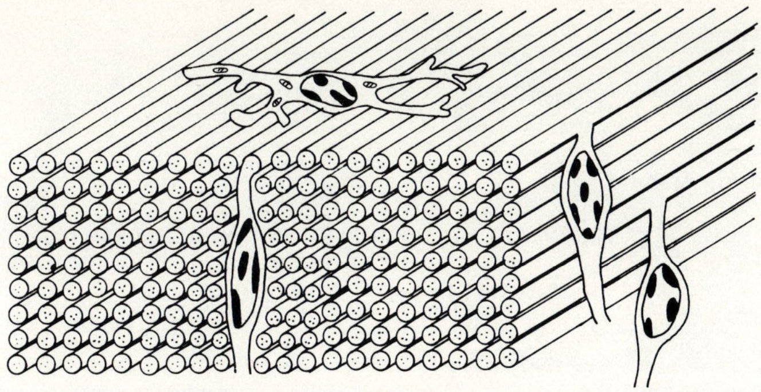

FIGURE 6. Illustration of the principle that the differentiating basket cells, whose dendrites are oriented at a right angle to the parallel fibers, are rendered immobile the moment they begin to differentiate. In contrast, the cell bodies of the differentiating granule cells can move downward between sheaves of parallel fibers. This migration is postulated to be guided by the processes of Bergmann glia cells that reach the surface of the cerebellar cortex (53). From Altman (4).

formed by trailing. Reference was made earlier to the fact that the basket cells do not migrate but differentiate *in situ*. The dendrites of the basket cells are oriented sagittally at a right angle to the stacks of parallel fibers which renders them immobile the moment they begin to differentiate (Figure 6).

Concurrently with the morphogenetic sculpturing that is in progress in the external germinal and molecular layers, the Purkinje cells also undergo morphogenetic changes (Figure 7). Several phases were distinguished in the postnatal differentiation of these prenatally formed elements (5). After the Purkinje cells have become dispersed and aligned in a monolayer, each develops a transient apical enlargement or cone filled with "growth" cytoplasm that is particularly rich in mitochondria. In the lateral aspect of the soma transient perisomatic processes are formed. In the next phase of development the perisomatic processes disappear and the apical cytoplasm streams upward into the growing apical dendrite that invades the formative molecular layer. The primary dendrite forms secondary and then tertiary branches, and gradually spines are formed which subsequently proliferate in great numbers. By this time permanent synapses have appeared on the soma of the Purkinje cells and are also seen in increasing numbers in the lower, or older part, of the molecular layer.

Postnatal Cerebellar Synaptogenesis

The early synaptogenic maturation of the cerebellar cortex has been studied recently by many investigators (among others, see 40,41,45,47,48,54). In one of our studies (3) we noticed round vesicles 400–1400 Å in diameter and furnished with an outer coat. We saw these in various parts of the cerebellar cortex in all young animals, but in particularly large numbers in rats aged

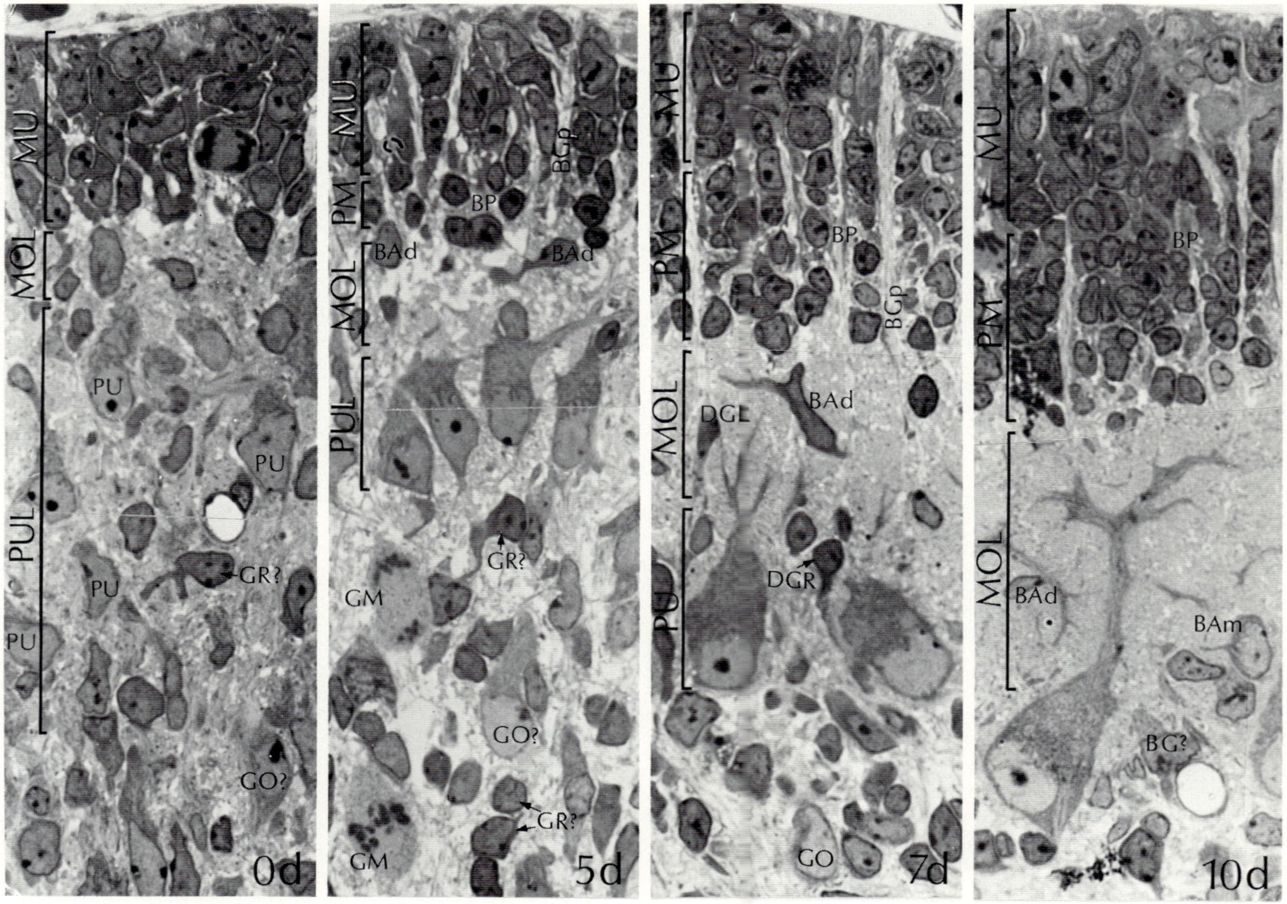

MU
MOL
PUL
PU
PU
PU
PU
GR?
GO?
0d
MU
PM
MOL
PUL
BAd
BP
BGp
BAd
GR?
GM
GO?
GR?
GM
5d
MU
PM
MOL
PU
BP
BGp
BAd
DGL
DGR
GO
7d
MU
PM
MOL
BP
BAd
BAm
BG?
10d

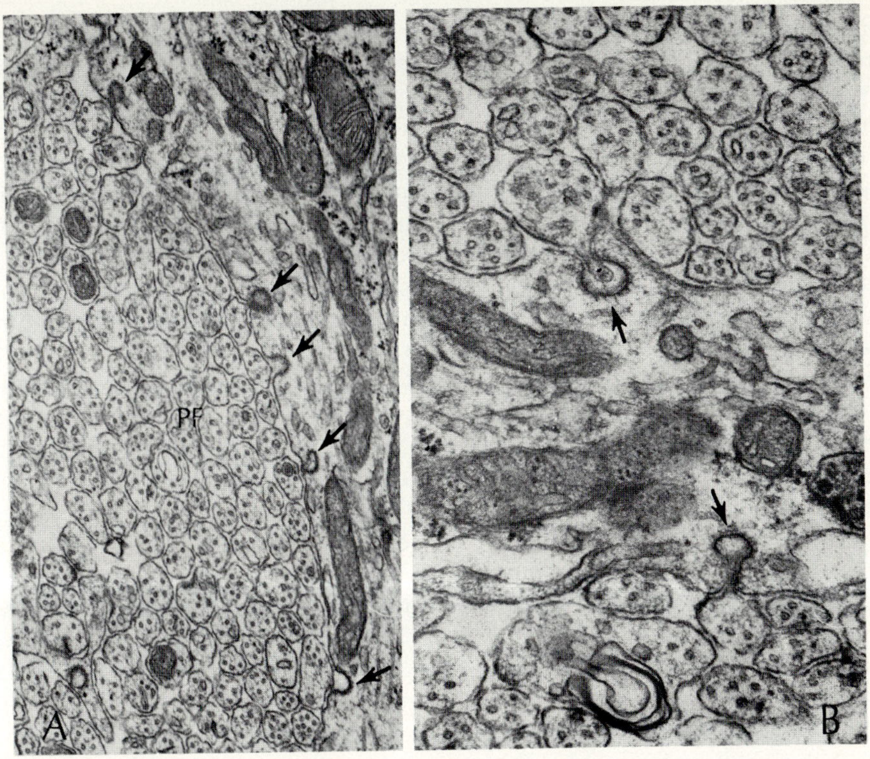

FIGURE 8. A. High concentration of open coated vesicles (arrows) in the primary dendrite of a Purkinje cell opposite parallel fibers (PF). B. Portion of the parallel fiber may be "sucked" into the open coated vesicle (arrows). Both electron micrographs from the pyramis of a 12-day-old rat. From Altman (5).

10–15 days (3). These vesicles were identified in closed (spherical), open (flasklike), and flattened forms. Closed coated vesicles were seen in large numbers in the vicinity of the Golgi apparatus and sometimes in direct continuity with its cisterns. Closed, open, and flat coated vesicles were seen on the surface of cells, and in neurons these were frequently opposite cell processes with which synapses are formed, such as in the dendrites of Purkinje cells opposite parallel fibers (Figure 8). Often, these open coated vesicles were situated

FIGURE 7. Photomicrographs of the cerebellar cortex from rats aged 0, 5, 7, and 10 days. At birth the Purkinje cells are still scattered throughout the cortex, by day 5 they form a distinct monolayer. In the 5- and 10-day-old rats the apical cone of Purkinje cells is very pronounced, heralding the imminent outgrowth of the apical dendritic system which is evident by day 10. Semi-thin sections embedded in Epon and cut in the sagittal plane. Stained with azure B; oil immersion, ×1600. Abbreviations: BAd, differentiating basket cells; BAm, mature basket cells; BG, Bergmann glia cell; BGp, Bergmann glia process; BP, bipolar cell in cross section; DGR, descending granule cell; GM, mitotic glia cell; GO, Golgi cell; GR, granule cell; MOL, molecular layer; MU, proliferative zone of the external germinal layer; PM, premigratory zone of the external germinal layer; PU, Purkinje cells; PUL, Purkinje cell layer; d, day. Slightly modified after Altman (4).

opposite cell processes which had dense membranes, and sometimes they were continuous with the dense membranes of early attachment sites, or presumptive synapses. Occasionally parts of the parallel fiber actually protruded into the cavity of the Purkinje cell coated vesicles suggesting an exchange of material between prospective pre- and postsynaptic elements. It was postulated that the coated vesicles are involved in the formation of early attachment sites or the dense membranes of synapses, and the following sequence of events was suggested. Through a budding process spherical, coated vesicles are formed from the membranes of the cisterns of the Golgi apparatus. These spherical vesicles migrate to the cell surface and after attachment to the membrane open up and unfold over its surface. When this unfolding becomes complete the flat dense membranes contribute material to or form the synaptic membranes. Coated vesicles may also contribute to the expansion of the dense membrane surface of already formed synapses.

Examination of the emergence with age of mature type of synapses around the somata of Purkinje cells and in the molecular layer (5) of the pyramis provided the following picture of the sequential steps in cerebellar synaptogenesis. Concurrently with the disappearance of perisomatic processes, the perikarya of Purkinje cells are surrounded by identifiable basket cell synapses. This is pronounced about 8–10 days after birth. A few days later parallel fibers begin to form synapses with outgrowing branchlets of Purkinje cells in the lower aspect of the molecular layer. During the next phase, which occurs after the disappearance of the external germinal layer about 20 days, parallel fibers establish synapses with dendritic spines in the upper molecular layer. The "march" of synaptogenesis in the molecular layer from the bottom upward is characterized by three successive events: an initial gradient in the appearance and disappearance of coated vesicles, heralding synaptogenesis; a similar subsequent trend in the formation of synapses; and finally, the interposition in the same sequence of glial processes between Purkinje cell dendrites and parallel fibers, marking the cessation of synaptogenesis. A summary of these events is presented in Figure 9.

The following were the salient events in the maturation of the granular layer (6). A large proportion of the granule cells is formed during the second week. But due to the time required for their migration and the lag in the formation of dendrites, few glomerular synapses with mossy fibers are formed before the beginning of the third week, and the process is still in progress at 30 days, long after the dissolution of the external germinal layer. The maturation of Golgi cells is a protracted process. Evidence was obtained that mossy fibers form synapses with the dendrites of Golgi cells and that Golgi cell axons synapse with granule cell dendrites as soon as the glomeruli begin to mature. These observations suggested that synaptogenesis succeeds the morphogenetic stage of maturation and that differentiating granule cells do not form synapses until their axons are formed and their cell bodies reach their final destination. However, in complex cells, as the Purkinje cell, the synaptic mat-

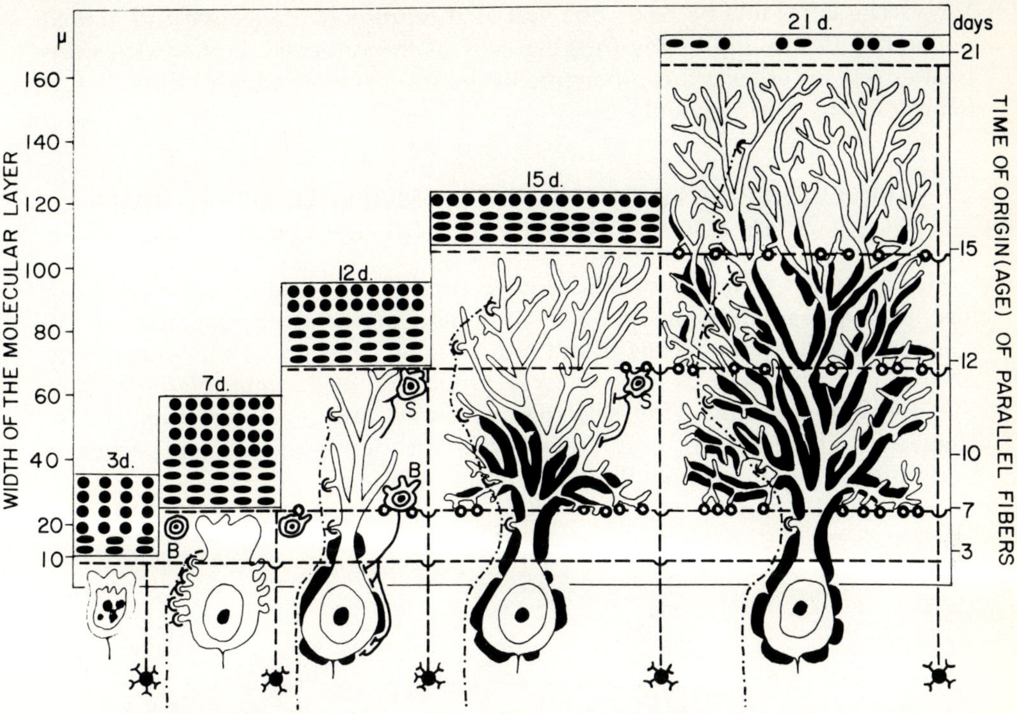

FIGURE 9. Diagrammatic illustration of some major events in the maturation of a Purkinje cell and of the molecular layer. The width of the molecular layer (left abscissa) as a function of the animal's age (5 discrete columns) is based on measurements [see Figure 4, in Altman (4)]. Considering the principle of the stacking of parallel fibers from the bottom upward, and disregarding the expansion produced by the invading dendritic processes during synaptogenesis, their location within the molecular layer indicates their "age" or time of origin (right abscissa). If the parallel fibers are traced through the columns from left to right it is seen that the fiber formed on day 7 has no synapses on that day but that it has synapses with basket cells on day 12, and increasing number of synapses from the fifteenth day onward with dendritic spines of Purkinje cells. Likewise, the parallel fiber formed on day 12 has no synapses at that time but it has synapses with a stellate cell on day 15 and with Purkinje cell dendritic spines on day 21. The parallel fiber formed on day 15 has synapses with Purkinje spines on day 21, but in the upper one-fourth of the molecular layer such synapses are still lacking at this age. The displacement and growth of a climbing fiber is indicated on the left side of the Purkinje cell. The upward "march" of glial sheathing of the Purkinje cell is also indicated. The cell width of the two zones of the external germinal layer [see Figure 1, in Altman (4)] is accurate but they are not drawn to scale. Slightly modified, after Altman (5).

uration of one region (the soma) may begin before the morphogenic maturation of the entire cell (the dendrites) is completed.

This analysis of the course of postnatal cerebellar neurogenesis served us with normative data for the proper assessment of the effects of various treatments that interfere with cerebellar development, such as undernutrition, the administration of hormones and drugs, and focal irradiation with low-dose

X-ray. The latter will be described first as it represents a selective and graded method of destroying newly forming cells of the cerebellar cortex with minimal effects on other cell components of the cerebellum and with little disturbance of neighboring structures.

INTERFERENCE WITH POSTNATAL CEREBELLAR DEVELOPMENT BY FOCAL LOW LEVEL X-IRRADIATION

Hicks and his collaborator (35,36) have studied for some time the effects of low level X-irradiation on the embryonic and perinatal development of the central nervous system. They found that a single exposure of the whole body of mice and rats to 200 R killed a large proportion of the multiplying cells of the developing brain. This selective action of low level radiation, Hicks suggested, should allow interference with the development of a particular brain region by appropriate timing of the irradiation.

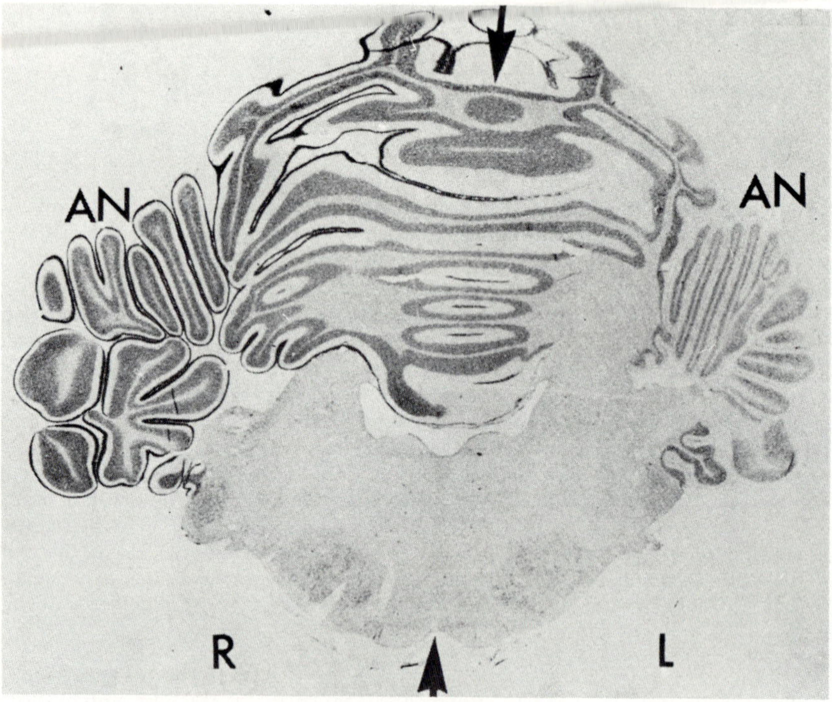

FIGURE 10. Photomicrograph of a section through the cerebellum of a kitten whose skull was irradiated on the left side (L) with five repeated doses of 200 R. AN, ansiform lobule; R, right nonirradiated side. Note absence of external germinal layer over entire left cerebellum. Arrows point to approximate midline. Magnification about ×6.6; cresyl violet. From Altman, Anderson, and Wright (13).

In a pilot study (13) we determined the optimal dose necessary for the selective destruction of the cells of the external germinal layer of the cerebellum. The heads of kittens were irradiated during the first 2 weeks of postnatal life with five repeated doses of X-ray with single doses ranging from 50 to 400 R in different animals. The effects on the irradiated and control sides were evaluated in the ansiform lobule (Figure 10). Repeated doses of 50–100 R reduced the cell population of the external germinal layer, 150 R produced a subtotal, and 200 R a total destruction of the entire layer. It was concluded, in agreement with Hicks' earlier results, that 200 R is the optimal X-ray dose for the selective destruction of precursors of the postnatally forming granule cells in the cerebellar cortex. The differential effects of single and multiple exposures were examined in subsequent studies.

Cell Reduction Coupled with Structural Disorganization

The morphological consequences of bilateral irradiation of the cerebellum in newborn rats were examined with the number of daily exposures ranging from 1 to 10 days (14,15). Within 24 hours after irradiation a single dose of 200 R reduced drastically the cell population of the external germinal layer, and maximal (subtotal) destruction could be obtained with an additional dose of 200 R (Figure 13). However, if 4 or more days elapsed between the end of the irradiation session and the killing of the animal the external germinal layer began to regenerate (Figures 11–13).

With up to 5 successive daily doses the speed of recovery of the external germinal layer was inversely related to the number of doses received (Figure 13). In all of these animals the external germinal layer was normal or supernormal in width by the tenth day after the last irradiation session. But planimetric studies revealed that the total area occupied by this germinal layer over the decreased cerebellar surface (or the total germinal cell population) was inversely related to the number of doses received. The regenerated external germinal cells retained their potential to differentiate but because fewer cells were available as a function of increased number of treatments, the result was a graded retardation in cerebellar growth (Figure 14).

When six or more doses of 200 R were delivered during infancy the external germinal layer failed to regenerate, presumably because the combination of prolonged exposure and delayed recovery prevented its recovery within the period that it is normally present (21 days after birth). The result of the extended treatment was the formation of a cerebellum devoid of granule cells and of the other postnatally formed neuronal elements (Figure 15).

Light and electron microscopic examination of the organization of the degranulated cerebellum (10,11) showed that the cell bodies of Purkinje cells were morphologically normal (Figure 16) but that there were changes in their dendritic configuration and that the circuitry of the cerebellar cortex was dras-

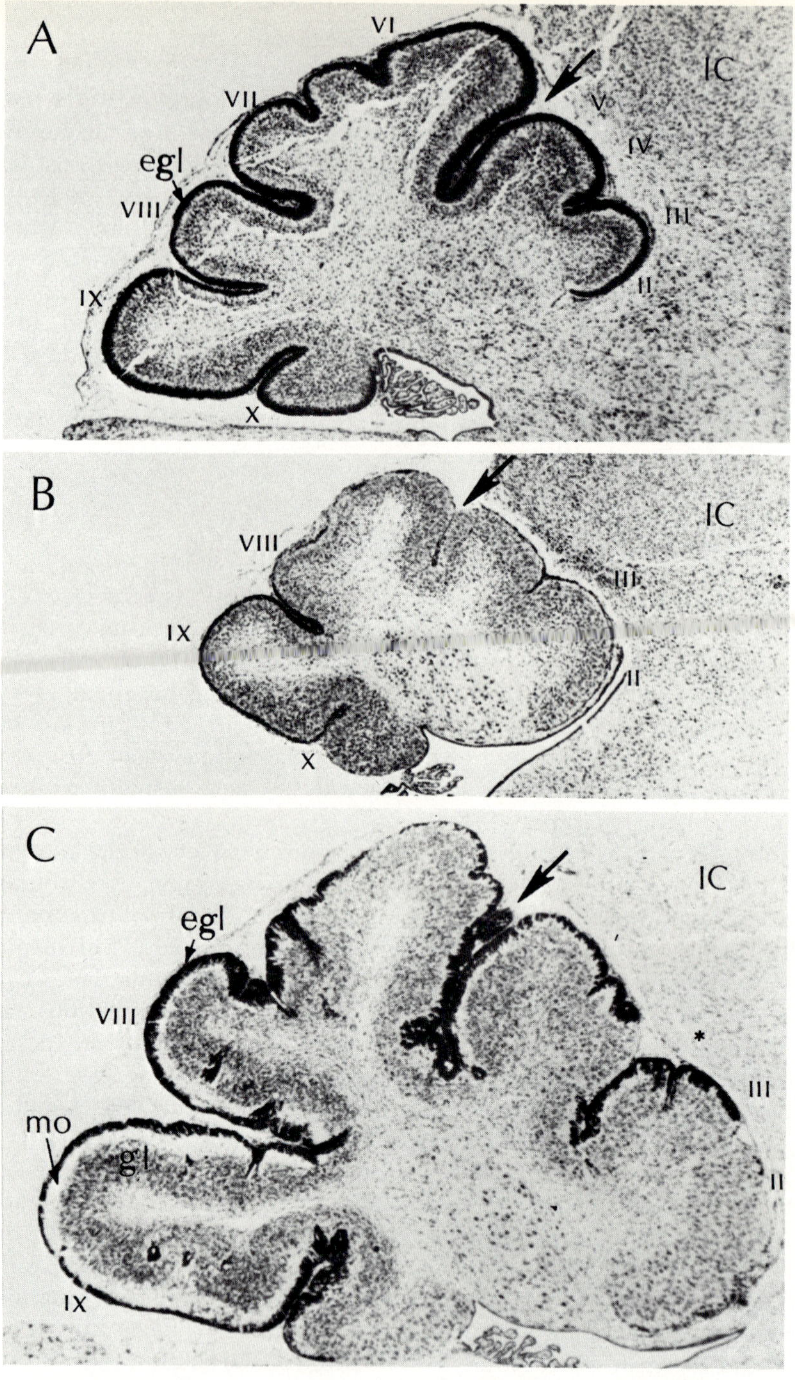

FIGURE 11. Low power photomicrographs of sagittal sections of the cerebellum (about 900 μm from midline). A. Cerebellar vermis of a normal 4-day-old rat; B, of a 4-day-old rat irradiated with 200 R on days 0, 1, 2, and 3 and killed 24 hours later. Note the absence of an external germinal

tically altered. The Purkinje cells had sprouted numerous massive dendrites (Figure 17) that were studded with thorns. But the dendrites were randomly oriented in space, and their arborization was different from normal and depended on the position of the cell body within the cortex. Postsynaptic membrane thickenings were prominent, even in the absence of apposed parallel fibers (the axons of granule cells). These observations indicated considerable autonomy in the morphological development of Purkinje cells in the cortex devoid of basket, stellate, and granule cells. However, the synaptic disorganization was profound. The mossy fibers, which normally terminate in the granular layer and contact granule cells, penetrated as far as the surface of the cortex and formed synapses with the soma and dendrites of Purkinje cells. In the absence of basket cells, basketlike synapses were formed on the cell bodies of Purkinje cells by terminals that were interpreted to belong to the recurrent axon collaterals of Purkinje cells (Figure 18). Postsynaptic membrane thickenings on the dendrites and thorns of Purkinje cells, which were seen to form contacts with climbing fibers (which is normal), were also abundant opposite other Purkinje dendritic thorns, and even glial processes (Figure 19). This suggested that many (probably the majority) of the "contacts" formed were abnormal or abortive. The observation of these mismatched connections made us conclude that the cellular depopulation of the cerebellum during the growth period results in profound morphogenetic and synaptogenetic disorganization. Similar observations were recently made by others in the degranulated cerebellum of mutant mice (37,55) and in a cerebellum degranülated by perinatal viral infection (34,43) or a drug (38).

Structural Disorganization without Substantial Cell Reduction

More attention has been paid recently to the phenomenon of nerve cell reduction as a consequence of interference with brain growth (e.g., 59,60) than to morphogenetic and synaptogenetic disorganization. But inappropriate connections formed by existing elements due to interference with the normal time course of neurogenesis might itself lead to faulty neural functioning.

Even though the direct effect of irradiation of the developing cerebellum is

---

layer excepting as a thin sheet over uvula; C, from a 10-day-old rat, irradiated as B. Note presence of a quasi-normal external germinal layer and developing molecular and granular layers caudally in uvula, to lesser extent in pyramis. More rostrally the external germinal layer is reconstituted excepting over centralis ventralis. There is no granular layer in the rostral lobules. Designation of vermian lobules, according to Larsell (41a): II, Centralis ventralis; III, centralis dorsalis; IV, culmen ventralis; V, culmen dorsalis; VI, declive; VII, tuber; VIII, pyramis; IX, uvula; X, nodulus. Large arrows point to fissura prima; egl, external germinal layer; IC, inferior colliculus; gl, granular layer; mo, molecular layer. Cresyl violet, ×100. Slightly modified after Altman, Anderson, and Wright (15).

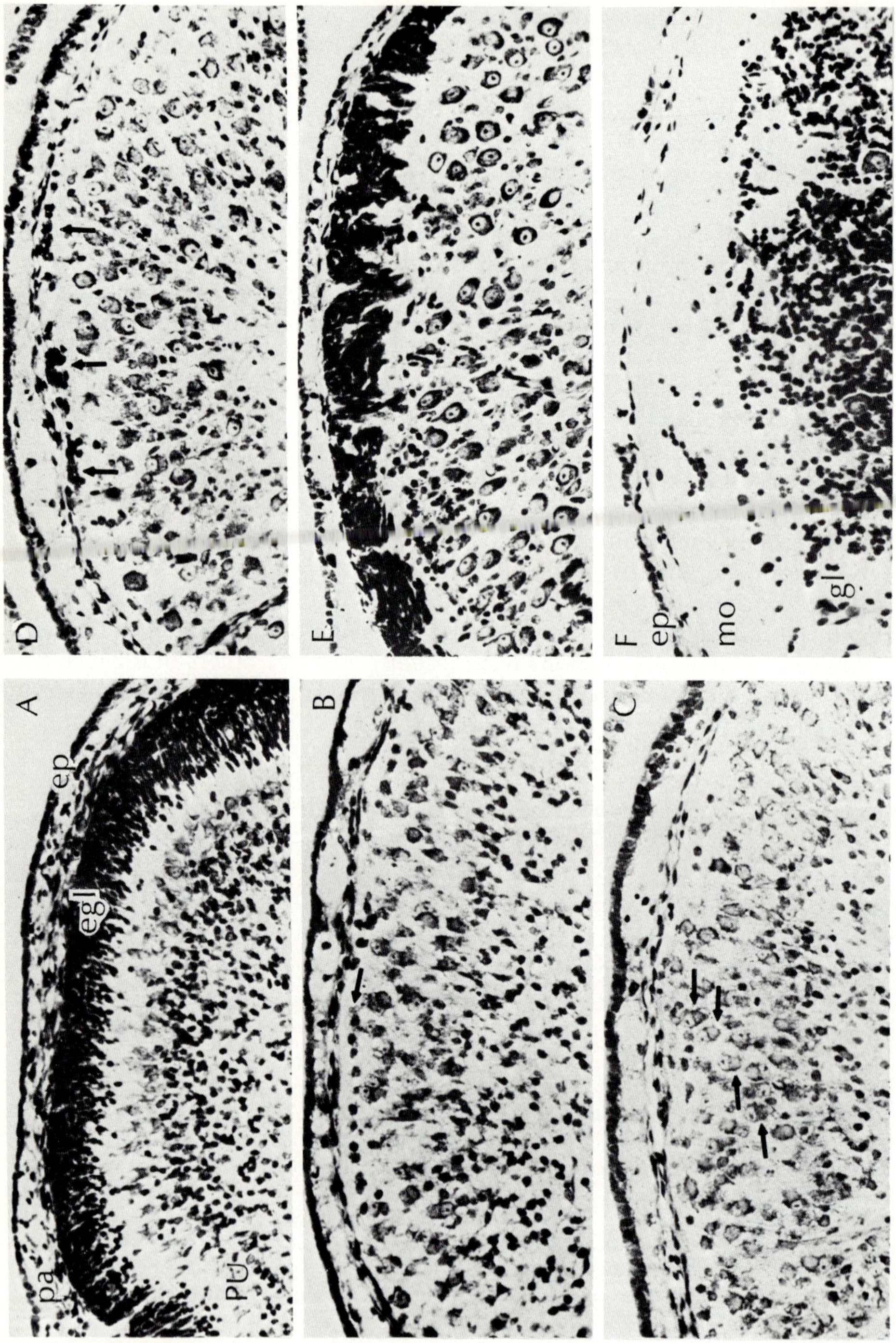
D
E
F
ep
mo
gl
A
pa
ep
egl
Pu
B
C

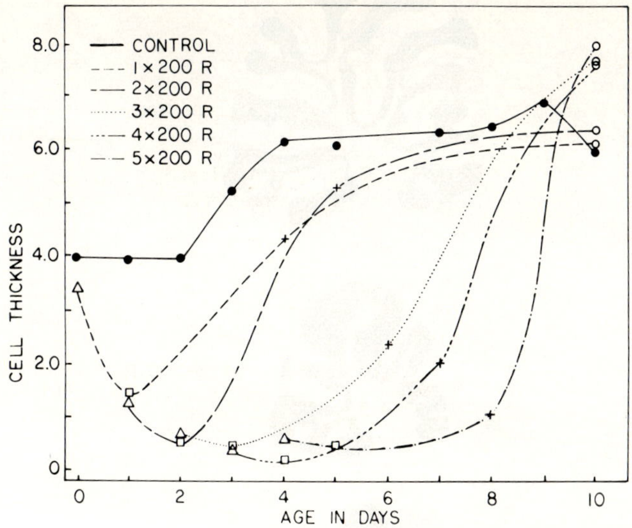

FIGURE 13. Cell thickness of the external germinal layer in the lobulus centralis dorsalis as a function of number of daily exposures, age, and the survival period after the last irradiation session. △, 2-hour survival (last experiment); □, 24-hour survival (last experiment); +, 4-day survival (last experiment); ○, 10 days of age. Slightly modified from Altman, Anderson, and Wright (15).

the decimation of the precursors of its postnatally forming neurons, some considerations suggested that this technique might be used to produce maximal structural disorganization with relatively little cell loss. For instance, in agreement with earlier observations (30,36) we found (7) that in rats irradiated with limited doses of 150 or 200 R from days 3 to 6 onward (but at no other times),

---

FIGURE 12. High power photomicrographs of matched regions of the lobulus centralis ventralis from a normal rat 4 days of age (A) and from rats that were focally irradiated with successive doses of 200 R on days 0, 1, 2, 3, and 4 and were killed at different periods thereafter. B. Survival time, 2 hours after last irradiation session. Note absence of external germinal layer (eg); the ependymal wall of the recess of the fourth ventricle (ep) and the pia-arachroid membranes (pa) are not visibly affected. Arrow points to some surviving radioresistant elements. C. Survival time, 24 hours after last irradiation. Arrows indicate the random orientation of the apical cones of Purkinje cells suggesting that, unlike in normal animals, the Purkinje cells are randomly oriented in space. Note also that the distribution of Purkinje cells into a monolayer (PU) has not taken place. D. Survival time, 4 days after last irradiation session. Arrows point to reappearing clusters of cells representing the regenerating external germinal layer. E. Survival time, 6 days after last irradiation (10 days of age). The regenerated external germinal layer forms a continuous sheet of cells. The layer is fragmented in appearance and the orientation of the cells of the external germinal layer is irregular. F. The appearance of portion of the lobus centralis ventralis from a rat that survived to 30 days of age. The external germinal layer is no longer present at this age but there is a cell-sparse molecular layer (mo) and a granular layer (gl). The location of Purkinje cells in the granular layer is abnormal. Cresyl violet, ×256. Slightly modified from Altman, Anderson, and Wright (16).

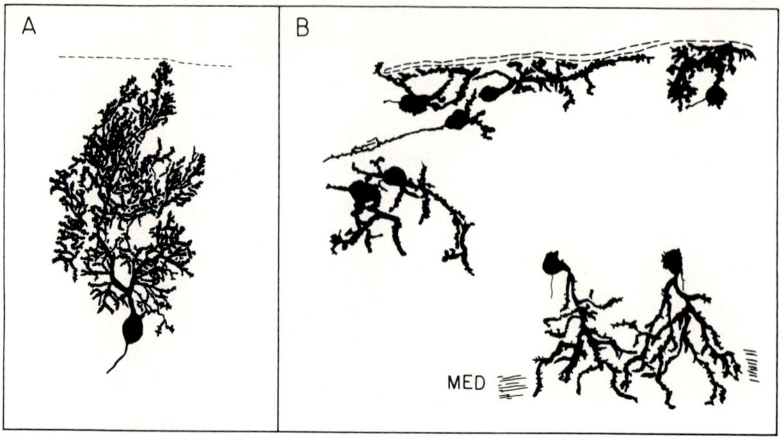

FIGURE 17. Camera lucida tracings of Purkinje cells impregnated with the Golgi technique. A. From the cerebellum of a normal adult rat (courtesy of Nancy Spivack). B. Purkinje cells at different depth of the degranulated cerebellar cortex. Note the prevalence of massive primary and secondary dendrites with thorns, and the absence of spiny branchlets. The orientation of the dendrites is varied. Those near the surface are often deflected sideways or downward; those in the depth of the cortex may have dendrites penetrating the medullary layer (MED). The absence of tertiary dendrites is associated with the absence of parallel fibers. Modified after Altman and Anderson (10).

the cells of the regenerated external germinal layer formed an "ectopic" zone of granule cells in the molecular layer (Figure 20). The morphological examination of the cerebellum of these rats indicated that the granule cells that were arrested in their migration through the molecular layer formed synapses with mossy fibers that penetrated into this layer. The position of the ectopic granule cell zone varied in different lobules as a function of the time of the commencement of regeneration and the estimated date of the descent of granule cells, and as a function of regional differences in cortical maturation and in the estimated upward growth of mossy fibers. Within the same lobule, the longer regeneration was delayed the higher in the molecular layer the differentiating and descending granule cells were "captured" by the apparently autonomously ascending mossy fibers. If regeneration started too early and allowed the descent of granule cells into the presumptive granular layer (early irradiation), or if regeneration of granule cells was prevented altogether (late irradiation), an ectopic zone was not formed. (This technique was used for estimating the normal autonomous growth pattern of mossy fibers in the different lobules.)

In the same and in similar experimental material another structural disorganization was noted (8). In the molecular layer the parallel fibers are normally oriented parallel to the long axis of the folium. But in the regenerated molecular layer they tended to be oriented randomly in various planes. In the cere-

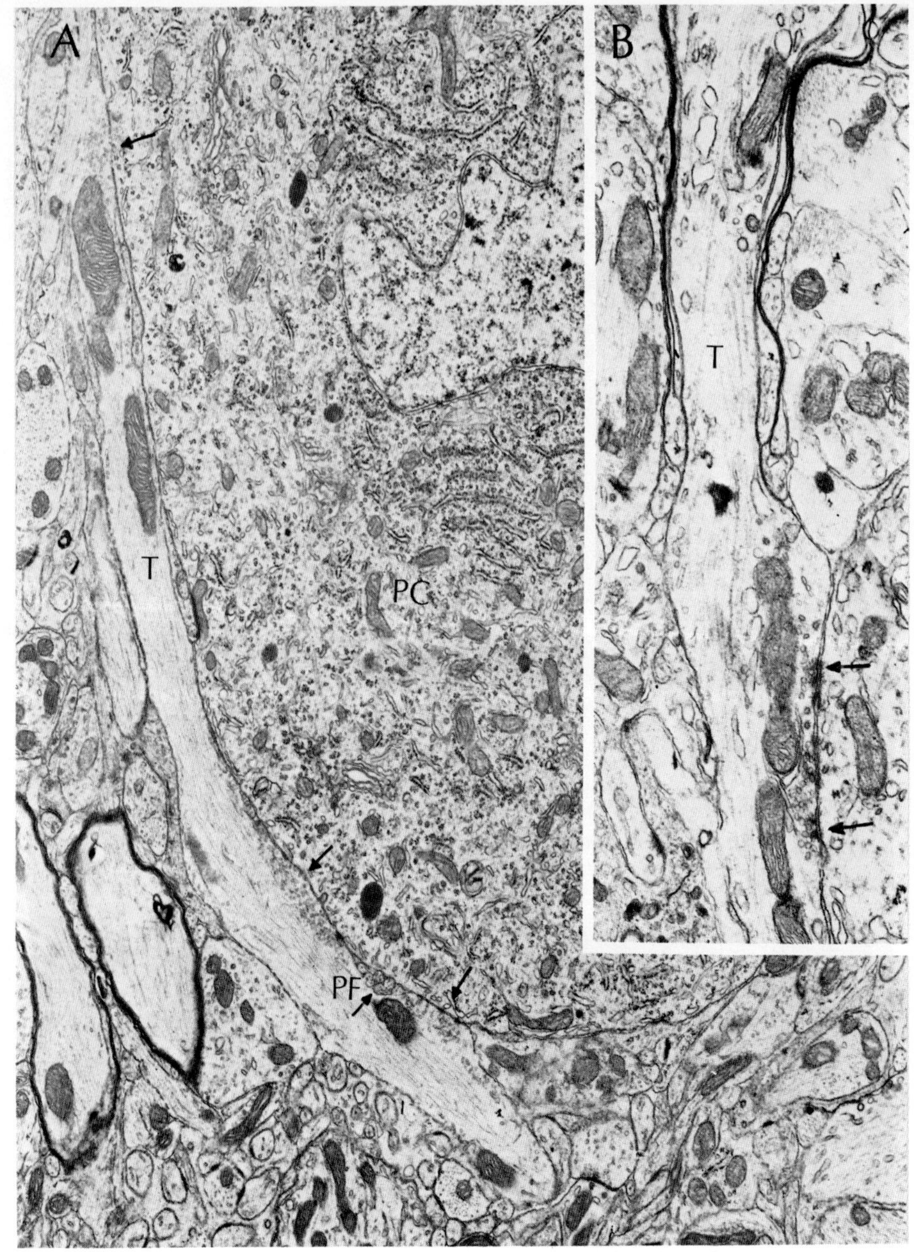

FIGURE 18. A. A very long axon terminal (T) on the lateral aspect of the soma of a Purkinje cell (PC) with *en passant* synapses (arrows). This terminal has all the characteristics of a basket cell and is often seen in the degranulated cerebella that are largely devoid of basket and granule cells. (A few parallel fibers, PF, are occasionally seen.) B. A similar axon terminal (T) from another irradiated animal. But this terminal is clearly not that of a basket cell because it is myelinated. It is assumed to be the terminal of a Purkinje cell recurrent axon collateral. A, ×13,680; B, ×25,080. From Altman and Anderson (10,11).

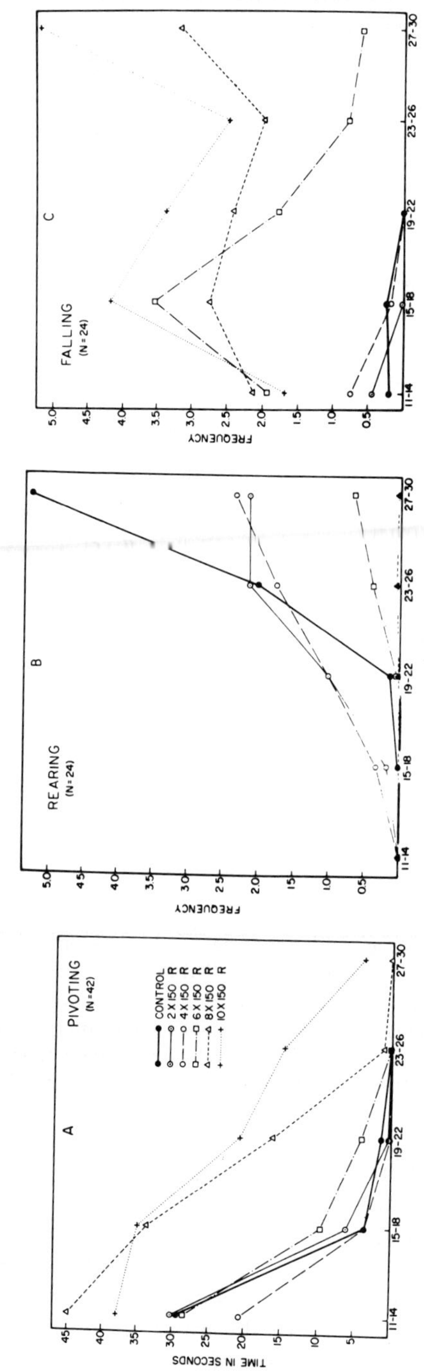

FIGURE 38. A. Persistence of the infantile trait of pivoting in the open field in normal and irradiated rats. B. Frequency of rearing without forelimb support. C. Incidence of falling during locomotion. After Altman, Anderson, and Strop (12).

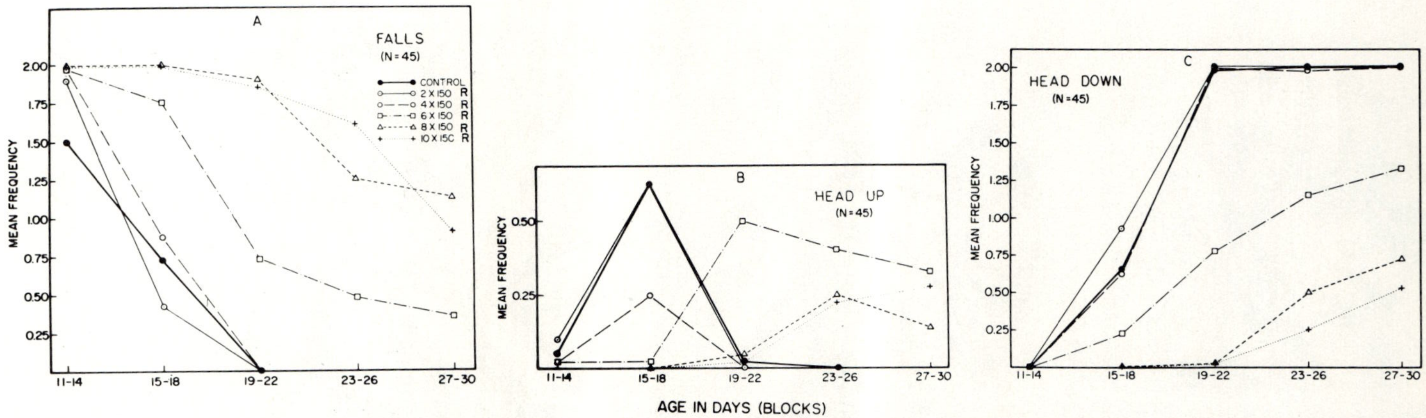

FIGURE 39. Mean frequency of falls (A), sliding down with head pointing upward (B), and turning around and descending with head in a leading position (C) when placed on a vertical rope. Note the longer persistence of falls and sliding in the groups that received 6–10 × 200 R and the slower acquisition of the mature descending posture. After Altman, Anderson, and Strop (12).

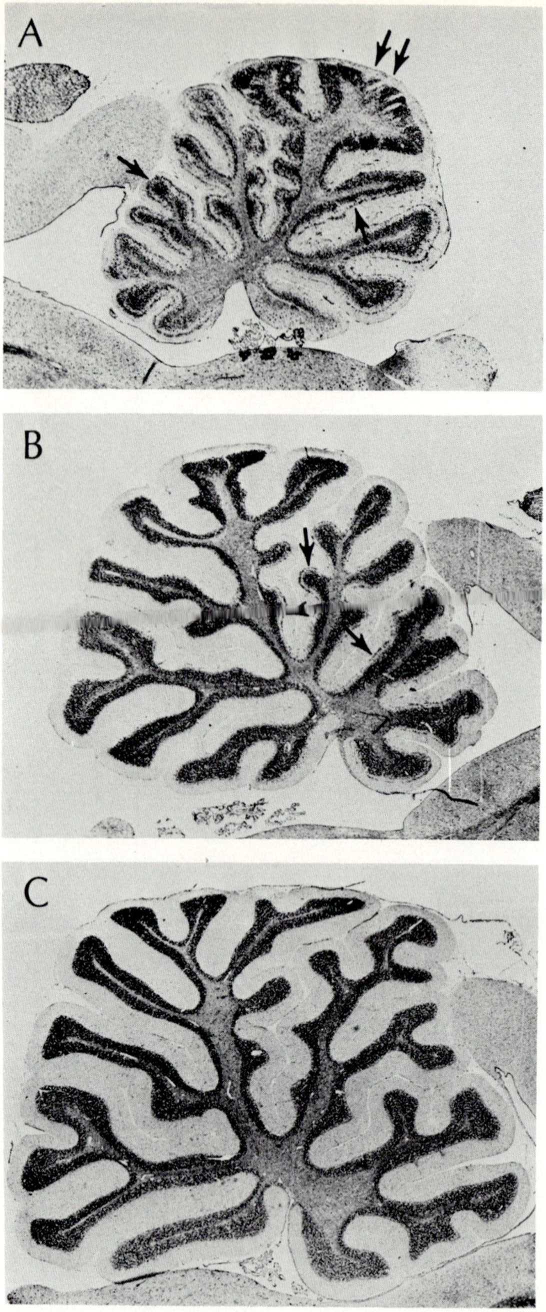

FIGURE 40. Low power photomicrographs of midsagittal cerebellar sections from 60-day-old rats that received 4 doses of X-ray (A), 2 doses (B), and of a control rat (C). Apart from the greater reduction in cerebellar growth there is evidence of laminar disorganization (double arrows) and ectopia (single arrows) in A; in B there is only mild ectopia (single arrows) present. From Brunner and Altman (24).

While these studies established a causal link between the disorganization and retardation of cerebellar development, on the one hand, and the maturation of motor skills, on the other, the exact role of the cerebellum was not clearly indicated. In a new series of studies, the first of which was recently published (24), we examined the locomotor capacity of adult rats that had received either two (2 × r) or four doses (4 × r) of cerebellar X-ray from day 4 on. These schedules produced, respectively, moderate or drastic interference with cerebellar development (Figure 40) with an estimated 49 and 72% reduction in granule cells in the vermis. Three classes of motor functions were examined in these rats when they became mature: various forms of locomotion (swimming, running on a treadmill, and traversing rotating rods), one type of jumping, and two types of climbing. Both irradiated groups equaled controls in swimming speed. Swimming, like running, requires the coordinated movement of forelimbs, hindlimbs, head, and tail for effective forward propulsion. It differs from locomotion on land in that the antigravity reactions are essentially suspended because rats tend to float in water. Moreover, because of the relatively stable hydrodynamic conditions on the surface of calm water, the need to utilize exteroceptive and proprioceptive feedback cues for adjusting the endogenous rhythmicity of swimming movements to changing external conditions may be minimal. We concluded tentatively, in line with an earlier observation in decerebellate dogs (44), that normal cerebellar functioning is not essential for coordinated swimming on the surface of water. From this the inference follows that a pattern of rhythmic progression which requires minimal concurrent postural adjustments and exteroceptive and proprioceptive feedback may be executed successfully by an animal with an underdeveloped cerebellum.

The task of running on a treadmill on a wide and level surface with good

Table I Extended Treadmill Running Tests

	Control $n = 18$	$2 \times r$ $n = 18$	$4 \times r$ $n = 18$
Experiment 2A (1000 ft)			
Horizontal best speed (ft/min)	286	272	256[a]
Uphill best speed (ft/min)	170	159	122[a]
Downhill best speed (ft/min)	353	364	275[a]
Distance (feet) endurance	5806	9389	5284
	Control $n = 12$	$2 \times r$ $n = 12$	$4 \times r$ $n = 6$
Experiment 2B (500 ft)			
Horizontal best speed (ft/min)	271	273	217[a]

[a] Refers to significance (t test) < 0.05.

traction (Table I) involves an additional performance variable, namely, the activation of antigravity responses to sustain the quadruped stance during ambulation. This did not handicap the 2 × r group either in terms of running speed or endurance. Even when another performance variable was added, namely, running on inclines, the performance of 2 × r group was not affected. The 4 × r group was handicapped minimally on the level running task, moderately on uphill and downhill maximal running speeds. These experiments suggested that the postural and feedback requirements in a simple running situation place minimal demands on cerebellar contribution and, therefore, moderate cerebellar retardation has no effect on running performance, and severe retardation has only a slight effect.

Accordingly, in the next series of tests (Table II), the demands for sensory and postural control were progressively increased and the deficits of the 4 × r animals and then also of the 2 × r group became apparent. Rats were required to cross rods of different width, texture, and speed of rotation to reach a goal box for food reward. On the rough-surfaced, stationary rods there were essentially no falls in any of the experimental groups at any of the widths tested, and only in terms of crossing speed (Figure 41) did the handicaps of the 4 × r group and then of the 2 × r group become evident. The combination of reduced width and slippery surface led to occasional falls and disqualifications in the 2 × r animals, to more in the 4 × r group. On the narrowest slippery rod the 2 × r group was as badly affected as the 4 × r animals in terms of speed of crossing. Because of the poor performance of both experimental groups on the narrowest slippery rod while stationary, rotation was not attempted.

In the other experimental situations, such as jumping and climbing, we did not use enough variables to attempt this type of an analysis. In general,

Table II Proportion of Falls and Disqualifications When Crossing on Rods of Different Texture, Width, and Speed of Rotation

			Falls (%)			Disqualified (%)		
Texture	*Width (inches)*	*Rotation (ft/min)*	*Co*	*2 × r*	*4 × r*	*Co*	*2 × r*	*4 × r*
Rough	4.25	Stationary	0	0	0	0	0	0
Rough	4.25	7.5	0	0	0	0	0	0
Rough	4.25	18.5	0	8	17	0	0	0
Rough	1.25	Stationary	0	0	0	0	0	0
Rough	1.25	7.5	0	0	0	0	0	0
Smooth	1.25	Stationary	14	16	39	0	10	40
Smooth	1.25	7.5	1	7	33	0	10	40
Rough	0.87	Stationary	0	0	4	0	0	0
Smooth	0.87	Stationary	5	7	20	0	10	40

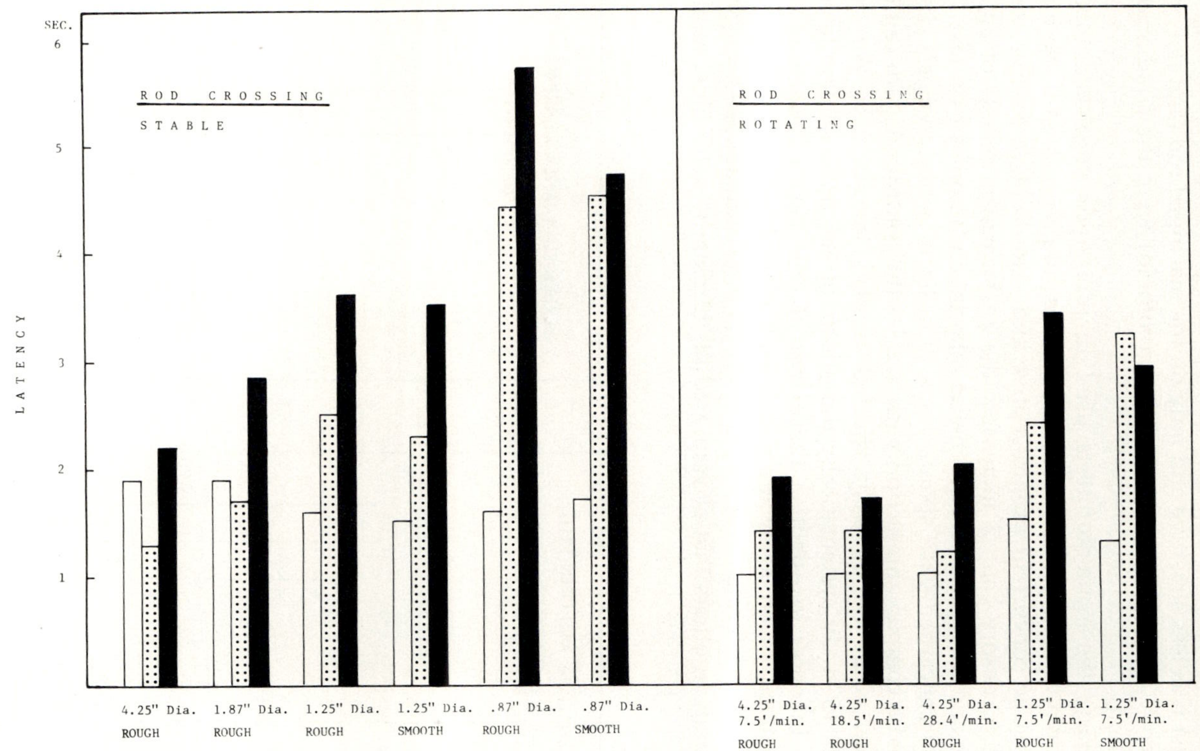

FIGURE 41. Average rod crossing latency for the control group (unshaded), group 2 × r (stippled), and group 4 × r (shaded). Texture and width of the rods and rotational speeds are indicated. From Brunner and Altman (24).

jumping, even in the simple form tested, appeared to be quite sensitive to cerebellar retardation. This may be due to the major role played by the hindlimbs which tend to be more severely affected than the forelimbs. The climbing test was less sensitive and only on the machined rod (and not on the screen-covered rod which offers sufficient foothold) were the irradiated animals deficient.

In summary, the locomotor tests used in this study suggested that full cerebellar involvement is not essential for successful progression if there is no need for precise concurrent proprioceptive and exteroceptive control. As the need for this sensory control increases, the performance deficits of animals with severe and then moderate cerebellar retardation becomes manifest.

The study concerned with spontaneous running in activity wheels (Figure 35) indicated a complex interaction with age, as the control rats reduced their activity level while the severely affected animals increased it. We began recently (25) to study systematically the effects of age on the infantile treatment used in order to establish the extent of "recovery of function." The animals received seven X-ray doses between days 4 and 15, and in some experiments the performance of juveniles (17–21 days) and adults (3–4 months) was compared, in others that of young adults (2 months) with older adults (8 months).

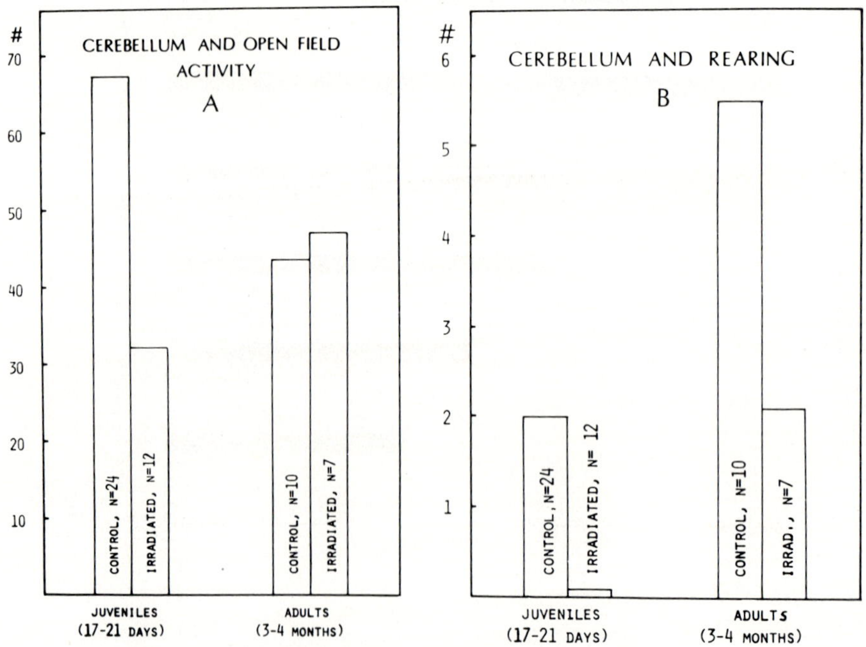

FIGURE 42. A. Mean number of squares traversed in the open field by nonirradiated control and irradiated rats of two ages. B. Mean frequency of rearing in the open field by the same group of animals. From Brunner and Altman (25).

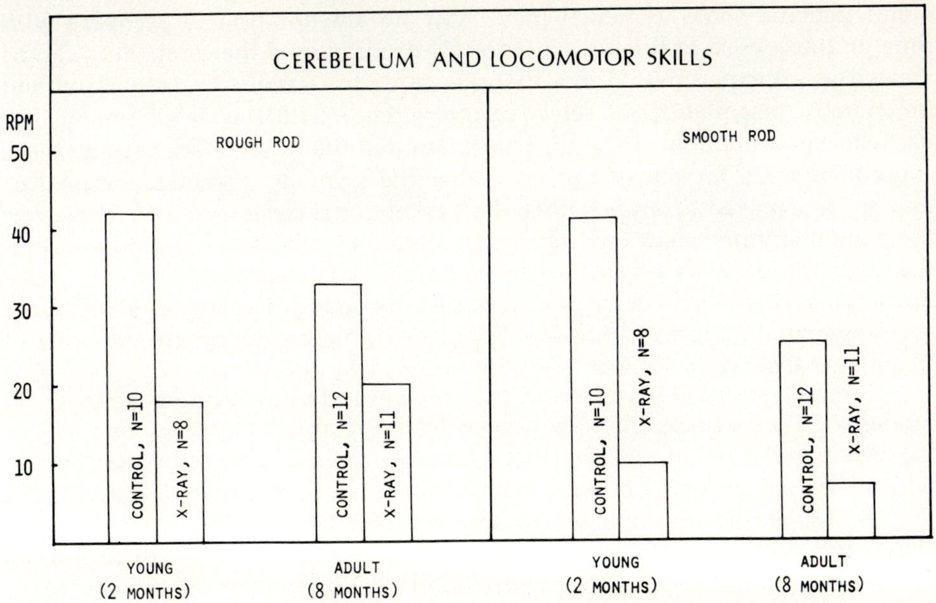

FIGURE 43. Maximal rotational speeds that control and irradiated rats of two ages could negotiate in crossing for food reward. This is a task which shows decrement in performance with age in normal animals, and there was no recovery of function in the irradiated animals. From Brunner and Altman (25).

In crossings in the open field (Figure 42A) there was a decline in the activity level of normal adults with respect to juveniles. In the irradiated animals this decline did not occur such that the performance of control and irradiated adults became similar. In the frequency of rearing (Figure 42B) there was an increase with age in both groups but the difference between the control and experimental animals remained substantial. Finally, no improvement was seen when 2- and 8-month-old animals were compared in their ability to traverse rough or smooth rotating rods (Figure 43). In summary, in some tests normalization of function did occur, in others there was some improvement, while still in others no recovery at all could be demonstrated. The tentative interpretation is that considerable recovery may occur in easy and general functions (the animal can traverse the open field in many ways) but little or no recovery in difficult and specific skills (such as balancing on a rotating rod).

PREWEANING TREATMENTS THAT INTERFERE WITH CEREBELLAR AND LOCOMOTOR DEVELOPMENT

The foregoing results established that interference with cerebellar development in rats by focal X-irradiation during the suckling period produces locomotor deficits, some of which may show no amelioration or recovery with time. In the context of this presentation, X-irradiation of the cerebellum can be viewed as an experimental tool that allows us to examine the structural and functional consequences of selective interference with the development of a particular brain region. It should be evident that the X-ray doses used in these experiments are far above the level that the growing organism, animal or human, is exposed to under other than exceptional circumstances. However, there are many prevalent environmental situations which can lead to substantial interference with cerebellar development. For example, cell loss in the developing cerebellar cortex was reported by many investigators following severe prenatal undernutrition (26–29,31,39,49). The following are examples of treatments that we have been studying in our laboratory.

In a recent study (22) we found that severe undernutrition of lactating rat mothers (50% diet restriction) produces in the retarded pups a severe loss in the cell population of the external germinal layer of the cerebellar cortex, which then results in a decrease in the number of differentiated granule cells (Figure 44). If the mothers are undernourished by the time they begin to suckle the neonates (which is achieved by fostering the newborn of normal mothers to mothers whose diet restriction was begun while they were pregnant), the effect on the young is comparable to that achieved with combined gestational–lactational undernutrition. The loss in the differentiated granule cell population persists after the rats have been rehabilitated during the postweaning period, but there is recovery in the area occupied by the granular layer (Figure 45). The latter finding, which is tentatively interpreted as a com-

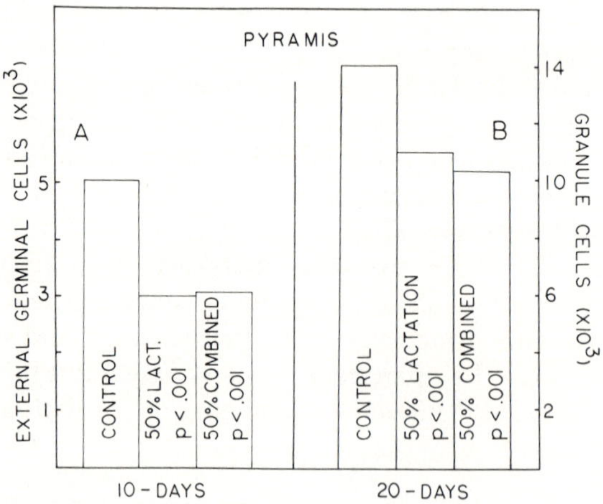

FIGURE 44. Effects of severe undernutrition of rat mothers during lactation or during gestation and lactation combined on the cell population of the external germinal layer in the pyramis at 10 days of age (A) and on the number of differentiated granule cells at 20 days (B). After Barnes and Altman (22).

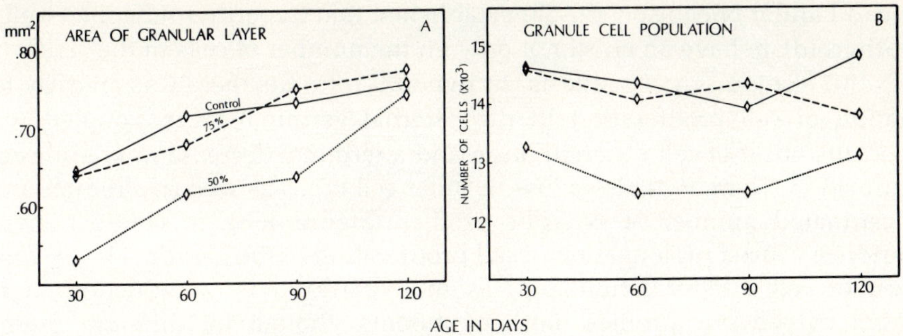

FIGURE 45. Effect of age on the area and cell population of the granular layer following rehabilitation of rats whose mothers were mildly (75%) or severely (50%) undernourished during the suckling period. After Barnes and Altman (23).

pensatory growth of the neuropil (perhaps increase in the size of mossy fiber terminals and granule cell dendrites), confirms a result that we obtained in an earlier study (18). The behavioral examination of these animals is still in progress. The results of an earlier study (20) indicated transient retardation in the development of different locomotor patterns (such as rearing, climbing, and descending) which disappeared after rehabilitation. Preliminary results of newer studies suggest that lasting deficits prevail when adult rats undernourished during infancy are tested on such skilled tasks as traversing smooth rotating rods for food reward.

Another example of a treatment that affects cerebellar cytogenesis is interference with thyroid hormone secretion (21,42). In our laboratory the studies of

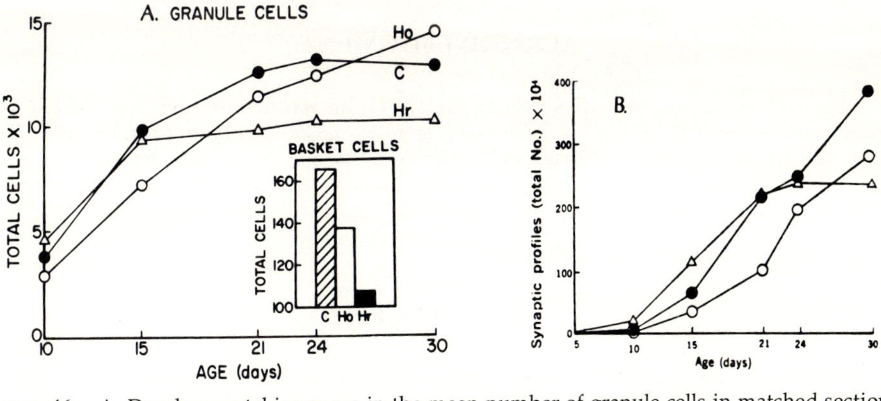

FIGURE 46. A. Developmental increases in the mean number of granule cells in matched sections of the pyramis in hypothyroid (Ho), hyperthyroid (Hr), and control (Co) rats. In inset mean number of basket cells in the three groups. From Nicholson and Altman (51). B. Estimated number of synaptic profiles in 96 μm^2 samples of the molecular layer in the three groups. From Nicholson and Altman (50).

Dr. Jean Lauder Nicholson (50–52) established that hyperthyroidism as well as hypothyroidism have an effect not only on the number of cells in the cerebellar cortex but also on synaptogenesis. In hyperthyroid rats there was an early termination of cell proliferation in the external germinal layer, coupled with precocious onset of cell differentiation and a terminal decrease in granule cells (Figure 46A). There was also a loss in other cell types as well as a reduction in the estimated number of synaptic profiles (Figure 46B). In contrast, hypothyroidism caused prolongation of cell proliferation in the germinal layer, retardation of cell differentiation and, as in hyperthyroids, a reduction in the number of synaptic profiles. Both treatments, though for different reasons resulted in a cerebellar cortex in which synapse formation was markedly interfered with.

CONCLUSION

It is hoped that these results support our belief that a combined analysis of the development of the cerebellum and locomotion under different rearing conditions can provide useful data about optimal conditions of neurobehavioral maturation. Not only is the growing cerebellum an extremely vulnerable brain structure, but harmful effects on its growth are relatively easy to assess. There is a large body of information at our disposal regarding the structural and functional organization of the cerebellum, and its direct link with clearly discernible overt motor activities offers the promise that some information will also be gained about conditions that adversely affect behavioral maturation.

ACKNOWLEDGMENT

I wish to thank all the individuals who cooperated in this research program over the last half-dozen years, in particular William J. Anderson, David Barnes, Robert L. Brunner, Gopal D. Das, Kiran Sudarshan, Robert B. Wallace, and Kenneth A. Wright. I am also thankful to Kunda Das, Zeynep Kurgun, and Donna Whitehurst for technical assistance. Support was provided by the National Institute of Mental Health and the U.S. Atomic Energy Commission.

REFERENCES

1. Altman, J. Autoradiographic and histological studies of postnatal neurogenesis. II. A longitudinal investigation of the kinetics, migration and transformation of cells incorporating tritiated thymidine in infant rats, with special reference to postnatal neurogenesis in some brain regions. *J. Comp. Neurol.*, 1966, **128:** 431–474.
2. Altman, J. Autoradiographic and histological studies of postnatal neurogenesis. III. Dating the time of production and onset of differentiation of cerebellar microneurons in rats. *J. Comp. Neurol.*, 1969, **136:** 269–294.

3. Altman, J. Coated vesicles and synaptogenesis. A developmental study in the cerebellar cortex of the rat. *Brain Res.*, 1971, **30:** 311–322.
4. Altman, J. Postnatal development of the cerebellar cortex in the rat. I. The external germinal layer and the transitional molecular layer. *J. Comp. Neurol.*, 1972, **145:** 353–398.
5. Altman, J. Postnatal development of the cerebellar cortex in the rat. II. Phases in the maturation of Purkinje cells and of the molecular layer. *J. Comp. Neurol.*, 1972, **145:** 399–464.
6. Altman, J. Postnatal development of the cerebellar cortex in the rat. III. Maturation of the components of the granular layer. *J. Comp. Neurol.*, 1972, **145:** 465–514.
7. Altman, J. Experimental reorganization of the cerebellar cortex. III. Regeneration of the external germinal layer and granule cell ectopia. *J. Comp. Neurol.*, 1973, **149:** 153–180.
8. Altman, J. Experimental reorganization of the cerebellar cortex. IV. Parallel fiber reorientation following regeneration of the external germinal layer. *J. Comp. Neurol.*, 1973, **149:** 181–192.
9. Altman, J., and Anderson, W. J. Irradiation of the cerebellum in infant rats with low-level X-ray. Histological and cytological effects during infancy and adulthood. *Exp. Neurol.*, 1971, **30:** 492–509.
10. Altman, J., and Anderson, W. J. Experimental reorganization of the cerebellar cortex. I. Morphological effects of elimination of all microneurons with prolonged X-irradiation started at birth. *J. Comp. Neurol.*, 1972, **146:** 355–406.
11. Altman, J., and Anderson, W. J. Experimental reorganization of the cerebellar cortex. II. Effects of elimination of most microneurons with prolonged X-irradiation started at four days. *J. Comp. Neurol.*, 1973, **149:** 123–152.
12. Altman, J., Anderson, W. J., and Strop, M. Retardation of cerebellar and motor development by focal X-irradiation during infancy. *Physiol. Behav.*, 1971, **7:** 143–150.
13. Altman, J., Anderson, W. J., and Wright, K. A. Selective destruction of precursors of microneurons of the cerebellar cortex with fractionated low-dose X-rays. *Exp. Neurol.*, 1967, **17:** 481–497.
14. Altman, J., Anderson, W. J., and Wright, K. A. Gross morphological consequences of irradiation of the cerebellum in infant rats with repeated doses of low-level X-ray. *Exp. Neurol.*, 1968, **21:** 69–91.
15. Altman, J., Anderson, W. J., and Wright, K. A. Early effects of X-irradiation of the cerebellum in infant rats: Decimation and reconstitution of the external granular layer. *Exp. Neurol.*, 1969, **24:** 196–216.
16. Altman, J., Anderson, W. J., and Wright, K. A. Reconstitution of the external granular layer of the cerebellar cortex in infant rats after low-level X-irradiation. *Anat. Rec.*, 1969, **163:** 453–472.
17. Altman, J., and Das, G. D. Autoradiographic and histological studies of postnatal neurogenesis. I. A longitudinal investigation of the kinetics, migration and transformation of cells incorporating tritiated thymidine in neonate rats, with special reference to postnatal neurogenesis in some brain regions. *J. Comp. Neurol.*, 1966, **126:** 337–390.
18. Altman, J., and McCrady, B. The influence of nutrition on neural and behavioral development. IV. Effects of infantile undernutrition on the growth of the cerebellum. *Develop. Psychobiol.*, 1972, **5:** 111–122.
19. Altman, J., and Sudarshan, K. Postnatal development of locomotion in rats. *Anim. Behav.*, (submitted for publication).
20. Altman, J., Sudarshan, K., Das, G. D., McCormick, N., and Barnes, D. The influence of nutrition on neural and behavioral development. III. Development of some motor, particularly locomotor patterns during infancy. *Dev. Psychobiol.*, 1971, **4:** 97–114.
21. Balázs, R., Kovács, S., Cocks, W. A., Johnson, A. L., and Eayrs, J. T. Effect of thyroid hormone on the biochemical maturation of rat brain: Postnatal cell formation. *Brain Res.*, 1971, **25:** 555–570.
22. Barnes, D., and Altman, J. Effects of different schedules of early undernutrition on the preweaning growth of the rat cerebellum. *Exp. Neurol.*, 1973, **38:** 406–419.

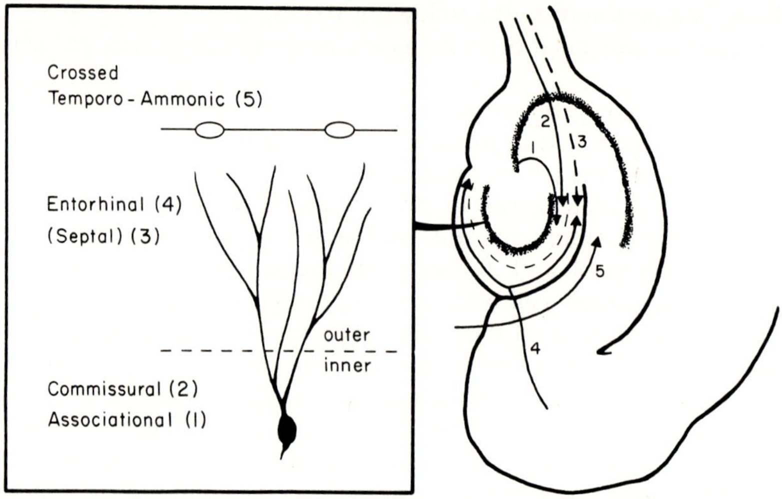

FIGURE 2. Schematic of the distribution of five afferent projections of the dentate gyrus and adjacent stratum moleculare of the regio superior. Note that the commissural (2) and associational (1) inputs are restricted to the inner molecular layer and do not overlap with the septal (3) and ipsilateral entorhinal (4) projections to the outer molecular layer. Thus the afferents to the molecular layer of the dentate form two nonoverlapping lamina (the inner and outer molecular layers). The fibers from the contralateral entorhinal cortex (5) end on the apical tips of the pyramidal cells and do not make contact with the granule cells.

ferents "sprout" and invade the deafferentated outer molecular layer. Specifically, the associational and commissural projections spread outward, the AChE-containing endings normally located in the outer molecular layer proliferate, and the axons from the contralateral entorhinal cortex establish contacts throughout the entire mediolateral extent of the outer molecular layer (Figure 3). [Detailed descriptions of these findings can be found in (1,10–13, 17,18,20).]

In the adult rat, these four systems do not grow randomly into the outer molecular layer but instead relaminate themselves; that is, CTA inputs do not overlap with the expanded commissural and associational system (Figure 3). Furthermore, there are important developmental differences in the degree of growth but these vary according to the afferent under consideration. The commissural and associational projections extend further into outer molecular layer after entorhinal lesions in young rats than after comparable lesions in adults (14,20) but the increase in AChE activity is more restricted. In contrast, we could find little developmental difference in the postlesion changes of the crossed entorhinal projections.

Turning now to the specific questions which in part prompted these experiments, we can now conclude that lesions of the ipsilateral temporo-ammonic tract cause responses in each of the afferents remaining to the dentate gyrus. However, there is considerable evidence that sprouting is not obtained in every situation [for examples, see Goodman and Horel (4) and Kerr (8)]. In other studies we have found that removal of the afferents to the inner molecular layer (that is, the commissural and associational systems) does not cause any major changes in the distribution of the entorhinal inputs in the dentate gyrus (15). Cotman and I have hypothesized that certain lesions create situations appropriate for postlesion growth and in these cases sprouting can occur in all appropriately placed intact afferents. Other lesions apparently do not produce conditions suitable for generalized sprouting.

It is also evident from the results obtained in the dentate gyrus that sprouting in adults is not a random process but instead is both regulated and guided. That is, the invading afferents form new layers with sharply defined boundaries between them. The situation after neonatal lesions is less clear. The changes in the AChE-containing afferents do not seem to overlap with the expanded commissural–associational systems, but the invading crossed entorhinal projections apparently do share dendritic space with these two projections. Relevant to this is the observation mentioned above that developmental

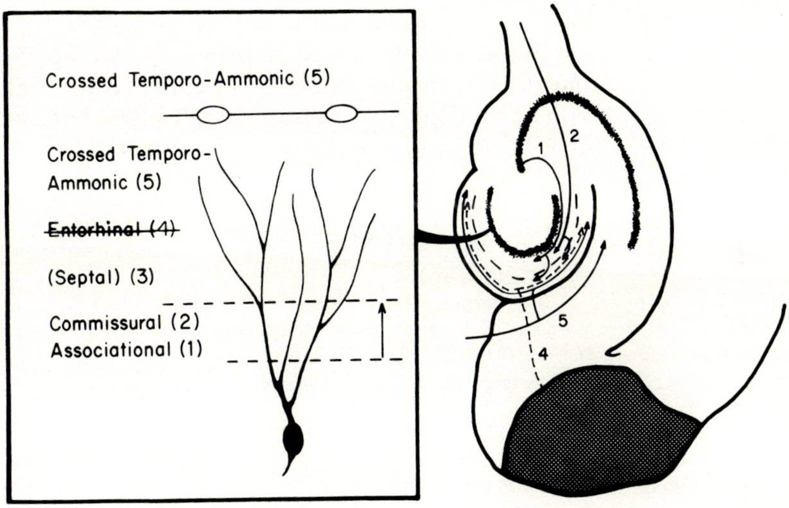

FIGURE 3. The distribution of remaining afferents to dentate gyrus after an ipsilateral entorhinal cortical lesion in an adult rat. The associational (1) and commissural (2) fibers sprout into the outer molecular layer (right panel) while the inputs from the contralateral entorhinal cortex (5) establish contacts throughout the outer molecular layer. The changes in the septal projections described in the text are not illustrated in this figure. The left-hand panel shows that despite extensive sprouting of its afferents the dentate gyrus retains a laminated organization; that is, the extended commissural and associational projections do not overlap with the sprouted crossed temporo-ammonic fibers. The arrow in the left-hand panel indicates that the boundary separating the afferent fields moves "out" the dendrites of the granules cells after the entorhinal lesion.

differences in the degree of postlesion growth seem to be different in the various afferents.

Finally, these results afforded us the opportunity to test the functional status of the aberrantly located terminal populations. We have found that electrical stimulation of either the CTA (17,18) or commissural projections (14,19) produce monosynaptic extracellular potentials in those outer molecular layer regions they invade after the entorhinal lesion. These physiological results were obtained in rats lesioned either as neonates or as adults.

The altered distribution of potentials in adults was first observed at 9 days postlesion indicating that this amount of time is required for postlesion growth to form effective synapses.

SUMMARY

It appears that aberrant but functional circuitry can rapidly develop after removal of particular afferent projections. The parameters describing this process appear to vary according to (1) the age at which the experimental manipulation was performed, (2) the specific afferent being studied, and (3) the particular input which is eliminated or possibly the brain region which is deafferented. It must also be emphasized that abnormal growth is not always found after lesions even in situations which a priori appear appropriate. Hopefully, these anatomical and physiological results obtained in a relatively "simple" brain system will be of help in evaluating the role played by abnormal wiring in the development of behavioral deficits.

REFERENCES

1. Cotman, C., Matthews, D. A., Taylor, D., and Lynch, G. Synaptic rearrangement: Histochemical evidence of post-lesion adjustments in the dentate gyrus of the immature and adult rat. *Proc. Natl. Acad. Sci. USA,* 1973, **70:** 3473–3477.
2. Eccles, J. C., Ito, M., and Szentágothai, J. *The Cerebellum as a Neuronal Machine.* Springer-Verlag, New York, 1967.
3. Edds, M. V. Collateral nerve regeneration. *Quart. Rev. Biol.,* 1953, **28:** 260–276.
4. Goodman, D. C., and Horel, J. A. Sprouting of optic tract projections in the brain stem of the rat. *J. Comp. Neurol.,* 1966, **127:** 71–88.
5. Hines, H. M. Effects of immobilization and activity on neuromuscular regeneration. *JAMA,* 1942, **120:** 515–517.
6. Hoffman, H. Local reinnervation in partially denervated muscle. A histophysiological study. *Aust. J. Exp. Biol. Med. Sci.,* 1950, **28:** 383–397.
7. Jerison, H. J. *Evolution of the Brain and Intelligence.* Academic Press, New York, 1973.
8. Kerr, F. W. L. The potential of cervical primary afferents to sprout in the spinal nucleus of V following long term trigeminal denervation. *Brain Res.,* 1972, **43:** 547–560.
9. Liu, C. N., and Chambers, W. W. Intraspinal sprouting of dorsal root axons. *Arch. Neurol. Psychiatr.,* 1958, **79:** 46–61.

10. Lynch, G., Deadwyler, S., and Cotman, C. W. Postlesion axonal growth produces permanent functional connections. *Science*, 1973, **180:** 1364–1366.
11. Lynch, G., Matthews, D., Mosko, S., Parks, T., and Cotman, C. Induced acetylcholinesterase-rich layer in rat dentate gyrus following entorhinal lesions. *Brain Res.*, 1972, **42:** 311–318.
12. Lynch, G., Mosko, S., Parks, T., and Cotman, C. W. Relocation and hyperdevelopment of the dentate gyrus commissural system after entorhinal lesions in immature rats. *Brain Res.*, 1973, **50:** 174–178.
13. Lynch, G., Rose, G., Gall, C., Stanfield, B., and Cotman, C. Sprouting by the dentate gyrus associational system: A horseradish peroxidase histochemical study. (Submitted for publication.)
14. Lynch, G., Stanfield, B., and Cotman, C. W. Developmental differences in post-lesion axonal growth in the hippocampus. *Brain Res.*, 1973, **59:** 155–168.
15. Lynch, G., Stanfield, B., Parks, T., and Cotman, C. W. Evidence for selective post-lesion axonal growth in the dentate gyrus of the rat. *Brain Res.*, 1974, **69:** 1–11.
16. Morest, D. K. A study of neurogenesis in the forebrain of opossum pouch young. *Z. Anat. Entwicklungs. Gesch.*, 1970, **130:** 265–305.
17. Steward, O., Cotman, C. W., and Lynch, G. Re-establishment of electrophysiologically functional entorhinal cortical input to the dentate gyrus deafferented by ipsilateral entorhinal lesions: Innervation by the contralateral entorhinal cortex. *Exp. Brain Res.*, 1973, **18:** 306–414.
18. Steward, O., Cotman, C. W., and Lynch, G. Growth of a new fiber projection in the brain of adult rats: Re-innervation of the dentate gyrus by the contralateral entorhinal cortex following ipsilateral entorhinal lesions. *Exp. Brain Res.*, 1974, **20:** 45–66.
19. West, J., Deadwyler, S., Cotman, C. W., and Lynch, G. Time course for changes in the distribution of commissural responses in the dentate gyrus following lesions of the entorhinal cortex in adult rats. (Submitted for publication.)
20. Zimmer, J. Extended commissural and ipsilateral projections in post-natally de-entorhinated hippocampus and fascia dentata demonstrated in rats by silver impregnation. *Brain Res.*, 1973, **64:** 293–311.

4

Physiological Properties of Vertebrate Nerve Cells in Tissue Culture

MARC A. DICHTER

*Department of Medicine, Beth Israel Hospital, Boston, Massachusetts**

The vertebrate central nervous system is a large, complicated collection of intimately interconnected systems. It has been studied at all levels—from the vantage of the whole system, as a "black box," to the vantage of individual molecular reactions within individual cells. Each of these approaches has added something to our understanding of basic mechanisms of mental retardation. Recently, advances in tissue culture technology have supported the development of a model system designed to facilitate the study of the development and function of small portions of the vertebrate nervous system at the cellular and synaptic level.

Vertebrate nervous tissue can be removed from a developing embryo and maintained *in vitro* for weeks or months. The neurons will grow and differentiate and form new connections *in vitro*. Such preparations are designed to accomplish two goals: (1) to simplify a highly complex system by separating it into smaller component parts, and (2) to allow more specific control over the environment in which the nervous tissue is developing and functioning.

There are three basic methods that are currently employed for maintaining primary cultures of neurons:

1. Explant culture. Small slices of nervous system are obtained from the region of interest (i.e., cortex, spinal cord, etc.) and are placed in a tissue culture vessel in nutrient broth. The local internal structure of the explant is undisturbed while many neurons are disconnected from distant areas of

* Present address: Department of Neurology, Beth Israel Hospital, Boston, Massachusetts.

nervous system. Hence, neurons have some degree of preexisting framework in which to develop and form new connections (5,17).

2. Reaggregate cultures. Cells from the relevant area of the nervous system are dissociated from one another by gentle enzymatic treatment or by mechanical means. A suspension of relatively spherical single cells is obtained which contains both neurons and nonneuronal elements. These cells are transferred to a nutrient broth in a flask and maintained on a shaker platform. The cells randomly collide in the vessel and appear to adhere preferentially to other cells in a relatively specific pattern. After several days of development, the cytoarchitecture of the explant may remarkably resemble that of the original intact nervous system. Such reaggregate cultures have been prepared from normal vertebrate nervous tissue and from animals with genetic defects which are manifest by abnormal nervous system development (7,8,14,17).

3. Dissociated cell cultures grown as modified monolayers. Cells from nervous tissue are dissociated as in reaggregate cultures, but are grown at relatively low density on cover slips or plastic petri dishes in such way as to keep the neurons separate from one another. In this system, the neurons grow and differentiate without physical contact with one another. They extend processes which form *de novo* connections. The culture grows up as a modified monolayer with the neurons often situated on top of a single layer of nonneuronal cells. In these dissociated cell cultures the original cytoarchitecture of the nervous system is totally disrupted, the cells are all freely exposed to the culture environment, and individual cells, or small groups of cells, can be observed as they develop. Moreover, in the mature culture, individual neurons can be visualized in the living state while detailed physiological and pharmacological experiments can be performed (2,6,9–12,15,16,18,21). Techniques are being developed to separate the initial population of dissociated cells into various components by either physical, or possibly functional, means (1). This may allow the comparison of the development and function of different classes of neurons separately in these cultures.

All of the tissue culture systems in present use are models which, at best, are approximations of phenomena in the intact nervous system. These systems can also be considered as two different kinds of models. In one case, these are models of the *process of development* of the nervous system. That is, the development of neuronal structure and function *in vitro*, the formation of synapses *in vitro*, and the development of a neuronal organization *in vitro* are thought to be analogous to similar events *in vivo*, or at least the two will share some general principles. In the second case, the system can be considered as a simplified model of the *function* of vertebrate central neurons. Studies of the physiology, pharmacology, and pathophysiology of the individual neurons in culture would be considered to apply to similar functions of the neurons *in situ*.

THE MODEL SYSTEM

Culturing Conditions and Cell Morphology

We have been growing a variety of vertebrate neurons and muscle cells in the dissociated cell system. Neurons from rat and mouse cortex, rat, human, and chick dorsal root (or sensory) ganglia, and chick spinal cord, and, in addition, skeletal muscle cells from rat and chick have been kept alive for as long as 4 months *in vitro*. Most of the work to be described dealing with chick spinal cord and dorsal root ganglion cells was done in collaboration with Dr. Gerald Fischbach (9–12). The cells are dissociated with trypsin and gentle mechanical agitation and are plated onto plastic petri dishes or glass cover slips which are covered with collagen or nonneuronal cells. They are grown in Eagle's Minimum Essential Medium with Earle's salts (Gibco), 5% fetal calf serum (for rat cells), or 10% horse serum plus 2% chick embryo extract (for chick neurons) and kept at pH 7.4 in a 5% CO_2 atmosphere. The individual cells settle onto the background within hours of plating (Figures 1A and B), and the neurons begin to extend processes shortly thereafter (Figure 1C). Within days the neurons have formed extensive networks of neurites. The neurons also differentiate from their initially spherical form to more characteristically "neuronal" morphology (Figure 1D and 2). There are also several types of nonneuronal cells which develop in these cultures including cells which resemble Schwann cells, glial cells, and ependymal cells.

Figure 2 illustrates the variety of morphologies which rat cortical neurons can develop. All of these cells were living at the time they were photographed using phase contrast microscopy. Cells shown in A–C are generally symmetrical with processes radiating in all directions. The cells in D–F have a more linear configuration. The cells in G–I have a pyramidal appearance with one long apical dendrite and shorter, branched basal dendrites. Interestingly, the three cells in I are aligned with their apical and basal dendrites oriented in parallel.

It can be shown that the neurons in these cultures can be stained with silver similar to neurons *in situ*. Figure 3 illustrates four cells from chick spinal cord and one from chick dorsal root ganglion cultures stained with silver. The spinal cord cells are of variable size and have multiple processes emanating from their somata. The dorsal root ganglion cell in culture retains its characteristic appearance as a spherical cell with one or a few processes coming abruptly out of the soma. Dorsal root ganglion cells, both from the chick and the rat, always maintain their characteristic morphology in culture and never differentiate into cells which resemble the spinal cord or cortical neurons. They may grow singly or in small groups, as illustrated in the phase contrast photomicrographs of Figure 4, and may be overgrown by the background non-

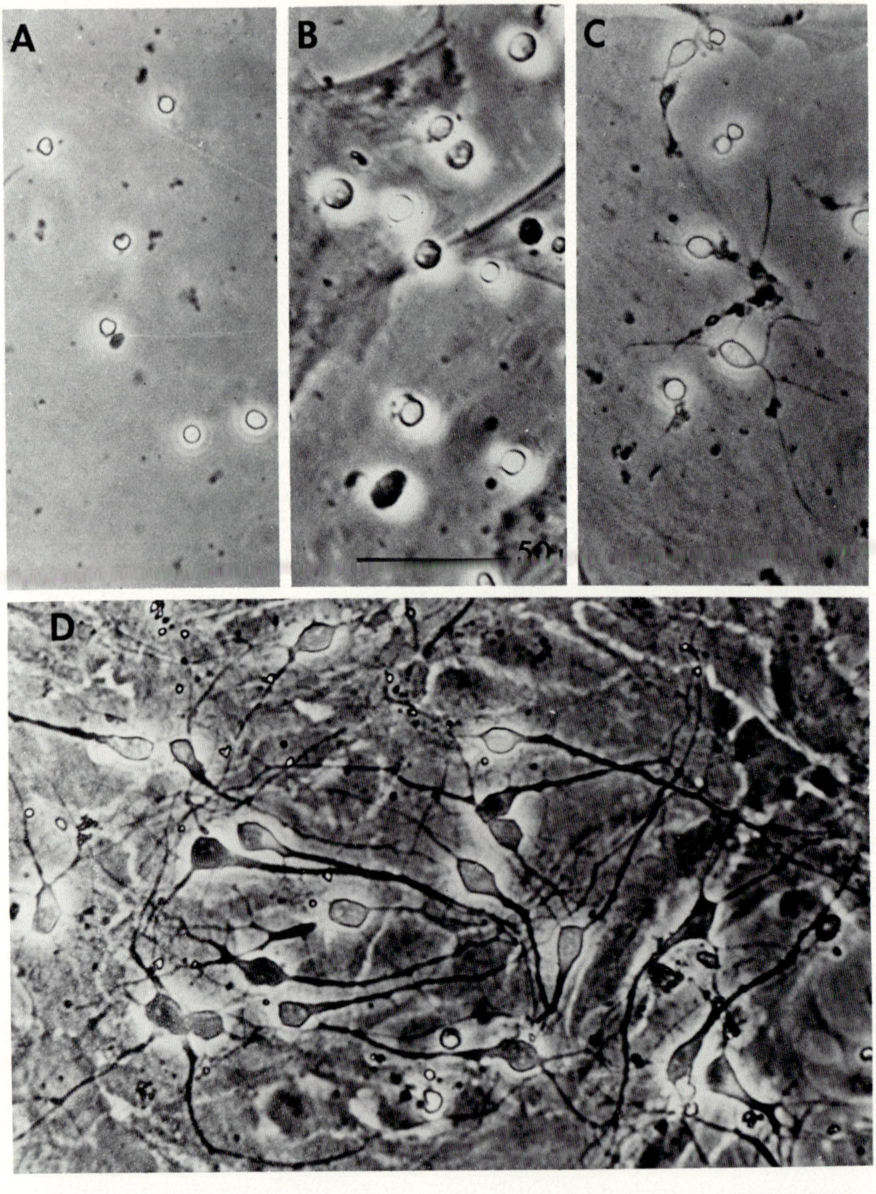

FIGURE 1. Rat cortical neurons in cell culture. A. Freshly dissociated cortical cells from 18-day rat embryo settling on collagen-coated plastic petri dish. B. Same as A but petri dish covered with flat, nonneuronal cells. C. Three hours after plating. Note several neurons have already begun sending out processes. D. Rat cortical neurons approximately 1 week in culture. Background nonneuronal cells have covered the surface of the dish.

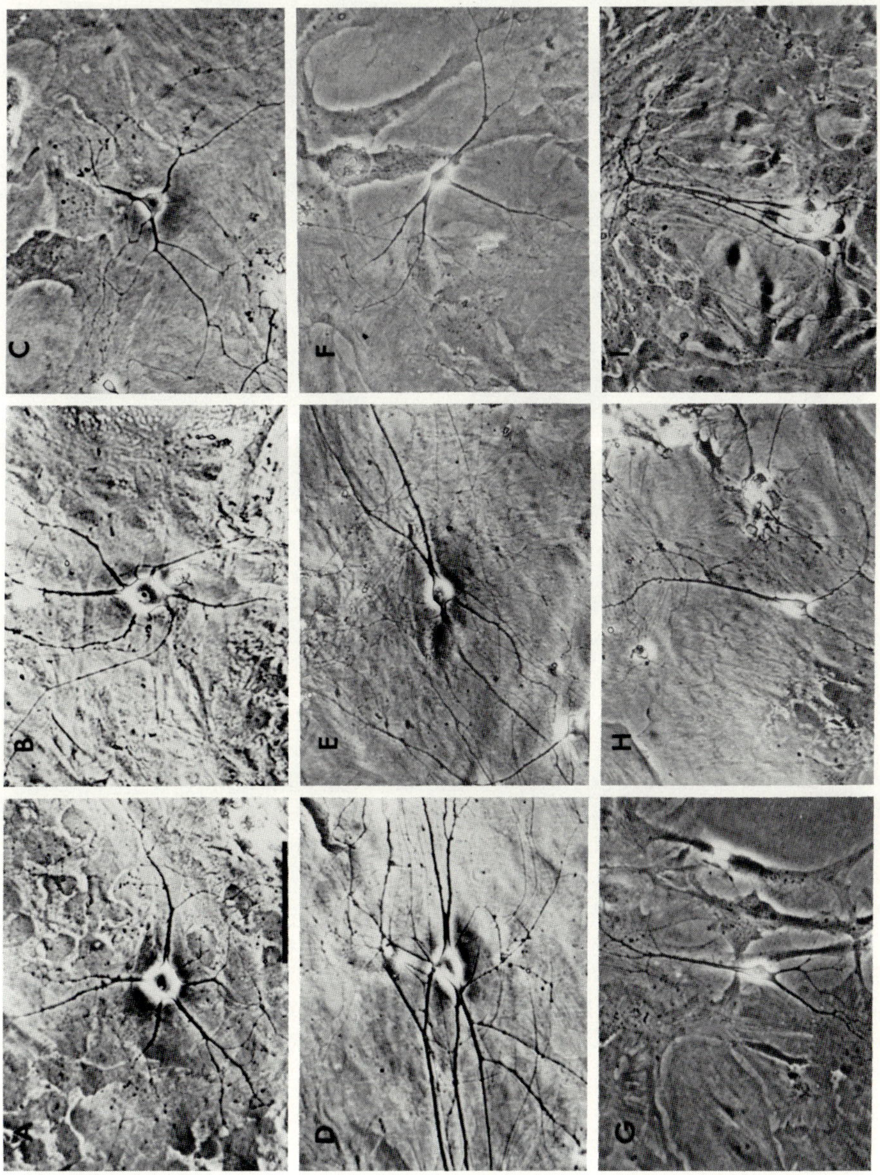

FIGURE 2. Living rat and mouse cortical neurons. A–E, H. Rat. F, G, I. Mouse. Ages *in vitro:* A, 19 days; B, 21 days; C, 15 days; D, 28 days; E, 28 days; F, 15 days; G, 15 days; H, 28 days; I, 12 days. Calibration: 100 μm.

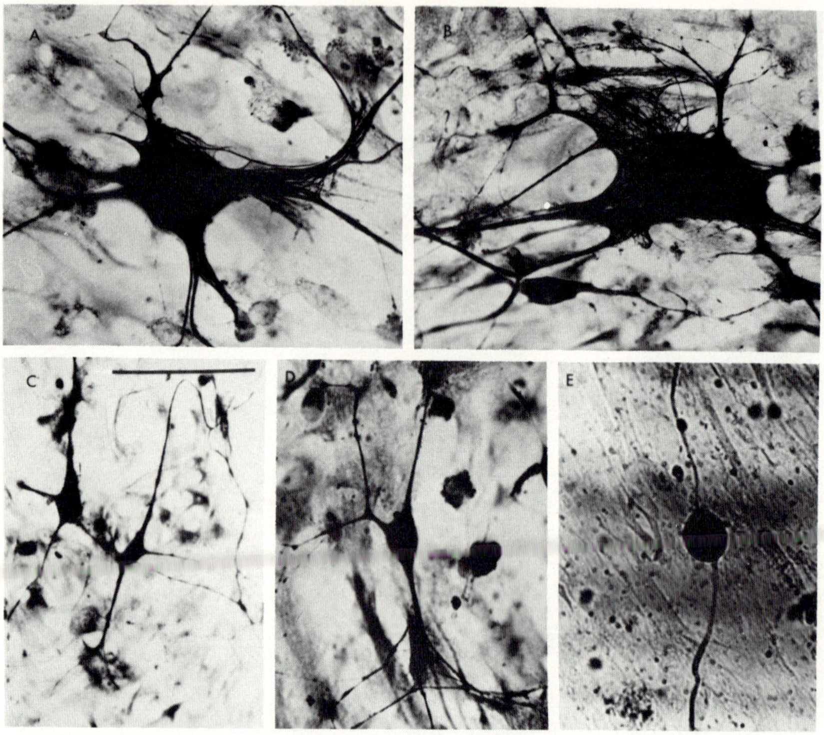

FIGURE 3. A–D. Silver stains of chick spinal cord. E. Dorsal root ganglion cell grown in cell culture. From Fischbach and Dichter (12).

neuronal cells. Occasionally, the ganglion cells appear to be surrounded by a capsule of satellite cells. Frequently, the axons of the ganglion cells are covered by a type of cell which resembles a Schwann cell.

Electron microscopic examination of these dissociated cell cultures indicates that many of the neurons lie uncovered by glial elements and are in direct contact with the bathing solution. The neurons contain the usual complement of intracellular organelles, including neurotubules and neurofilaments and small synaptic vesicles. Synapses can be seen which resemble synapses in the intact nervous system, with their pre- and postsynaptic membrane modifications and collections of synaptic vesicles near the presynaptic membrane (Figure 5).

Physiological Studies

The neurons in these cultures can be penetrated under direct visual control with microelectrodes. The cells have resting potentials ranging from approximately -40 to -75 mV, have input resistances of 2 to 60 mΩ, and can

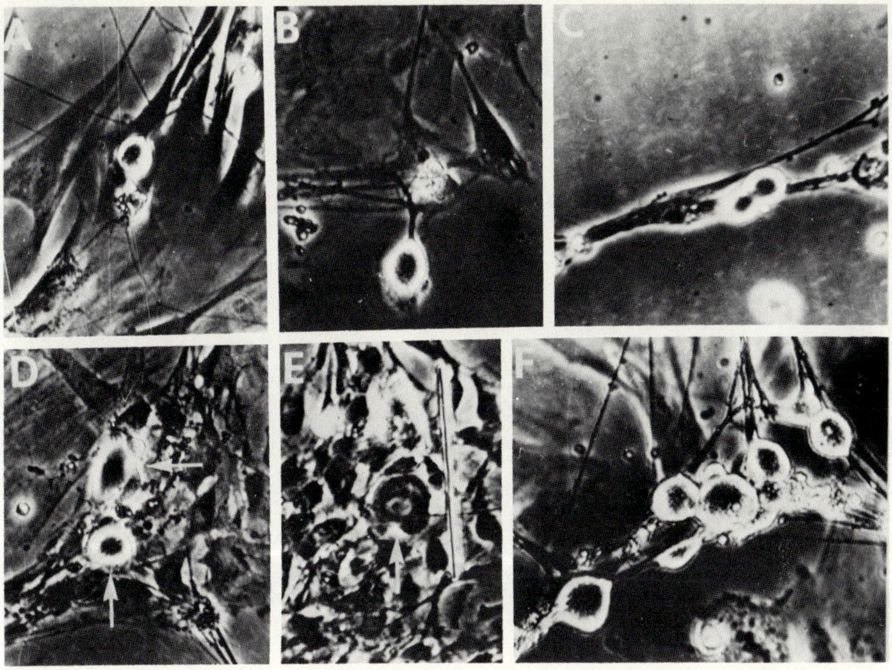

FIGURE 4. Living rat dorsal root ganglion cells. A and B. Isolated, ovoid neurons with one process seen emanating from soma. C. Two neurons lying opposed to one another. D. Two neurons (arrows) enmeshed in background cells and partially buried. E. Dorsal root ganglion cell buried and flattened (arrow). Processes of this cell and those in D not visible. F. Group of approximately six neurons in a cluster with numerous neuronal processes projecting in several directions. The relatively spherical neurons become bright in the phase contrast microscope and when photographed appear to have a halo.

generate all-or-nothing overshooting action potentials. Different cells produce action potentials with different properties. For example, Figures 6A and B illustrate two action potentials from two chick spinal cord cells which both had resting potentials of −53 mV. The action potential in 6A has a more rapid rate of rise, larger overshoot, and more rapid fall than the spike in 6B. Another characteristic which differs from cell to cell is the degree of repetitive firing produced by a long pulse of current. The cell in 6C produced a train of spikes while the cell in Figure 6D could only produce one action potential before accommodating. Action potentials from all the cells studied in chick spinal cord cultures or rat cortical cultures were very sensitive to tetrodotoxin, an agent known to block the active sodium spike mechanism.

When neurons from chick spinal cord or rat cortex cultures are impaled, many of the cells exhibit small spontaneous depolarizing or hyperpolarizing potentials. These potentials have the appearance of typical excitatory postsynaptic potentials (EPSPs) or inhibitory postsynaptic potentials (IPSPs) seen

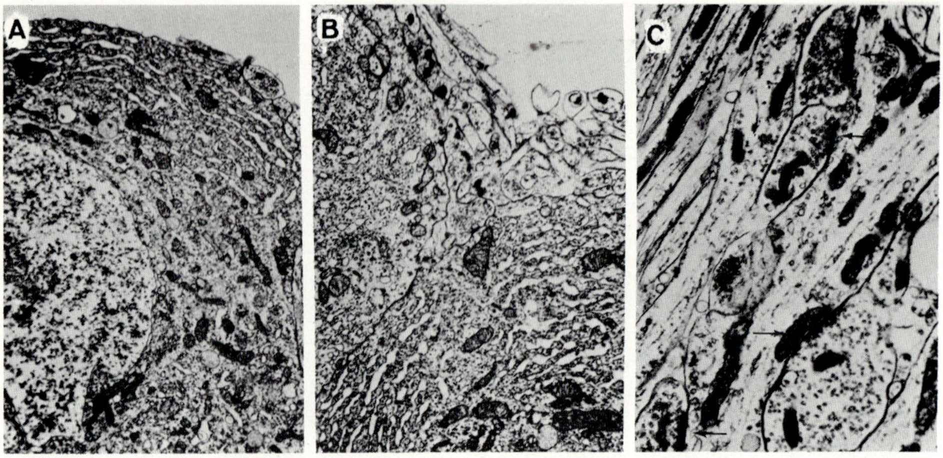

FIGURE 5. Electron microscopy of chick spinal cord neurons. A. View of portion of cell surface. Note lack of glial covering for much of the surface. B. Two neuronal somata and contacting processes. Note that at the junction of the two cells a process forms a synapse with the cell on the right (arrow) and contacts the other cell also (although without a synaptic ending). C. Neuropil of culture. The process running vertically across the figure receives several synaptic inputs from other processes (arrows). Fixed in OsO_4. Electron micrographs kindly provided by Dr. John Heuser.

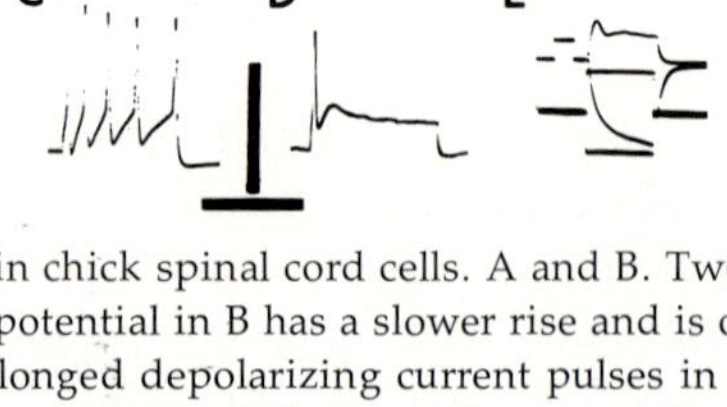

FIGURE 6. Action potentials in chick spinal cord cells. A and B. Two cells with steady resting potentials of 53 mV. The action potential in B has a slower rise and is of longer duration than that in A. C and D. Response to prolonged depolarizing current pulses in two cells. C. Repetitive firing for as long as the current persists. D. Cell fires only one action potential despite continued suprathreshold stimulation. E. Abolition of action potential following addition of tetrodotoxin (10^{-7} gm/ml) to the media. The bump in the depolarizing potential is due to delayed rectification and is not an active response. Calibration: A–D, 50 mV; A, B, 5 msec; C, D, 50 msec; E, 10 mV, 5 msec. From Fischbach and Dichter (12).

in situ. Figure 7A illustrates spontaneously occurring EPSPs in chick spinal cord neurons. The EPSPs occasionally reach threshold and produce an action potential. Figure 7B shows recordings from two cells which had spontaneously occurring IPSPs (one of which also had spontaneous EPSPs). The PSPs were of varying sizes and time courses. The larger PSPs disappear when tetrodotoxin is added to the medium indicating that they probably arise as a result of spontaneous action potential activity in the presynaptic cell. The smaller PSPs remain even in the presence of tetrodotoxin and are probably due to spontaneous release of transmitter from the presynaptic cell, that is, they are miniature PSPs.

Most postsynaptic potentials in the vertebrate central nervous system are a result of a permeability change to specific anions or cations in the postsynaptic membrane. One of the critical characteristics of such a change in permeability is that the size of the postsynaptic potential is proportional to the difference between the resting potential of the cell and the equilibrium potential of the ion(s) whose permeability has just been increased. Therefore, if the resting potential of the cell is increased, that is, if it is moved further from the EPSP equilibrium potential, the size of an EPSP should increase. On the other hand, since the equilibrium potential of the IPSP is more negative than the resting potential, hyperpolarization of the cell will cause the IPSP to decrease in size. In either case, if the resting potential is changed sufficiently to go beyond the PSP equilibrium potential, the EPSP or IPSP would invert. Figure 8 illustrates two cells with spontaneous EPSPs and IPSPs. In Figure 8A the EPSPs get smaller as the cell is depolarized and invert to negative potentials as the cell is depolarized beyond −5 mV. Figure 8B illustrates spontaneous IPSPs which invert when the cell is hyperpolarized beyond the IPSP equilibrium potential. Thus, the spontaneous potentials which resemble PSPs also demonstrate physiological characteristics consistent with chemical synaptic potentials.

Using one intracellular microelectrode and a mobile extracellular stimulating microelectrode or two intracellular microelectrodes, the network properties of

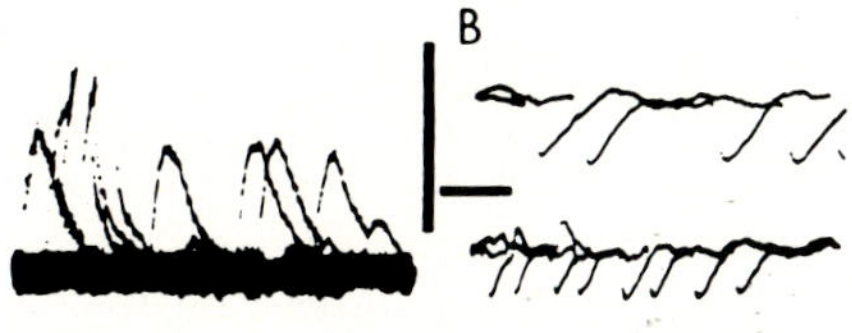

FIGURE 7. Spontaneous postsynaptic potentials in chick spinal cord cells. A. Recurrent, high gain oscilloscope sweeps showing spontaneous EPSPs which occasionally reach threshold and trigger action potentials (off screen). B. Recurrent oscilloscope sweeps illustrating spontaneous IPSPs (top) in one cell and both spontaneous EPSPs and IPSPs in another cell (bottom). Calibration: Vertical bar = A, 10 mV; B, 12 mV. Horizontal bar = A, 5 msec; B, 10 msec. From Fischbach and Dichter (12).

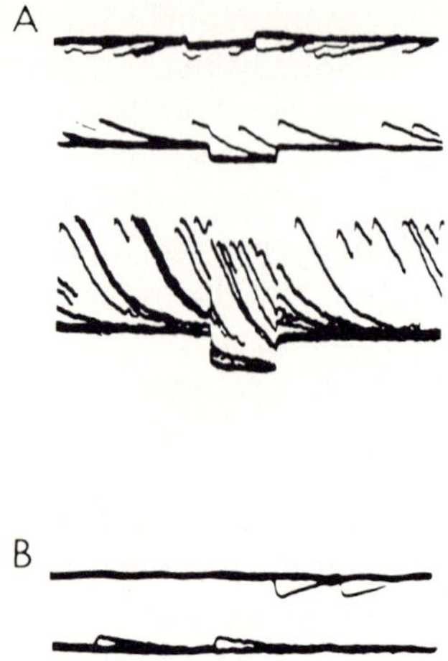

FIGURE 8. Inversion of synaptic potentials. A. Repetitive oscilloscope sweeps showing decrease in EPSP size with cell depolarization from Vm = −44 mV (bottom) to −22 mV (middle) and inversion with depolarization beyond the EPSP equilibrium potential (VM = +4 mV − top trace). A constant pulse of current was injected in the middle of each sweep. B. Inversion of an IPSP with cell hyperpolarization from Vm = −28 mV (top) to Vm = −40 mV (bottom). From Fischbach and Dichter (12).

the neurons *in vitro* can be studied. Some neurons in spinal cord or cortex cultures form synaptic connections back on themselves—either directly or through an interneuron. Recurrent connections, both excitatory and inhibitory, are fundamental building blocks in the vertebrate CNS and can be seen from spinal cord to cortex in the intact animal.

Although the neurons can connect with one another in culture they do not form functional synapses with every other neuron they contact. In fact, proximity is not a necessary requirement for formation of connections. Some cells have synaptic connections with another cell hundreds of micrometers away in the dish but not with several in a nearby cluster. Some of the neuron pairs in the cultures are reciprocally connected while many are not. There are frequent examples of several neurons being innervated by one common neuron.

Sensory ganglion cells in culture form synapses with spinal cord neurons but only rarely have synapses been found between two sensory ganglion cells. Spinal cord neurons form functional synapses with skeletal muscle cells in culture. Dorsal root ganglion cells have never been seen to form functional synapses with muscle cells. It is not known if the patterns of synapse formation seen in these cultures are due to the preservation of intrinsic specificity in the cultures or to nonspecific factors.

USE OF THE CULTURE SYSTEM AS A MODEL OF NEURONAL FUNCTION

Dorsal root ganglion cells from both chick and rat maintain their morphological differentiation in the culture system. This is not a function of the culture conditions but rather appears as a maintenance of the differentiation which takes place *in vivo*. There are also physiological functions which serve to distinguish sensory ganglion cells from central neurons. Despite the fact that these cells are large, are fairly accessible to physiologists, and are rather important as the neurons which are interposed between the external world and the central nervous system, their cellular properties have been little studied by physiologists.

Chick dorsal root ganglion cells in culture have an unusual action potential (3,4,9,18,21). Figure 9 compares a typical chick spinal cord cell action potential with that from a chick sensory ganglion cell. Note the slightly slower rate of rise and, more significantly, the break in the falling phase of the action potential. This is seen in the majority of chick sensory ganglion cells studied and is not correlated with cell injury. Such a spike is never seen in a chick spinal cord neuron or in a rat cortical neuron. On further analysis, this action potential is generated by a different mechanism than that of spinal cord neurons. Tetrodotoxin does not abolish this spike, but does lower the rate of rise. Removal of all external Na ions similarly does not abolish the spike. However, if all external Ca is also removed, or if an inhibitor of Ca spikes (i.e., $CoCl_2$) is added to the Na-free or tetrodotoxin medium, the spike is abolished. Removal of Ca alone or addition of $CoCl_2$ alone causes the disappearance of the break in the falling phase and makes the spike thinner (resembling now a spinal cord

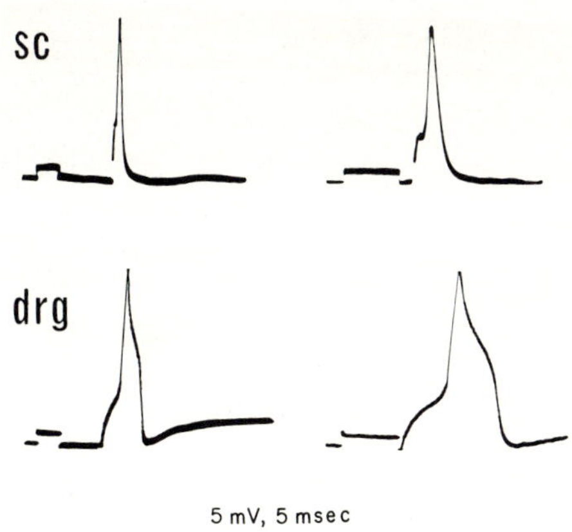

FIGURE 9. Chick spinal cord (SC) and dorsal root ganglion (DRG) cell action potentials illustrated at two sweep speeds.

neuron spike). The remaining thin spike is then sensitive to tetrodotoxin. Thus, the chick dorsal root ganglion cell soma action potential is produced by both a Na and Ca mechanism together. Further confirmation of this obtained by measurements of action potential properties in solutions containing different concentrations of one of the active ions, in the absence of the other (Figure 10).

Interestingly, it can be shown that although the sensory ganglion cell soma spike-generating mechanism consists of both a Na and Ca component, the axons of these cells utilize exclusively, or predominantly, a Na mechanism. The axon is capable of firing high frequency, repetitive discharges of thin spikes while the soma can only fire at lower frequencies and with fatter spikes. Since the soma is situated in such a position in this pseudounipolar cell that impulses do not have to pass through it, the relevance of such an arrangement in the intact animal is not known.

Another interesting, and perhaps unique, property of these cells is that in some, but not all, chick sensory ganglion cells the soma action potential is followed by a prolonged large depolarizing potential (4,9). This potential is generated by a large conductance increase and disappears when Ca is removed from the medium. It is associated only with the Ca component of the soma action potential. It remains in Na-free medium or tetrodotoxin medium even when the axon is unable to generate an action potential. The exact origin of this potential is not known, but it does not appear to be a synaptic potential. Its occurrence in the intact adult ganglion is not known.

The presence of both a relatively prolonged action potential and a prolonged late depolarizing wave in the somata of chick dorsal root ganglion cells has the potential for significantly affecting the transmission of impulses along the

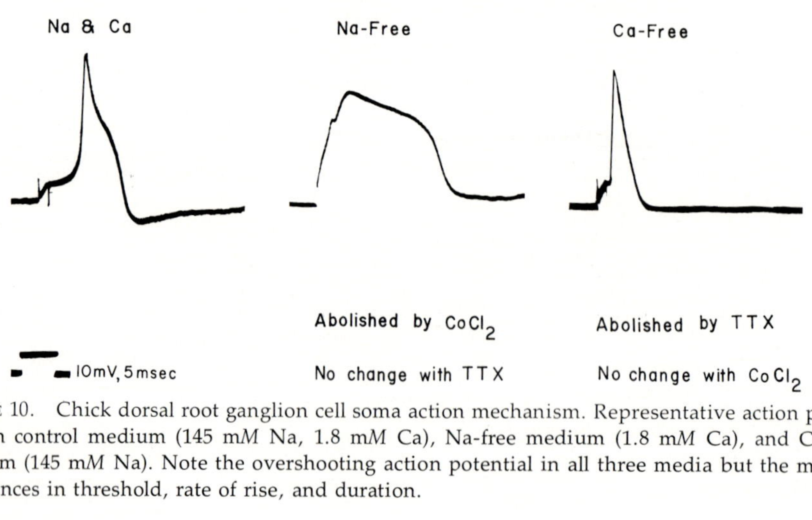

FIGURE 10. Chick dorsal root ganglion cell soma action mechanism. Representative action potentials in control medium (145 m*M* Na, 1.8 m*M* Ca), Na-free medium (1.8 m*M* Ca), and Ca-free medium (145 m*M* Na). Note the overshooting action potential in all three media but the marked differences in threshold, rate of rise, and duration.

ganglion cell axon from the periphery to the spinal cord. In adult dorsal root ganglia the soma gives off one axon which then branches into a centrally and peripherally directed branch (pseudounipolar). As impulses travel up the axon from the periphery at relatively high frequencies, there is a variability in the conduction of these impulses past the branch point such that, above certain frequencies, the impulses do not invade the branch to the cell body and at other frequencies transmission to the spinal cord is blocked (13,19,20). The characteristics of transmission through this branch point are dependent on the physical characteristics of the axon, the electrophysiological characteristics of the axon spike (i.e., duration of spike, duration of refractory period, spike afterpolarizations, etc.) and transmission in nearby fibers. A long-lasting depolarizing current originating from the soma late depolarization could obviously affect such a mechanism. The adult chicken dorsal root ganglion cell has not been studied and it is not known if the action potential characteristics of these cells *in vitro* will be found in the cells in the adult.

SUMMARY

Vertebrate neurons in tissue culture are providing us with a new model system for studying the complex events which occur during neuronal differentiation, synaptogenesis, and neural network formation. It is already apparent that dissociated embryo neurons are capable of differentiating both morphologically and physiologically along predetermined lines in the absence of external influences. These neurons can form new connections with one another but retain some specificity in their selections. Both simple and complex neural networks can be seen.

At the present time, the development of the *in vitro* model system is just being explored. The potential value of a system of this kind at a variety of investigative levels should be appreciated. Questions of a fundamental nature in neurobiology, such as how synapses form, what rules govern such interaction, how cells recognize one another, and the nature of the basic two-, three-, or four-cell circuits that comprise the more complex nervous tissue can be approached with this system. Studies of the neurons and synapses themselves can lead to a more basic understanding of vertebrate nervous system functioning. The development of certain pathophysiological processes and the effects of neuroactive drugs on vertebrate neurons may be studied at the cellular level. Finally, the basic mechanism of some genetic abnormalities which produce abnormal nervous structure and function may be more easily determined in a simplified *in vitro* model than in the intact central nervous system.

The value of any model is not inherent in the elegance of the model itself, but only in its ability to suggest answers to fundamental questions about the system being modeled. Many fundamental questions about brain mechanisms in mental retardation remain unanswered. Perhaps some day the model of nerve cells in tissue culture will bring us closer to the answers to these questions.

REFERENCES

1. Barkley, D., Rakic, L., Chaffee, J., and Wong, D. Cell separation by velocity sedimentation of postnatal mouse cerebellum. *J. Cell. Physiol.*, 1973, **18:** 271–280.
2. Cavanaugh, M. W. Neuron development from trypsin dissociated cells of differentiated spinal cord of the chick embryo. *Exp. Cell Res.*, 1955, **9:** 42–48.
3. Crain, S. Resting and action potentials of cultured chick embryo spinal ganglion cells. *J. Comp. Neurol.*, 1956, **104:** 285–329.
4. Crain, S. Intracellular recordings suggesting synaptic functions in chick embryo spinal sensory ganglion cells isolated *in vitro*. *Brain Res.*, 1971, **26:** 188–191.
5. Crain, S. Tissue culture models of developing brain functions. In: *Studies on the Development of Behavior and the Nervous System*. Vol. 2. (G. Gottlieb, Ed.). Academic Press, New York, 1974: 69–114.
6. Crain, S., and Bornstein, M. Organotypic bioelectric activity in cultural reaggregates of dissociated rodent brain cells. *Science*, 1972, **176:** 182–184.
7. De Long, G. R. Histogenesis of fetal mouse isocortex and hippocampus in reaggregating cell cultures. *Dev. Biol.*, 1970, **22:** 563–583.
8. De Long, G. R. and Sidman, R. Alignment defect of reaggregating cells in cultures of developing brains of reeler mutant mice. *Dev. Biol.*, 1970, **22:** 584–600.
9. Dichter, M., and Fischbach, G. Physiological properties of chick dorsal root ganglion cells grown in dissociated cell cultures. (In preparation.)
10. Fischbach, G. Synaptic potentials recorded in cell cultures of nerve and muscle. *Science*, 1970, **169:** 1331–1333.
11. Fischbach, G. Synapse formation between dissociated nerve and muscle cells in low density cultures. *Dev. Biol.*, 1972, **28:** 407–429.
12. Fischbach, G., and Dichter, M. Electrophysiologic and morphologic properties of neurons in dissociated chick spinal cord cells cultures. *Dev. Biol.*, 1974, **37:** 100–116.
13. Ito, M., and Saiga, M. The mode of impulse conduction through the spinal ganglion. *Jap. J. Physiol.*, 1959, **9:** 33–42.
14. Moscona, A. Recombination of dissociated cells and the development of cell aggregates. In: *Cells and Tissue in Culture*. Vol. 1, (E. N. Willmer, Ed.). Academic Press, New York, 1965: 489–529.
15. Peacock, J., and Nelson, P. Synaptogenesis in cell cultures of neurones and myotubes from chickens with muscular dystrophy. *J. Neurol. Neurosurg. Psychiatry*, 1973. **36:** 389– 398.
16. Peacock, J., Nelson, P., and Goldstone, M. Electrophysiologic study of cultured neurons dissociated from spinal cords and dorsal root ganglia of fetal mice. *Dev. Biol.*, 1973, **30:** 137–152.
17. Sato, G. (Ed.) *Tissue Culture of the Nervous System*. Plenum, New York, 1973.
18. Scott, B., Engelbert, V., and Fisher, K. Morphological and electrophysiological characteristics of dissociated chick embryonic spinal ganglion cells in culture. *Exp. Neurol.*, 1969, **23:** 230–248.
19. Tagini, G. Aspetti del potenziale di azione nelle cellule dei gangli spinali di rana. *Boll. Soc. Ital. Biol. Sper.*, 1971, **47:** 130–132.
20. Tagini, G. Risposta delle cellule di gangli spinali di rana a stimoli di diversa frequenza. *Boll. Soc. Ital. Biol. Sper.*, 1971, **47:** 132–133.
21. Varon, S., and Raiborn, C. Excitability and conduction in neurons of dissociated ganglionic cell cultures. *Brain Res.*, 1971, **30:** 83–98.

4A

Discussion: Biochemical Studies in Various Culture Systems of Neural Tissues

J. de VELLIS, G. A. M. BREEN,* and J. F. McGINNIS

Mental Retardation Research Center and Department of Anatomy, University of California Los Angeles, Los Angeles, California

The electrophysiological studies presented by Dr. Dichter provide clear evidence that dissociated neurons from a variety of embryonic nervous tissues survive for several weeks in low density cultures and form functional excitatory and inhibitory synapses. The similarity often observed between the electrophysiological properties of neurons in culture and *in vivo* validates tissue culture as a model to study synapse formation and differentiated bioelectric properties. Before proceeding to the discussion of biochemical properties of neural tissues in culture it is worthwhile to describe briefly the various methods of tissue culture available and then the advantages and limitations of each.

There are four basic types, classified according to how the tissue is processed and maintained in culture. First, an explant culture consists of small pieces of tissue (0.5 to 1 mm^3) dissected from the organ. Numerous techniques have been used to grow them in culture. Recently we devised a simple method to grow large numbers of explants between strips of perforated cellophane (7,9). The second system is called dissociated cell culture because the tissue is dissociated enzymatically or mechanically to a suspension of single cells. The dispersed cells are cultured on the pretreated surface of a dish either at low density or at high density. At low density the cell bodies will remain separated from each other as seen in Dr. Dichter's cultures. On the other hand, at

* Present address: Molecular Biology Department, Roswell Park Memorial Institute, Buffalo, New York.

high density, cells will form small clusters on top of a background layer. The third type of tissue culture provides conditions that will promote the formation of aggregates. Dissociated cells are placed in a rotating flask. As a result, within a few hours small round aggregates (0.6 to 2 mm) are formed (14,22,23, 32). The fourth system is clonal cell lines established by culturing the progeny of a single cell. The culture, therefore, consists of cells genetically homogeneous. The cell line does not need to be subcultured continuously since it can be kept frozen for long periods of time, thus preserving the original genetic makeup. During continuous culture, mutations and chromosomal loss may occur which sometimes can provide useful mutants. Unlike connective tissue from which fibroblast cell lines have been established, it has not yet been possible to obtain cell lines from normal neural tissues but only from tumors [for review, see McMorris *et al.* (26)].

Each of the systems described has the advantage of providing the experimenter with a broader range of control of the physical and chemical environment of the cells than is possible with the intact animal. Substances can be quickly added or withdrawn from the culture medium allowing a precise temporal analysis of the sequence of events which for instance occur in hormone action or cell differentiation. Tissue culture also circumvents the problem of the blood–brain barrier. Each of the types of culture systems offers particular advantages. Dissociated cell cultures allow the visualization of individual living cells which can be monitored during culture morphologically and electrophysiologically. Although not yet achieved it should also be possible to obtain and correlate biochemical, morphological, and electrophysiological data from a single cell. An alternative to observing and quantitating variables in a single cell is to separate into pure fractions the cell types present in the suspension of cells and then culturing each fraction separately or in various combinations (2). This would greatly facilitate, for instance, the study of the role of heterotypic cell–cell contacts in cell differentiation (36) and of the specificity of synapse formation. Enriched but not totally pure cell cultures can be obtained by selective plating (38,39) or selective media (6,24). One of the advantages of aggregate cultures over dissociated cell cultures is to provide tridimensional growth. The cells inside the aggregate are first distributed at random then they sort out into patterns often resembling the organization seen *in vivo* (9,14,15,32,36). In aggregates the visualization of individual cells is lost. This preparation does not present real advantages for the electrophysiologist. As for dissociated cultures, cell types can be separated before aggregation. Unlike the two types of tissue culture just described, explants conserve the original tissue organization. It is assumed that normal cell–cell contacts are maintained. Of course, the organization can be disturbed by death of cells and possibly by new cell contacts arising in long-term cultures. The importance of tridimensional tissue organization is illustrated by the observation that glutamine synthetase, a marker of retinal differentiation, is inducible by hydro-

(cf. 21,36, for extensive references to this literature) to the human neonate. Our previous attempts to account for the electrographic features of primary evoked potentials in immature cortex have emphasized the early development of synaptic inputs to dendritic elements subtending the most superficial layers of cortex as likely generators of the predominantly surface-negative component of these responses (38,40,44,49). In contrast the appearance of prominent initial surface-positivity of the primary response in older animals has been attributed to the maturation of synaptic activities in deeper layers of cortex. Preliminary observations address the question of a possible approach to the functional maturation of primary projection cortex from examination of visual evoked potentials and neuronal morphology in the human infant.

MATERIAL AND METHODS

Small blocks of unfixed or formalin-fixed tissue cut normal to the longitudinal axis of the hippocampal formation were removed from 70 brains studied at autopsy in the Department of Pathology, Albert Einstein College of Medicine. Samples of other brain areas were also removed for studies similar to those described in this report. Specimens were obtained from spontaneous and induced abortions, preterm infants, full-term neonates, and young infants and children up to the age of 10 years. Clinical, general pathological, and neuropathological data were available on all cases with the exception of early stillborn fetuses.

Cajal and/or Bodian silver stains, the latter modified according to Weinzimer (64) were prepared in all cases for examination of axons and axonal plexus in the hippocampus (see below). Forty of the 70 cases were also studied with the rapid Golgi and/or Golgi-Cox methods which yielded satisfactory results in approximately 30 cases.

DENDRITIC DIFFERENTIATION IN HIPPOCAMPAL NEURONS OF HUMAN FETUS

The major morphological characteristics of dendritic growth processes in the subprimate mammalian brain have been detailed in Golgi preparations most recently by Morest (31–33). For present purposes it is sufficient to indicate that many of the characteristics of dendritic differentiation emphasized in Golgi studies of laboratory animals can be identified in the human fetal hippocampus between 18 and 26 weeks gestational age (g.a.). Satisfactory rapid Golgi preparations of several fetal brains 20–22 weeks g.a. illustrate the most prominent morphological aspects of dendritic differentiation observed in the human hippocampus.

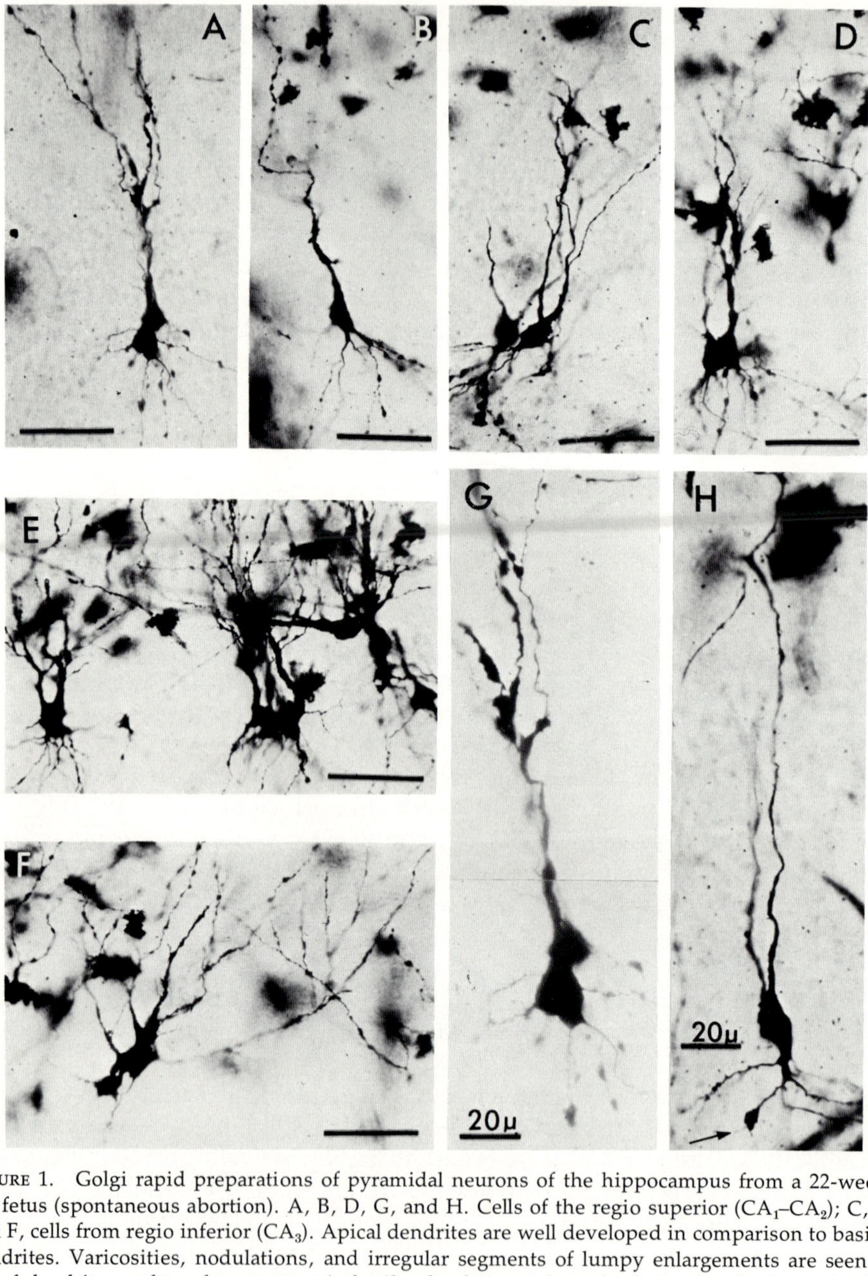

FIGURE 1. Golgi rapid preparations of pyramidal neurons of the hippocampus from a 22-week-old fetus (spontaneous abortion). A, B, D, G, and H. Cells of the regio superior (CA_1–CA_2); C, E, and F, cells from regio inferior (CA_3). Apical dendrites are well developed in comparison to basilar dendrites. Varicosities, nodulations, and irregular segments of lumpy enlargements are seen in apical dendrites and to a lesser extent in basilar dendrites. A branch of a basilar dendrite of cell H exhibits a terminal enlargement which gives rise to two fine filopodia (at arrow). Further description in text. Magnification marker, 50 μm unless noted otherwise.

Examples of the overt characteristics of pyramidal neurons of the hippocampus from a 22-week-old fetus are shown in Figure 1. Cells of the regio superior (CA_1–CA_2) are shown in Figures 1A, B, G, and H. Apical dendrites of these elements are well developed whereas basilar dendrites are thin, few in number, and short in length. Irregular expansions of the apical dendrites and their branches are observed in Figures 1A and G. Regularly spaced varicosities in a branch of the apical dendrite in Figure 1B are also frequently encountered. It is not uncommon for fine thin branches to arise from rather large expansions of more proximal dendritic segments (Figures 1C, D, and G). Some neurons of the regio superior have apical dendrites which are of uniform diameter and lack the irregularities and varicosities of neighboring neurons. Such a cell exhibiting more mature apical dendritic characteristics is seen in Figure 1H. Apical dendrites of neurons in regio inferior (CA_3) are shorter, more irregular and generally exhibit varicosities (Figures 1E and F).

Basilar dendrites of hippocampal pyramidal neurons in the 22-week-old fetus typically exhibit prominent irregularly spaced enlargements or varicosities which may give rise to one or two filopodia (Figure 1H, arrow). Details of these and other growth processes are summarized in Figure 2.

A laterally growing dendritic branch emerging from the cell body of a CA_3 neuron is seen in Figure 2A. A large expansion of the dendrite occurs distal to its origin. From this expansion arise several thick and irregularly small branches with varicose and lumpy enlargements. An apical branch of a dendrite in Figure 2B terminates in an expanded process (single arrow) which at higher magnification (Figure 2C) is seen to consist of a growth cone with several finer filopodia-like processes. To the right, another terminal dendritic process has the form of a bulbous enlargement (double arrows). Figure 2D shows an unusual formation of a fine process with a terminal bulb arising directly from a bifurcation point of a dendritic tree. Irregular, thick dendritic segments characterize the other limb of the apical process. Figures 2E and F illustrate the morphological differences between the varicose and irregular enlargements of growing basilar dendrites and the smooth, regular contour of the axon arising from a pyramidal neuron. Details of a basilar dendrite of this element are shown in Figure 2F. The primary branch point presents an expanded segment from which a fine spicule emerges. Similar spicules and filopodia are seen on varicosities distal to the branch point (Figure 2F). Several additional examples of spicules and filopodia emerging from varicose and lumpy enlargements of apical dendrites are noted in Figures 2G–N. These figures illustrate the wide variation in the characteristics of these dendritic growth processes found in different hippocampal neurons. While no difficulty is encountered in identifying filopodia in Figure 2K, it is not certain whether the fine dendritic processes in Figures 2M and N represent filopodia, dendritic spicules, or incipient dendritic spines. Finally, Figure 2O is an enlargement of a fine dendritic process which terminates in a clawlike expansion.

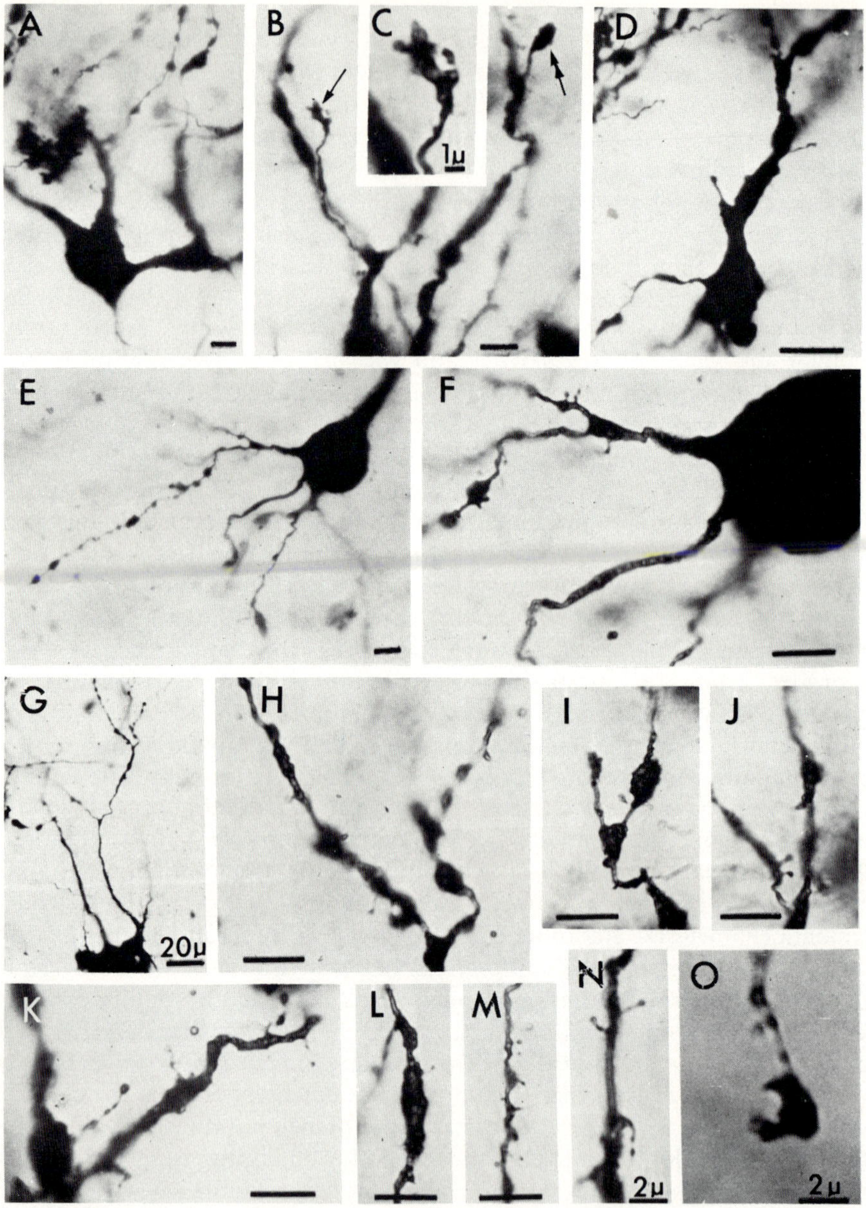

FIGURE 2. Details of dendritic growth processes seen in rapid Golgi preparations of hippocampal neurons from a 22-week-old fetus. A. A cell has a lateral dendrite with a large distal expansion that gives rise to several branches and branchlets. B. Two forms of dendritic growth cones (at single and double arrows) observed in a single field. Inset (C) at higher magnification shows that multiple fine processes arise from the terminal process. D. Asymmetrical formation of dendritic branches from main apical stem. E. Basilar dendrite of well-developed pyramidal neuron exhibits multiple varicosities. F. Higher magnification of E. Note spicules and filopodia arise from varicos-

Dendritic growth processes similar to those illustrated in Figures 1 and 2 from a 22-week-old fetus were observed in somewhat younger (18–20 weeks) as well as older fetuses (up to 25–26 weeks). In five cases spanning the period of 28–33 weeks of gestation, prominent dendritic varicosities, lumpy enlargements, and terminal and preterminal growth cones or filopodia arising from varicose swellings were not observed in pyramidal neurons of the hippocampus. Indeed in the 33-week-old infant dendritic growth appears to occur in a more uniform fashion (Figures 3D–G), since most major dendritic systems appear to have attained their general branching characteristics. At this stage some fine excrescences are detectable on dendrites of CA_3 neurons (Figures 3D,E, and F) particularly on proximal segments that are in relation to mossy fiber projections. Soma and dendritic spicules and spines in apparent synaptic relation with a mossy fiber are evident on a neuron in CA_4 (Figure 3C). In the 33-week-old infant basilar dendritic growth of hippocampal pyramidal neurons has progressed at a much slower rate than apical dendritic elaboration and in some cells nodulation is evident on thin basilar dendrites (Figure 3G).

No attempt will be made to describe the characteristics of dendrites of cells of the fascia dentata. It is of interest, however, that the variety of growth processes observed in hippocampal pyramidal neurons in the 20–29-week-old fetus are not prominently displayed in dentate granule cells. Either such growth processes occur at an earlier gestational age than that examined here or dendrites of most granule cells grow and differentiate by simple linear extension of terminal processes and diffuse increment in dendritic volume. It is significant that in the 33-week-old infant some granule cells may exhibit dendrites that are thick and mature in overt features (with the exception of spines (Figure 3B), whereas others in the same area may be thin and exhibit varicosities (Figure 3A). More detailed study of the growth and differentiation of fascia dentata neurons in the human fetal brain is an obvious necessity in order to evaluate structural features observed in Golgi studies of later developing pathological processes (54).

The observations summarized in Figures 1–3 suggest that the period spanning 20–28 weeks of gestation is a phase of maximum dendritic growth and differentiation of pyramidal neurons of the hippocampus. The data also indicate that many of the features which characterize dendritic growth as described in immature laboratory animals (31–33) are detectable in the cerebral cortex of the human fetus at midgestation. Although cells in different sections of the hippocampus exhibit different temporal patterns of dendritic growth and differentiation during the period defined in this study no evidence has

---

ities and nodules. The initial axonal segment is smooth and of relatively uniform diameter. G. Segments of apical dendrites show varicosities and nodulation. H. Higher magnification of branching segment of cell in G. I–N. Examples of primitive spines, spicules, and filopodia-like processes, some of which arise from lumpy enlargements (K and L). O. Fine dendritic branch exhibits a clawlike terminal expansion. Magnification markers, 5 μm unless noted otherwise.

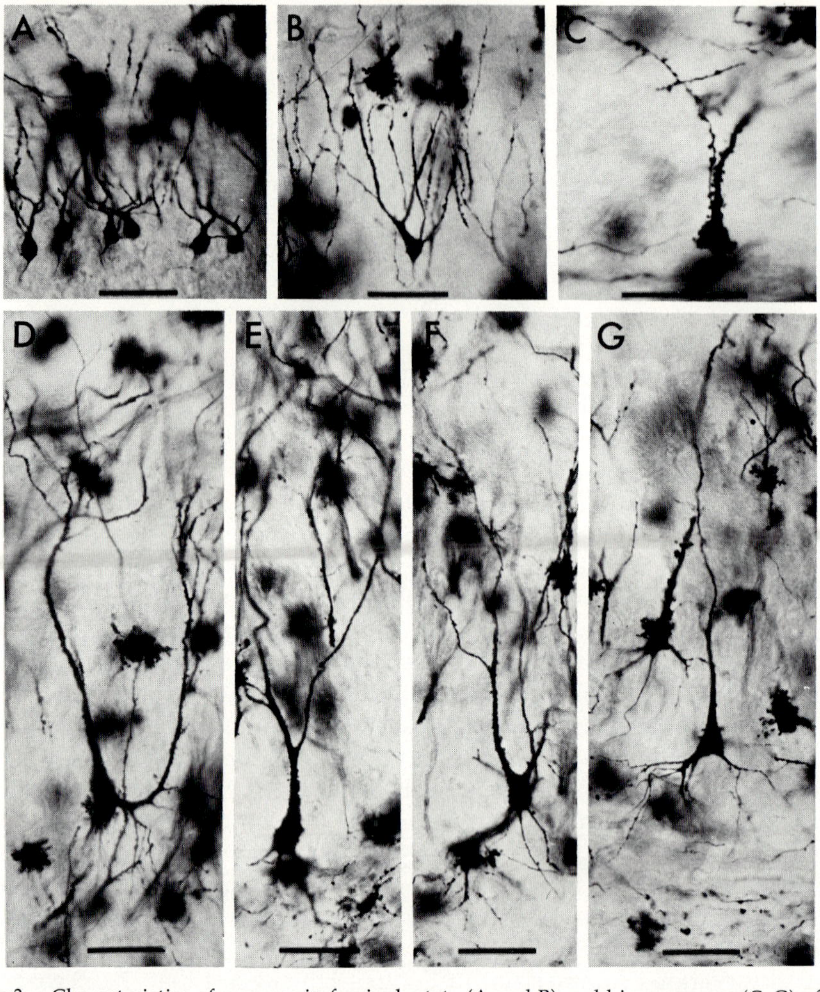

FIGURE 3. Characteristics of neurons in fascia dentata (A and B) and hippocampus (C–G) of a 33-week-old premature infant (respiratory distress syndrome) Golgi-Cox preparation. Fascia dentata granule cells are well developed at this stage. C. Neuron in CA_4 (hilus of the fascia dentata) has pronounced somadendritic spines which appear to be contacted by a large mossy fiber. D, E, and F. Large pyramids of CA_3. Note remarkable expansion of apical dendritic and lateral dendritic branches in D. Proximal segments of cells in E and F have thornlike excrescences suggestive of mossy fiber termination sites. Basilar dendrites of all cells shown are poorly developed at this stage and some show fine modulation. Spines are detectable in some apical dendrites. Magnification markers, 50 μm.

been obtained for a second phase of dendritic differentiation of pyramidal neurons after 30 weeks. This suggests that the maturational cycle of hippocampal pyramidal neurons is relatively synchronous throughout the hippocampus and argues against significant addition of newly formed pyramidal neurons to the hippocampus at later stages of human fetal brain development.

AN APPROACH TO THE COMPARATIVE DEVELOPMENT OF AXOSOMATIC AND AXODENDRITIC SYNAPTIC PATHWAYS IN IMMATURE HUMAN HIPPOCAMPUS

There is no substitute for quantitative electron microscopic studies of the development and distribution of synaptic contacts on different parts of the somadendritic membrane of a neuron in any meaningful investigation of synaptogenesis. There are, however, approaches to this problem which permit reasonable extension of available morphological data from laboratory animals to light microscope studies of the human immature hippocampus. For example, the appearance and elaboration of dendritic spicules and spines on hippocampal neurons which occur at about 22–26 weeks g.a. (Figures 4A and B) and proceed rapidly thereafter to completion by the end of the fifth to sixth postnatal month (Figure 4C) provide indirect (light microscopy) evidence for the relatively precocious development of axospinodendritic synapses. But it must be borne in mind that electron microscopic data are available which indicate that cortical axodendritic synapses related to dendritic trunks make their appearance before dendritic spines are detectable in the kitten (62). Similar types of cortical axodendritic synapses in the human fetus are detectable as early as 8.5 weeks (postovulation) (30). The question arises, what can be inferred concerning the

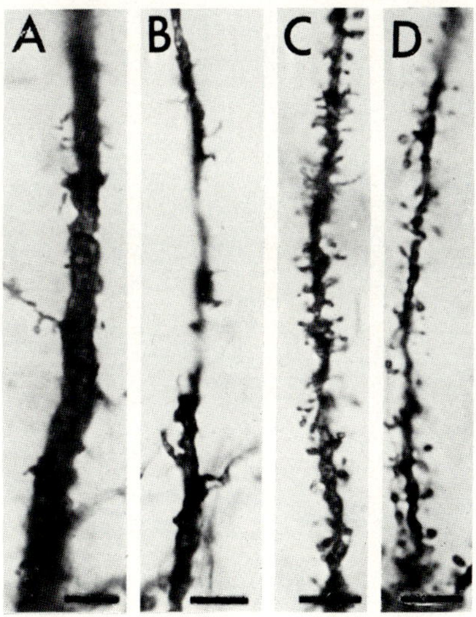

FIGURE 4. General appearance of fine dendritic processes of apical dendrites of hippocampal pyramidal neurons at different developmental stages. Golgi rapid preparations. A and B. Twenty-six-week-old fetus. A. A thick dendrite shows a fine branchlet and several spines clustered distally. B. A thin dendrite shows a variety of branchlets, spicules, and filopodia-like processes. C. Thin dendrite from a 6-month-old infant, normal brain. Some heterogeneity in spine morphology is evident. D. Example of spine distribution on a fine dendritic process from a 7-year-old child, accident case, normal brain. Magnification markers, 5 μm.

development of prominent axosomatic synaptic pathways? In this regard the hippocampus is a particularly favorable structure for analysis.

It has long been established (9,27) that the axons and axon collaterals that form a dense fibrillar plexus in the stratum pyramidale of the hippocampus derive from intrinsic neurons (interneurons) located above, in the stratum radiatum-lacunosum, and below the pyramidal layer in the stratum oriens. A

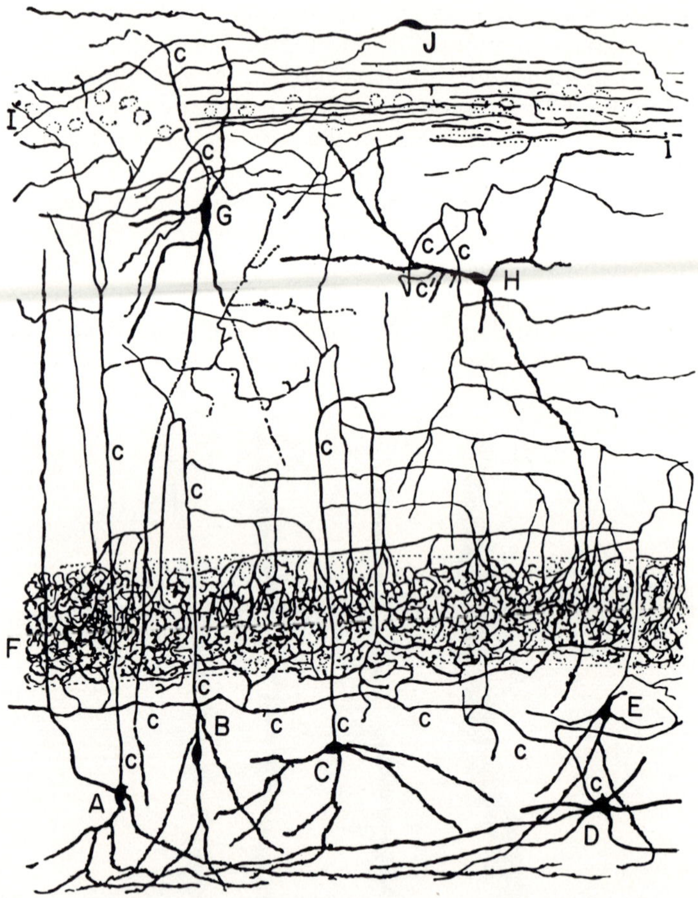

FIGURE 5. Summary diagram from Cajal (9) of the location and axonal distribution of intrinsic neurons (interneurons) of the hippocampus of the 1-month-old rabbit. Cells A, B, C, D, and E are located in the stratum oriens. Axons (C) enter the stratum pyramidale (F) and either collateralize profusely in the stratum pyramidale or pass through (F) and send recurrent collaterals back into the stratum pyramidale. The basketlike network of axon terminals of these cells is readily appreciated. It is estimated that the axon of a single neuron (e.g., B or E) may be in synaptic relation with 200–500 pyramidal cell bodies of the stratum pyramidale [cf. Andersen (1)]. The morphological nature of the plexus in relation to the cell body of a single pyramidal neuron is well illustrated in Figures 6H and H_1.

reproduction of a summary drawing from the classic studies of Cajal (9) amply illustrates the general nature and origin of the plexus of the stratum pyramidale in the 1-month-old rabbit (Figure 5). Typically the axons of interneurons terminate in pericellular basket arrangements on many pyramidal cell bodies. Electron microscopy has confirmed that the terminals of the pericellular basket plexus constitute the major axosomatic input to hippocampal pyramidal neurons (1,11). Of particular significance for the present problem are the observations that axosomatic synapses on hippocampal pyramidal neurons in the kitten develop postnatally when axodendritic pathways are well established (46,55). Additionally, unpublished studies from our laboratory indicate that the period of maximum axosomatic synaptogenesis in the feline hippocampus coincides with the elaboration of the pericellular basket plexus. These different lines of evidence suggest that the density of the axonal plexus of the stratum pyramidale of the hippocampus in the developing human brain reflects in a general sense the number of preterminal axosomatic synaptic processes formed by axons of hippocampal interneurons. One assumption is necessary if there is to be a serious attempt to utilize axon–plexus density as a parameter of maturation of synaptic subsystems. This is that the failure to detect the pericellular plexus in Cajal or Bodian silver stains is not due to failure of the histological methods per se. Fortunately, in all the material utilized in the present series no difficulty was encountered in staining axons bordering the upper and lower limits of the stratum pyramidale, as well as the fiber systems of the stratum oriens and stratum-lacunosum, even in the most immature brains (18 weeks g.a.).

A summary of the observations on the development of the axonal plexus of the stratum pyramidale is shown in Figure 6 in samples of Cajal silver preparations of the hippocampus. In all the cases in Figure 6 general neuropathological examination of the brains indicated normal brain for age (Figures 6A–G) or no neuropathological findings in the case of the adult brain of Figure 6H.

The stratum pyramidale of the hippocampus from a 22-week-old stillborn fetus is illustrated in Figures 6A and A_1. No fibers are detectable in more superficial laminae of the stratum pyramidale (Figure 6A), but a few coarse fibers penetrate the lower borders of the pyramidal layer (Figure 6A). Figures 6B–D were obtained from premature infants who survived for a few hours to a few days after the onset of respiratory distress.

At 27 weeks g.a. (Figures 6B and B_1) axons are more frequently encountered in relation to pyramidal neurons deep in the stratum pyramidale and some are noted about major dendritic branches (at arrow in Figure 6B). Axons passing through the more superficial parts of the stratum pyramidale exhibit close apposition to pyramidal neurons (arrow in Figure $6B_1$) but lack fine collaterals and branches. Essentially similar findings are noted at 28 weeks g.a. (Figure 6C and C_1). By 33 weeks g.a. a greater density of axons appears in relation to deep lying hippocampal pyramidal neurons (Figure 6D). Essentially no change

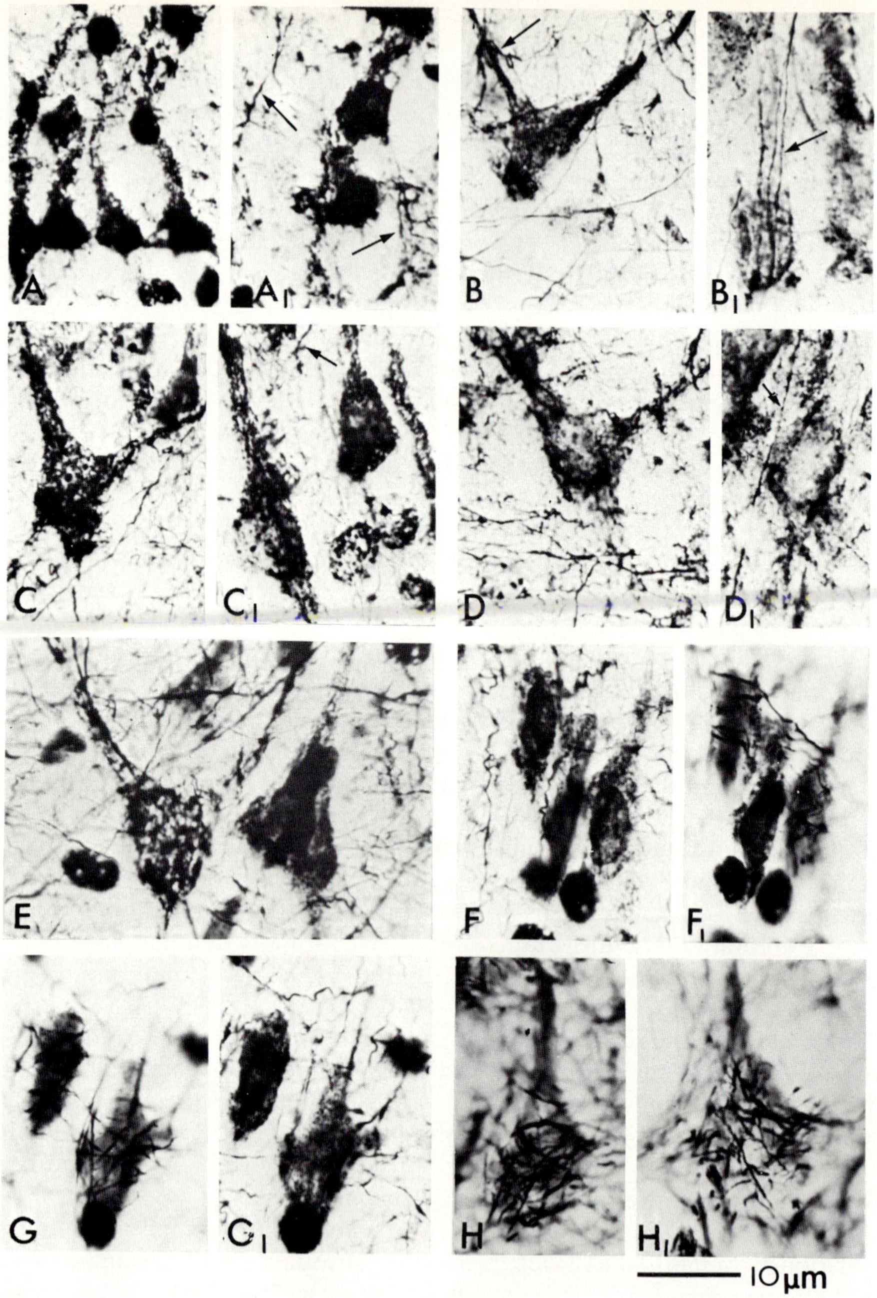

FIGURE 6. Development of the axon plexus of the stratum pyramidale of the hippocampus in the human brain. Cajal preparations. A and A_1. Twenty-two-week-old fetus; B and B_1, 27-weeks, preterm infant. E, F, F_1, G, and G_1. Two weeks postnatally, full-term infant. H and H_1. Normal adult. Note that in very immature hippocampus only a few axons are detectable, especially in relation to deeper lying pyramidal neurons (B, B_1, C, C_1, and D, D_1). There is a dramatic increase in the density of the axon plexus in the 2-week-old full-term infant. In the adult the dense basketlike plexus consists of many very fine axons and axon terminals with fine boutons. The apical dendrite is free of the plexus (H and H_1). Further description in text.

has occurred in the appearance of axons related to superficial cells in the 33 weeks g.a. infant from that at 28 weeks g.a. However, between 36 weeks g.a. and for several weeks after birth in the full-term infant there is a remarkable increase in the caliber and density of the axonal plexus of the stratum pyramidale (Figure 6E). Careful examination at different focal planes reveals many pericellular arrangements of axons which collateralize among several pyramidal neurons (Figures 6F, F_1, G, and G_1). While there is considerable maturation of the plexus in the immediate postnatal period the pericellular network still lacks the density and characteristics of the plexus observed in the adult brain (Figures 6H and H_1).

To the extent that the progressive appearance in silver preparations of the axonal plexus in the stratum pyramidale of the immature human hippocampus provides indirect evidence for the elaboration of preterminal axosomatic synaptic processes it may be inferred from the studies summarized above that these synaptic inputs develop relatively late in human gestation in comparison to axodendritic and particularly axospinodendritic synaptic projections to pyramidal neurons. This inference is consonant with previous findings in the immature feline brain (46,49,55,62). The results of Figure 6 also provide a useful and relatively simple light microscopical approach to evaluation of the "maturational status" of the hippocampus from the standpoint of development and elaboration of axon collaterals and preterminal processes in a well-defined cortical location. In the final analysis the number of axosomatic synapses on pyramidal neurons must be a function of the number of axonal preterminals that constitute the presynaptic element of these synapses. And since there is no difficulty in resolving axons in the range of 1 μm (and possibly less) in good Cajal or Bodian preparations of the immature hippocampus it may be argued that the number of such small diameter axons bears a direct relationship to the number of fine axonal preterminal processes.

The foregoing inferences are worthy of consideration in attempts to identify factors which could conceivably delay, modify, or interrupt the process of axonal invasion, growth, and axon collateral proliferation in the stratum pyramidale during the third trimester and in the immediate postnatal period. Obviously such factors as metabolic or cardiorespiratory disturbances with or without underlying genetic determinants are likely to exert widespread alterations in developmental processes. The problem here, however, is one of detection of developmental events particularly vulnerable to such disturbances. Several illustrations serve to define the problem as it relates to the development of the axonal plexus of the stratum pyramidale.

Examples of Cajal silver preparations of the stratum pyramidale in four cases representing two pairs of age-related infants are shown in Figure 7. The normal appearance of the axonal plexus in a 2-week-old full-term infant who succumbed following acute respiratory distress (Figure 7A) is compared with the appearance of the stratum pyramidale in a 1.5-week-old infant with Down's syndrome and Tetralogy of Falot (Figure 7B). Apart from the reduction

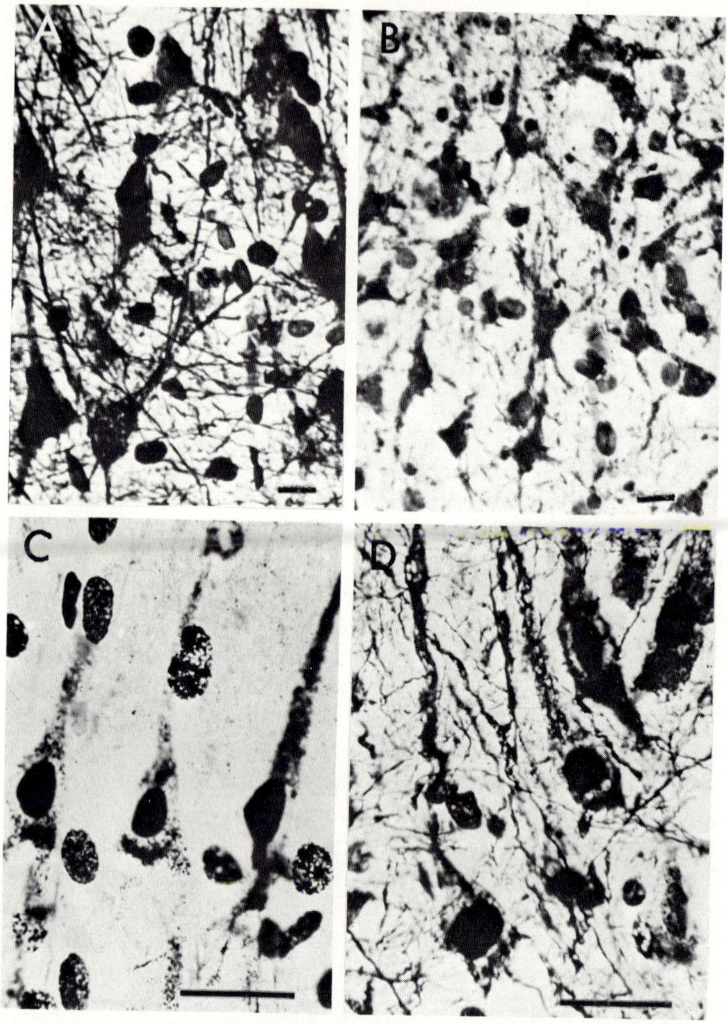

FIGURE 7. Comparison of the density of the axonal plexus of the stratum pyramidale in different clinical conditions. (Cajal preparations.) A. Relatively normal density of the plexus of the hippocampus in a 2-week-old full-term infant who succumbed following acute respiratory distress. B. Absence of the axonal plexus in a 2-week-old full-term infant with Down's syndrome and Tetralogy of Falot. C. Absence of the axonal plexus in a 6-week-old full-term infant with cyanotic heart disease. D. Development and persistence of the axonal plexus in a 6-week-old full-term infant with cerebro-hepatorenal syndrome. Note twisted appearance of dendrites of some pyramidal neurons in this condition. Magnification markers, 10 μm.

in neuron cell size there is no significant difference in the density of neurons in the section from the Down's case (Figure 7B) and in the age-related "control" (Figure 7A). In contrast there is a striking absence of the axonal plexus in the infant with Down's syndrome and associated multiple congenital anomalies. It cannot be concluded from available data that the decreased density or loss of the axonal plexus of the stratum pyramidale seen in Figure 7B is a direct expression of the genetic abnormality of Down's syndrome. It should be noted that one of a number of possible factors contributing in the Down's case was the presence of congenital cyanotic heart disease which could conceivably influence the perinatal development of the axonal plexus. That prolonged and unremitting cyanotic heart disease alone could retard or prevent the growth and proliferation of axons in this subsystem is clear from the findings in another case shown in Figure 7C from a 6-week-old infant (full-term). Despite the presence of well-developed pyramidal neurons in this infant the axonal plexus is virtually absent. However, such is not the situation in an age-related case of cerebro-hepatorenal syndrome (Figure 6D) that was studied extensively in regard to the metabolic defect responsible for this syndrome (18). While the density of the axonal plexus in the stratum pyramidale in the 6-week-old infant with cerebro-hepatorenal syndrome is less than expected for this age, it is clear that the peroxisomal and mitochondrial defects underlying this disorder have not had a major influence on axon plexus development. Rather, it is suggested from examination of all available cases to date that the factor of prolonged cerebral hypoxemia (and probably associated blood and tissue pH changes) is a significant deterrent to the relatively late development of synaptic pathways, such as those subserved by the axonal plexus of the hippocampal stratum pyramidale. This raises the question as to what relation exists between changes in the characteristics of this axonal plexus and the maturation of dendritic spines of pyramidal neurons in the hippocampus in cases of developmental retardation in young infants?

OBSERVATIONS ON DENDRITIC SPINES AND FINE DENDRITIC PROCESSES IN DEVELOPMENTAL RETARDATION

There is now a growing body of data that dendritic branching patterns as seen in Golgi preparations are significantly different in the cerebral cortex of some, but not all, cases of profound mental retardation (cf. Huttenlocher, Chapter 5, this volume). Marin-Padilla (28,29) has applied the rapid Golgi method in a detailed study of dendritic spines of cortical neurons in two cases of chromosomal abnormalities known to be associated with mental retardation. In one case, that of an 18-month-old retarded female with confirmed trisomy 21, motor cortex dendrites exhibited variable reduction in spines with many segments completely free of spines. Other segments might be covered with small spines possessing fine pedicles and barely visible terminal heads (28). In the second case, that of a newborn female with confirmed D_1 (13–15) trisomy, reduction, nonuniform distribution and bizarre abnormalities were observed in dendritic spines of motor cortex neurons (29). Emphasis was placed by Marin-Padilla on the very long (hairlike), thin, irregular, tortuous, and disoriented appearance of dendritic spines in the D_1 (13–15) trisomy case.

We have examined the hippocampal formation for changes in dendritic spines in three infants of similar age each of whom had clinical evidence of developmental retardation. Two infants, ages 8 and 9 months, were confirmed cases of trisomy 21 with classic stigmata of Down's syndrome and associated multiple cardiac anomalies. A third infant, (8 months) with a clinical history of intractable generalized seizures, spastic quadraplegia, and failure to attain any motor or behavioral milestones is presented as a case of severe developmental retardation of unknown etiology.

Routine neuropathological examination of the cerebral cortex in the 8-month-old infant with seizures and failure to develop revealed nonspecific reactive meningitis, focal, mild. Otherwise no alterations were found. Studies of the hippocampal formation disclosed marked loss of neurons in the Sommer sector which was sharply demarcated from the regio inferior (Figure 8A). (It is possibly significant that although an Apgar score of 9 was recorded at birth the infant required positive pressure oxygen and resuscitation for 5 minutes in the delivery room.) Examination of the stratum pyramidale of the preserved CA_3 sector failed to disclose the axonal plexus characteristic of this cell layer (Figure 8B). In general, neurons in CA_3 had dendrites with well-developed and numerous spines (Figure 8C). Rarely some segments of these dendrites showed uneven distributions of spines or spine loss. Surviving neurons in the CA_1 sector, outside the region of maximum cell loss, possessed dendrites with a paucity of branches. Such dendrites exhibited varicosities and segments with considerable spine loss (Figure 8D). In some segments clusters of dendritic spines, spicules, and bizarre filopodia-like processes were observed. The filopodia-like processes were extremely fine and could sometimes be identified only by virtue of the terminal heads (Figure 8D, arrow). Dendrites of neurons in the subiculum and presubiculum exhibited bizarre and pleomorphic spines, spicules, and filopodia-like processes (Figures 8E–G). The abnormal characteristics of these dendritic processes are readily appreciated by comparison with dendritic spines of hippocampal neurons in a normal 6-month-old infant with a negative neurological history and normal brain for age (Figures 8O–Q). It is of interest that the dendritic spine characteristics in the 8-month-old infant with seizures and developmental retardation resemble in many respects the descriptions of abnormal spines reported by Marin-Padilla (29) in a case of trisomy D_1 (13–15).

Two cases of confirmed trisomy 21 with stigmata of Down's syndrome emphasize the problem of further defining the developmental alterations in dendritic spines and axonal plexus of the stratum pyramidale in a chromo-

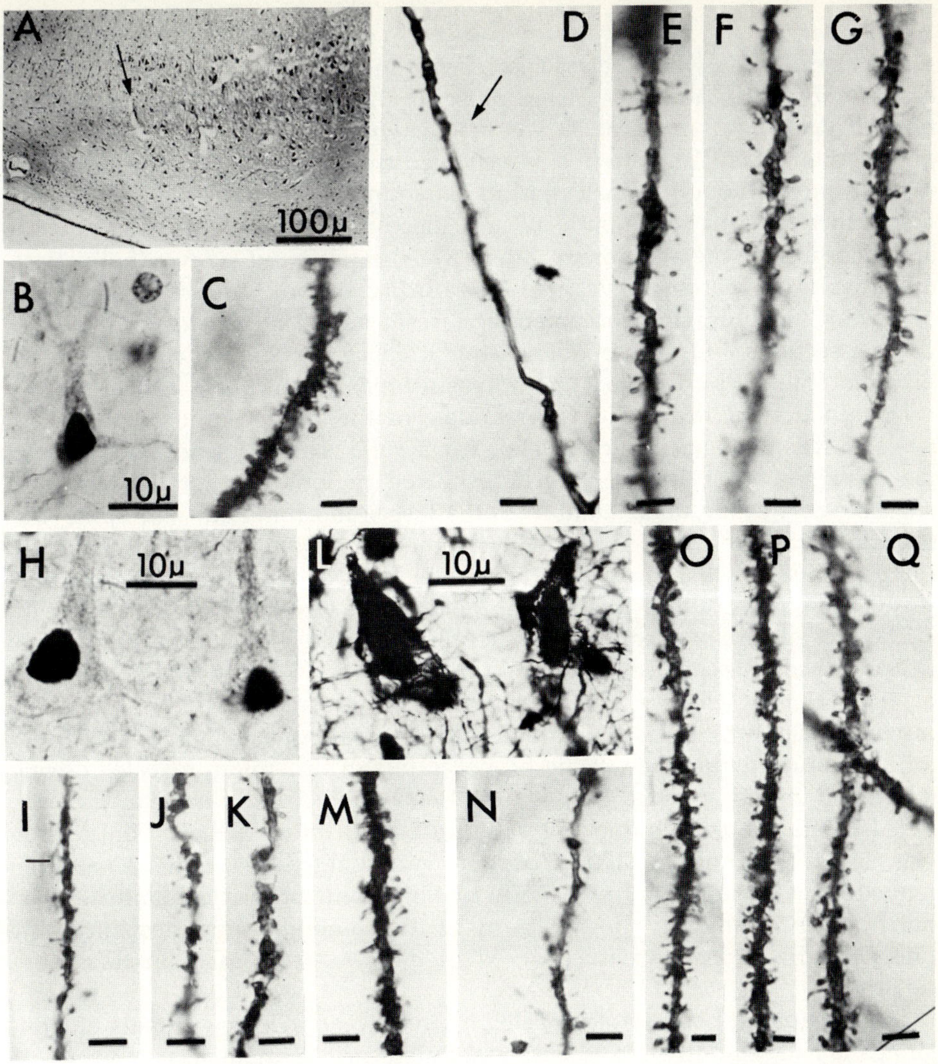

FIGURE 8. A–G. Examples of neuronal elements of the hippocampal formation of an 8-month-old infant with intractable seizures and developmental retardation. A. Nissl preparation, at arrow, beginning of region of maximal neuronal loss in the Sommer sector. B. Bodian preparation for neurofibrils. Cell in the surviving CA_3 region. The axonal plexus is not observed in the entire stratum pyramidale. C. Large dendrite of a CA_3 neuron. D. Dendrite of a neuron in CA_1 with a paucity of abnormal spines and spicules. A fine filopodia-like process is barely detectable (at arrow) but the terminal head is visible. E–G. Abnormal appearing fine dendritic processes of pyramidal neurons in the subiculum and presubiculum. H–K. Elements of the hippocampus of an 8-month-old infant with confirmed trisomy 21 (Down's syndrome). H. Bodian preparation shows absence of axonal plexus of the stratum pyramidale. I–K. Abnormal appearance of dendrites and dendritic fine processes of hippocampal pyramidal neurons. L–N. Hippocampal elements of a 9-month-old infant with confirmed trisomy 21. L. Cajal preparation. The axonal plexus is well developed. M. Apical dendrite with some reduction in spine density. N. Basilar dendrite with paucity of spines and spine abnormalities. O–Q. Dendrites of hippocampal pyramidal neurons of a 6-month-old infant with negative neurological history, normal brain. Magnification markers, 2.5 μm, unless noted otherwise.

somal disorder known to be associated with mental retardation. In both cases congenital cardiac anomalies were present. One infant, 8 months old at the time of death, was born at 33 weeks g.a. with A-V communis and patent ductus anteriosus. The patient never showed clinical signs of cardiopulmonary insufficiency although a small right to left shunt was noted at the time of cardiac catheterization at 5 months of age. Elective ligation of the patent ductus and banding of the pulmonary artery were carried out uneventfully. Postoperatively the patient developed low cardiac output, suffered generalized myoclonic seizures, and three cardiac arrests before a fatal fourth. Multiple coronal sections and microscopic examination of the cerebral cortex revealed no abnormalities in hematoxylin and eosin preparations.

Examination of the stratum pyramidale of the hippocampus in this case revealed well-developed pyramidal neurons but a virtual absence of the axonal plexus (Figure 8H). Many dendrites showed regions of poor impregnation suggestive of cystic degeneration. Spine loss was prominent and spine distribution was irregular. Additionally, spines were fine and hairlike and resembled filopodia-like processes (Figures 8I–K). Dendritic branching patterns were not significantly different from those of the 6-month-old normal infant.

The second case of trisomy 21 was a full-term male with external stigmata of Down's syndrome and Tetralogy of Falot. The patient was admitted at the age of 9 months for elective cardiac catheterization which was complicated by common iliac thrombosis. Death occurred 10 days thereafter.

The stratum pyramidale of the hippocampus in this infant revealed a well-developed axonal plexus (Figure 8L). Remarkably few abnormalities were noted in the dendritic branching pattern or dendritic spines. The impression was gained that most apical dendrites of pyramidal neurons exhibited a minor reduction in spines (Figure 8M). In striking contrast basilar dendrites had much fewer spines and showed many of the spine abnormalities, including fine filopodia-like processes observed in the two other cases in this series (Figure 8N).

The foregoing two examples of Down's syndrome in young infants of similar age (8 and 9 months), both with associated cardiac anomalies, showed significant alterations in dendritic "spine" structure of hippocampal neurons. These observations are consistent with the findings of Marin-Padilla (28,29) in cases of chromosomal abnormalities known to be associated with mental retardation. One of the two infants with Down's syndrome also exhibited a marked attenuation of the axonal plexus of the stratum pyramidale. The other did not, even though cardiac abnormalities (Tetralogy of Falot) were more severe. Perhaps it is significant that the infant with the attenuated axonal plexus was born at 33 weeks g.a., thus compounding the risk factor of Down's syndrome and congenital heart disease on developmental processes regulating axon plexus maturation.

None of the stigmata of Down's syndrome was observed in the 8-month-old infant with intractable seizures and developmental retardation. Yet dendritic spine abnormalities on hippocampal neurons were prominent and more impressive than in the two cases of Down's syndrome of similar age. In view of these observations it seems unlikely that specific abnormalities in dendritic spine structure characterize the dendritic spines in cases of specific chromosomal abnormalities known to be associated with mental retardation. The same may be said in regard to the development of the axon plexus of the hippocampus. Prematurity and associated cardiac anomalies and/or prolonged neonatal hypoxemia may be more important in influencing the development of the axon plexus than the presence of Down's syndrome per se.

It must be emphasized that the three infants studied in this series were approximately the same age at the time of death (8–9 months). Conceivably, had they lived to attain early childhood or adolescence, the early changes in dendritic processes noted here might have progressed to the stage described by Marin-Padilla in an 18-month-old infant with trisomy 21 (28). There is an important implication in this, namely, that in such conditions as Down's syndrome cortical neuronal growth and differentiation including early synaptogenesis may proceed with some temporal delays through the last phases of antenatal development and perhaps through most of the first year of infancy. Thereafter degenerative changes in elements of the neuropil (axonal terminals, axodendritic and axospinodendritic synapses) may occur at a variable tempo with consequent loss of or bizarre alterations in dendritic spines, the appearance of dendritic branching pattern abnormalities, and attenuation and degeneration of axonal terminals. Much work will be required to further define specific stages in this continuum of morphological alterations and their various interrelations.

MORPHOLOGICAL SUBSTRATE OF VISUAL EVOKED POTENTIALS IN THE PRETERM INFANT

There appears to be some agreement that the visual evoked response (VER) to photic stimulation in preterm infants ranging in age from 24 weeks g.a. to about 30 weeks g.a. is characterized by an initial surface-negative deflection of variable duration (15,16,23,24,61,63). According to published data at approximately 32 weeks g.a. (± 2 weeks) the prominent negativity is preceded by a smaller positive deflection whose development heralds the progressive development of the early positive–negative component of the VER that is characteristically observed in the full-term neonate (15,16,23,24). Few investigators concerned with the maturation of the VER in the human infant have resisted speculation as to the possible developmental changes in neuronal and synaptic organizations responsible for these dramatic changes in the early components of the VER. Some have sought clues to the maturational status of the visual cortex in the preterm infant in the studies of Conel (14) and Rabinowicz (51,52) despite the fact that these authors have not reported neurohistological observations in preterm infants in the sixth and seventh months of gestation. Other investigators have relied heavily upon comparative morphophysiological data obtained in different species of laboratory animals (21,36,49). No studies have been reported in which the morphology of the visual cortex was examined with the rapid Golgi method in preterm infants in which electrophysiological data on the characteristics of the VER were obtained prior to death of the infant. Such correlative morphophysiological studies are currently being pursued in the anticipation that the morphogenetic events underlying the transition in early components of the VEP in the preterm infant may be better defined.

At this time only the basic plan of approach and some preliminary observations can be reported to indicate the potential value of the method. The case selected for discussion is that a preterm infant born at 29 weeks g.a. (birth weight 1330 gm), with respiratory distress requiring assisted respiration and oxygenation. Three weeks after birth (32 weeks g.a.) the photic evoked potentials (VEP) shown in Figure 9 were recorded. Death occurred several days later

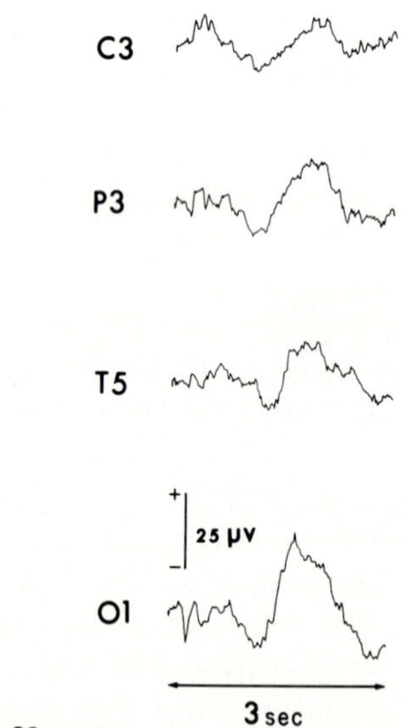

FIGURE 9. Averaged visual evoked potentials recorded from central, parietal, temporal, and occipital sites, referred to the ipsilateral ear. Stroboscopic stimulation, ISI 8 seconds. Infant 32 weeks estimated gestational age (3 weeks postpartum). Prominent early negativity at occipital lead (01) is preceded by a small positivity. Late components are especially noteworthy and indicative of considerable complexity in the VEP at this age. Golgi preparations of the visual cortex from this infant are illustrated in Figure 10. (From M. Eisengart, M. W. Kremenitzer, J. A. Kreuzer, and H. G. Vaughan, Jr., unpublished data.)

after brief repeated episodes of cardiac arrest. VEP's recorded at 32 weeks from the occiput exhibited a prominent early negativity preceded by a small surface positivity. Remarkably complex long latency wave-forms were also observed in this infant following the positive–negative initial components. The VEP's recorded at this age may represent a transitional stage from the more immature configuration (i.e., initial large surface negativity) to the early mature form (i.e., diphasic positive–negative initial components).

The general morphological features of several of the most prominent types of neurons encountered in the visual cortex are illustrated in Figure 10 in examples from rapid Golgi preparations obtained from the 32-week preterm infant whose VEP's are shown in Figure 9. Small and medium pyramidal and pyramidal-like cells of the superficial layers of the visual cortex are illustrated in Figures 10A–C. Apical dendrites of these elements are in a state of continuing growth as indicated by the presence of many fine processes, varicosities, and lumpy enlargements on shafts and branches of the apical dendritic system. Basilar dendrites, in contrast to apical dendrites, are poorly developed and in many instances are represented by a few protoplasmic extensions from cell bodies (Figures 10B and C). Basilar dendrites of deeper lying medium pyramids appear somewhat more developed (Figure 10D) but they do not exhibit the extensive development of the basilar dendrites of layer V pyramids (Figure 10M) or Meynert cells (Figure 10P).

A most striking finding is the presence of well-developed neurons termed by Cajal (9) *cellules à double bouquet dendritique* (Figures 10E–H). Characteristically these are fusiform cells with groups of dendrites originating from both poles and subtending layers superficial and deep to the cell body (11,59). The dendrites exhibit a vertical orientation and not infrequently the superficially directed dendrites penetrate through the molecular layer (Figures 10G and H). The fine axons of these cells are difficult to visualize in their entirety but in general they conform to the "horse-tail" description applied recently by Szentágothai (59) who has suggested their important involvement in cartridge-like climbing fiber axodendritic synapses on apical dendrites of deep lying pyramids. It is of interest that the cell body of the *cellule à double bouquet dendritique* was most frequently encountered in the superficial half of the visual cortex. Descending dendrites of these elements terminated as deep as the layer of Meynert cells (layer V). Cells of layer VI with arciform ascending axons were also identified in the present case (Figures 10I and M). Stellate cells of the subgennarian layer were found to have extensive, well-developed dendrites (Figures 10N and O) that were often longer than the basilar dendrites of layer V and VI pyramids.

Dendritic spines were not observed on the vast majority of apical dendritic shafts or side branches of pyramidal neurons whose cell bodies were located in layers III–VI. However, occasionally small localized segments of apical dendritic shafts passing through layers IV and V possessed primitive dendritic spines, spicules, or filopodia-like processes (Figures 10J–L). Surprisingly, the

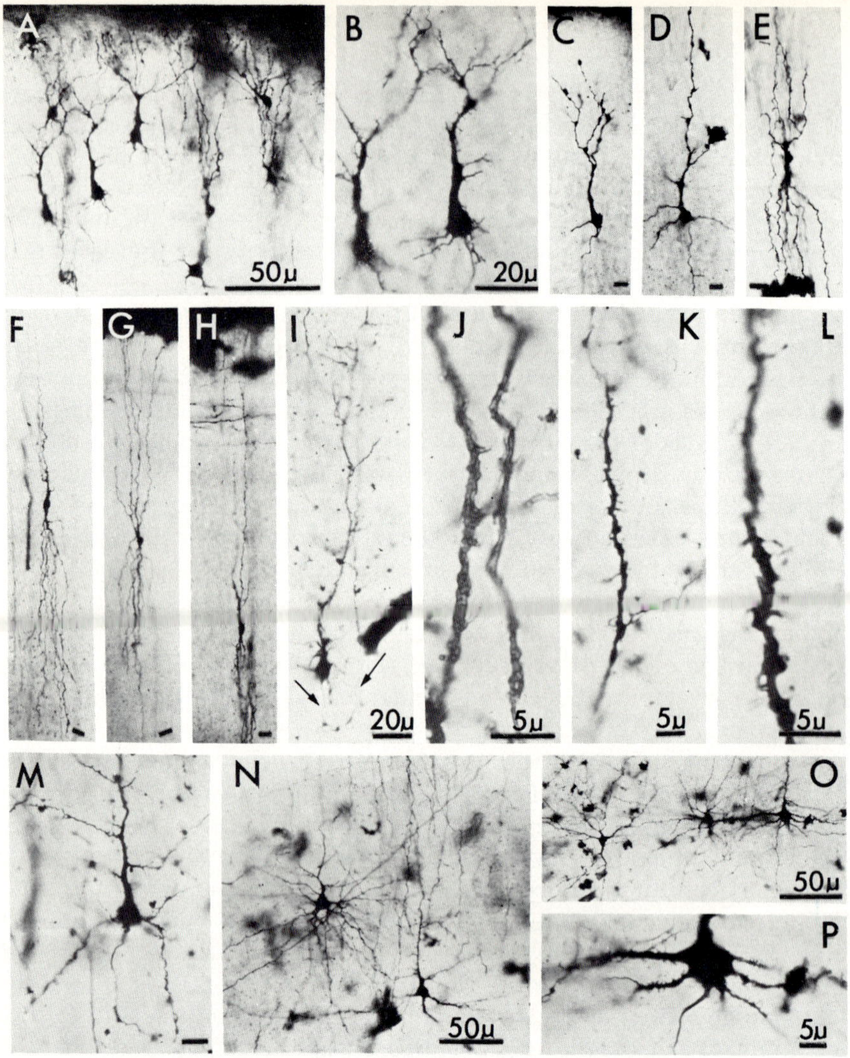

FIGURE 10. Morphological characteristics of some prominent neuron types in the visual cortex of a 33-week-old preterm infant (born at 29 weeks g.a.) Golgi rapid preparations. A–C. Small and medium pyramids of layers II and III. Dendritic growth processes are detectable on apical dendrites of most of these elements. Basilar dendrites are poorly developed. D. Pyramidal neuron of layer III. E–H. Examples of Cajal's *cellules à double bouquet dendritique*. Note, in G and H superficially directed dendrites of these cells penetrate the molecular layer. I. Neuron of layer VI with arciform axon ascending in close relation to its apical dendrite (arrows). J. Higher magnification of midapical region (axon on the right). The dendrite is free of typical spines. K and L. Low and higher magnification, respectively, of an apical dendrite of a layer V cell. A localized cluster of primitive dendritic fine processes (spines?) is evident in the higher magnification photo (L). M. Pyramidal neuron of layer VI with axon collateral well-visualized. Basilar dendrites well developed. N–O. Large stellates and pyramidal neurons of layers V and VI. P. Meynert cell with thorny excrescences on proximal segments of basilar dendrites. Magnification markers, 10 μm, unless noted otherwise.

basilar dendrites of Meynert cells exhibited conspicuous thorny processes.

The foregoing summary description of several types of visual cortex neurons encountered in a 32-week-old preterm infant should be considered only a first approximation to the main problem which lies ahead in categorizing relations between developmental changes in cortical neurons and maturational changes in the VEP. Many types of cells such as the cells with double dendritic bouquet, which are thought to play an important role in translaminar columnar operations in visual cortex (11,59), as well as pyramidal neurons and stellate cells of the subgennarian layer appear remarkably well-developed in the present case. On the other hand superficial pyramids are in a state of active dendritic differentiation. The absence of spines on dendritic shafts of most varieties of pyramidal neurons is striking. The finding that small segments of dendritic shafts in layers IV and V exhibited small clusters of spines and spicules is of interest from the standpoint of the relation of these dendritic processes to the possible proliferation of axon collaterals of stellate cells (59). A more intriguing question, however, is how do the geniculocortical afferents engage cortical neurons at this developmental stage? There is good evidence that in adult animals lateral geniculocortical afferents terminate predominantly in relation to dendritic spines of elements in layers IV and III (10,13,17,59) probably avoiding the apical dendrites of pyramidal neurons (59). If this is the case in the mature cortex, what can be inferred concerning the mode of termination of geniculocortical afferents in the immature brain when dendritic spines are not prominent, as in the material illustrated in Figure 10. Since well-localized VEPs are detectable at this time [and much earlier (15,23,61,63)] it may be suggested that the immaturity of the VEP (i.e., prominence of early negative component) is related in some obscure fashion to the type of synaptic engagement of geniculocortical afferents as well as the mode of distribution of these afferents. This problem has been dealt with previously in connection with the immature feline visual cortex (26) and awaits further examination.

COMMENT: TOWARD A DEVELOPMENTAL NEUROBIOLOGY OF MENTAL RETARDATION?

The present studies have explored several approaches to developmental events in the immature human brain that have been useful in ontogenetic investigations in laboratory animals. While the observations have provided additional information on the morphological features of immature neurons in the hippocampus and visual cortex in preterm infants they have contributed little to the problem of the relationship of aberrant development to mental subnormality. Nor should this be otherwise; for this problem is not likely to yield to the minimal effort exemplified here by attention to a few aspects of neuronal development in two selected areas of the human brain. Nevertheless the problem has been engaged with strategies that have some merit in their appeal to questions of general neurobiological interest. Several findings summarized above illustrate this viewpoint.

Definition of the period in human fetal development during which dendritic differentiation occurs is clearly of interest in specifying events of considerable importance in cortical development (9). Dendrites of cortical neurons provide more than 90% of the surface area for synaptic inputs to cortical neurons (58) even though the total area occupied by postsynaptic membrane is a very small fraction of the available somadendritic surface area (12,13). Notwithstanding this, dendritic growth and dendritic branching patterns are generally considered to be essential parameters of the probability of neuronal interaction in normal and pathological situations (cf. Huttenlocher, Chapter 5, this volume).

Unfortunately it remains to be established whether significant deviations from "normal" branching patterns necessarily imply abnormal neuronal interaction. Other critical factors are likely to be the number, distribution, and geometry of dendritic spines, which are morphological reflections of the major mode of synaptic engagement of cortical neurons by extrinsic afferents (13,17,25,59). Significant changes in the number, distribution, and geometry of dendritic spines should have important consequences for neuronal operations (54,65) providing of course that all dendritic spines are sites of synaptic contacts. This is probably true in normal mature brain but does not necessarily hold for conditions in which dendrites exhibit abnormally appearing spines, spicules, or filopodia-like processes, as in the present studies and those of Marin-Padilla (28,29). Thus, physiological implications of dendritic spine abnormalities observed in Golgi material can only be fantasized until it is established in electron microscope studies that abnormal dendritic "spines" in immature cortex are in synaptic relation with axonal processes. Recent electron microscope studies of dendrites and dendritic spines of neurons in pathological specimens of hippocampal tissue removed at the time of surgery for temporal lobe epilepsy are relevant to this problem (8).

The present studies have emphasized another strategy for analysis of neuronal development in the human brain. This approach recognizes the usefulness of fiber stains for determining the maturational features of a remarkable axonal plexus well-characterized in comparative neuroanatomical studies of the hippocampus (9,27). The fact that the vast majority of axons in this plexus terminate in basketlike networks that envelop pyramidal cell bodies has already been noted (1,4). More importantly, physiological observations suggest that axosomatic synapses formed by this basket plexus are inhibitory in function (1,3). Indeed it has been proposed that the basketlike plexus of axosomatic terminals onto hippocampal pyramidal neurons constitutes one of the most powerful inhibitory systems in the cerebral cortex (1). Hence the significance of attempts to define its temporal pattern of development and the possible factors influencing axon terminal proliferation. Data on this point are far from complete.

Available information suggests that the axon plexus of the hippocampus may be exquisitely sensitive to a variety of factors which place the preterm and full-term infant at risk. What effect attenuation of inhibitory synaptic events might exert on the normal functional operations of the hippocampus is not known, since so little is understood about the nature of these operations to begin with. It is probably no coincidence that the axonal plexus of the hippocampus was found to be severely attenuated in the case described above with infantile seizures and developmental retardation. Conceivably the loss of axosomatic inhibitory input subsequent to attenuation of the axonal plexus might provide one mechanism for hippocampal involvement in seizures of infancy (43). Clearly this problem is amenable to experimental inquiry in immature laboratory animals and is worthy of close pursuit for its relevancy to the problem of the pathogenesis of temporal lobe seizures in early childhood.

Another approach to the study of developmental events in the immature human brain has been illustrated by preliminary observations on the morphological features of visual cortex neurons in a preterm infant in which visual evoked potentials (VEPs) were recorded several days prior to death. The specific aim of this approach is to correlate morphological changes in cortical neurons with developmental changes in early components of VEPs. A formidable task considering that experimental studies have yielded few unequivocal data concerning the morphological substrate of any variety of evoked cortical potential in laboratory animals. Nevertheless experimentally derived data must continue to provide the basis for analysis of structure–function relations in the human brain.

Registration of VEPs and examination of the maturational status of visual cortical neurons in infants who fail to survive can provide a wealth of data on several important questions. The issue of the mode of synaptic engagement of cortical elements by primary geniculocortical afferents in preterm infants prior to the elaboration of dendritic spines is of no little importance as noted previously. The relationship between temporal patterns of apical and basilar dendritic growth in neurons at different cortical depths to characteristics of VEPs in early and late preterm infants is another question that is amenable to investigation. Finally, there remains the problem of providing a satisfactory description of the maturation of certain spectacular elements such as the *cellules à double bouquet dendritique,* which may play a central role in the morphological substrate for functional columnar organizations (11,59).

The several approaches described in this report obviously reflect the special interest of the author and therefore hold no claim to priority of importance. Hopefully they may be viewed as the most tentative gropings toward a developmental neurobiology of the human brain which will have as one of its primary objectives an adequate understanding of the morphophysiological basis of mental retardation.

SUMMARY

Several approaches utilized in ontogenetic investigations in laboratory animals have been explored in preliminary studies of morphogenetic events in the human cerebral cortex.

1. Golgi studies of dendritic growth cones, filopodia, and other developmental processes have permitted specification of the maximal phase of dendritic growth and differentiation of pyramidal neurons in the hippocampus. This period spans the twentieth to twenty-eighth week of fetal development.

2. Studies of the temporal pattern of appearance of the axonal plexus of the stratum pyramidale suggest that axosomatic synaptic pathways in the hippocampus develop relatively late in respect to the appearance of axospinodendritic inputs.

3. Dendritic spine development is evident at 26 weeks g.a. in the hippocampus but not in the visual cortex. Most hippocampal pyramidal neurons have acquired a full complement of spines by 6 months postnatally. The presence of severe metabolic and cardiorespiratory disturbances and/or chromosomal abnormalities significantly influences dendritic spine morphology and development.

4. The general morphological features of several varieties of neurons in the visual cortex of a 32-week-old preterm infant are considered in respect to the electrographic characteristics of this infant's visual evoked responses. The observations in this and other cases illustrate the manner in which ontogenetic problems susceptible to inquiry in laboratory animals can serve to guide similar morphophysiological studies of normal and aberrant developmental events in the human brain.

ACKNOWLEDGMENTS

The expert technical assistance of Mrs. Marie Buschke in the preparation of the histological material is gratefully acknowledged. Mr. Stanley Brown contributed greatly to the photographic work illustrated in this report. This study could not have been carried out without the dedicated services of these two fine persons.

This work was supported in part by grants from the NINDS NS-07512, NICHD HD-01799, and the Alfred P. Sloan Foundation.

REFERENCES

1. Andersen, P. Correlation of structural design with function in the archicortex. In: *Brain and Conscious Experience.* (J. C. Eccles, Ed.), Springer-Verlag, Berlin and New York, 1966: 59–79.

2. Andersen, P., Blackstad, T. W., and Lømo, T. Location and identification of excitatory synapses on hippocampal pyramidal cells. *Expl. Brain Res.*, 1966, **1:** 236–248.
3. Andersen, P., Eccles, J. C., and Løyning, Y. Location of postsynaptic inhibitory synapses on hippocampal pyramids. *J. Neurophysiol.*, 1964, **27:** 592–607.
4. Blackstad, T., and Flood, P. Ultrastructure of hippocampal axo-somatic synapses. *Nature (Lond.)*, 1963, **198:** 542–543.
5. Blackstad, T., and Kjaerheim, A. Special axo-dendritic synapses in the hippocampal cortex: Electron and light microscopic studies on the layer of mossy fibers. *J. Comp. Neurol.*, 1961, **117:** 133–159.
6. Blackstad, T. W. On the termination of some afferents to the hippocampus and fascia dentata. An experimental study in the rat. *Acta Anat.*, 1958, **35:** 202–214.
7. Blackstad, T. W., Brink, K., Hem, J., and Jenne, B. Distribution of hippocampal mossy fibers in the rat. An experimental study with silver impregnation methods. *J. Comp. Neurol.*, 1970, **138:** 433–450.
8. Brown, W. J. Structural substrates of seizure foci in the human temporal lobe. In: *Epilepsy. Its Phenomena in Man.* (M. A. B. Brazier, Ed.). UCLA Forum in Medical Sciences, No. 17. Academic Press, New York, 1973: 339–374.
9. Cajal, S. Ramón Y. *Histologie du Système Nerveux de l'Homme et des Vertébrés.* Maloine, Paris, 1911. Reprinted by Conseju Superior de Investigaciones Cientificas, Madrid, 1955.
10. Colonnier, M. L. Experimental degeneration in the cerebral cortex. *J. Anat.*, 1964, **98:** 47–53.
11. Colonnier, M. L. The structural design of the neocortex. In: *Brain and Conscious Experience.* (J. C. Eccles, Ed.). Springer-Verlag, Berlin and New York, 1966: 1–23.
12. Colonnier, M. L. Synaptic patterns on different cell types in the different laminae of the cat visual cortex. An electron microscope study. *Brain Res.*, 1968, **9:** 268–287.
13. Colonnier, M. L., and Rossignol, S. Heterogeneity of the cerebral cortex. In: *Basic Mechanisms of the Epilepsies.* (H. H. Jasper, A. A. Ward, and A. Pope, Eds.). Little, Brown, Boston, Massachusetts, 1969: 29–40.
14. Conel, J. L. *The Postnatal Development of the Human Cerebral Cortex.* Vol. 1. Harvard Univ. Press, Cambridge, Massachusetts, 1941.
15. Ellingson, R. J. Cortical electrical responses to visual stimulation in the human infant. *Electroenceph. Clin. Neurophysiol.*, 1960, **23:** 663–667.
16. Engel, R. Electroencephalographic responses to sound and light in premature and full-term neonates. *Lancet*, 1967, **87:** 181–186.
17. Garey, L. J., and Powell, T. P. S. An experimental study of the termination of the lateral geniculo-cortical pathway in the cat and monkey. *Proc. R. Soc., Lond.* [*Biol.*] 1971, **179:** 41–63.
18. Goldfischer, S., Moore, C. L., Johnson, A. B., Spiro, A. J., Valsamis, M. P., Wisniewski, H. K., Ritch, R. H., Norton, W. T., Rapin, I., and Gartner, L. M. Peroxisomal and mitochondrial defects in the cerebro-hepato-renal syndrome. *Science*, 1973, **182:** 62–64.
19. Hamlyn, L. H. The fine structure of the mossy fibre endings in the hippocampus of the rabbit. *J. Anat.*, 1962, **96:** 112–120.
20. Hamlyn, L. H. An electron microscope study of pyramidal neurons in the Ammon's horn of the rabbit. *J. Anat.*, 1963, **97:** 189–201.
21. Himwich, W. A., Ed. *Developmental Neurobiology.* Thomas, Springfield, Illinois, 1970.
22. Hjorth-Simonsen, A. Hippocampal efferents to the ipsilateral entorhinal area: An experimental study in the rat. *J. Comp. Neurol.*, 1971, **142:** 417–438.
23. Hrbek, A., Karlberg, P., and Olsson, T. Development of visual and somatosensory evoked responses in preterm newborn infants. *Electroenceph. clin. Neurophysiol.*, 1973, **34:** 225–232.
24. Hrbek, A., and Mareš, P. Cortical evoked responses to visual stimulation in full-term and premature newborns. *Electroenceph. clin. Neurophysiol.*, 1964, **16:** 575–581.
25. Jones, E. G., and Powell, T. P. S. An electron microscopic study of the laminar pattern and node of termination of afferent fibre pathways in the somatic sensory cortex of the cat. *Philos. Trans. Soc. Lond.* [*Biol. Sci.*], 1970, **257:** 45–62.

26. Laemle, L., Benhamida, C., and Purpura, D. P. Laminar distribution of geniculo-cortical afferents in visual cortex of the postnatal kitten. *Brain Res.*, 1972, **41:** 25–37.
27. Lorente de Nó, R. Studies on the structure of the cerebral cortex. II. Continuation of the study of the ammonic system. *J. Psychol. Neurol.*, 1934: **46:** 113–177.
28. Marin-Padilla, M. Structural abnormalities of the cerebral cortex in human chromosomal aberrations. A Golgi study. *Brain Res.*, 1972, **44:** 625–629.
29. Marin-Padilla, M. Structural organization of the cerebral cortex (motor area) in human chromosomal aberrations. A Golgi study. I. D1 (13–15) trisomy, Patau syndrome. *Brain Res.*, 1974, **66:** 375–391.
30. Molliver, M. E., Kostović, I., and Van Der Loos, H. The development of synapses in cerebral cortex of the human fetus. *Brain Res.*, 1973, **50:** 403–407.
31. Morest, D. K. The differentiation of cerebral dendrites: A study of the post-migratory neuroblast in the medical nucleus of the trapezoid body. *Z. Anat. Entwicklungsgesch.*, 1969, **128:** 271–289.
32. Morest, D. K. The growth of dendrites in the mammalian brain. *Z. Anat. Entwicklungsgesch.*, 1969, **128:** 290–317.
33. Morest, D. K. A study of neurogenesis in the forebrain of opossum pouch young. *Z. Anat. Entwicklungsgesch.*, 1970, **130:** 265–305.
34. Nafstad, P. H. J. An electron microscope study on the termination of the perforant path fibres in the hippocampus and the fascia dentata. *Z. Zellforsch. Mikrosk. Anat.*, 1967, **76:** 532–542.
35. Pappas, G. D., and Purpura, D. P. Electron microscopy of immature human and feline neocortex. *Progr. Brain Res.*, 1964, **4:** 176–186.
36. Persson, H. E. Development of somatosensory cortical functions. *Acta Physiol. Scand., Suppl.* 1973: **394:** 5–64.
37. Poliakov, G. I. Some results of research into the development of the neuronal structure of the cortical ends of the analyzers in man. *J. Comp. Neurol.*, 1961, **117:** 197–212.
38. Purpura, D. P. Morphophysiological bases of elementary evoked response patterns in the neocortex of the newborn cat. *Ann. N.Y. Acad. Sci.*, 1960, **92:** 840–859.
39. Purpura, D. P. Ontogenetic analysis of some evoked synaptic activities in superficial neocortical neuropil. In: *Nervous Inhibition.* (E. Florey, Ed.). Pergamon, Oxford, 1961: 424–446.
40. Purpura, D. P. Analysis of axodendritic synaptic organizations in immature cerebral cortex. *Ann. N.Y. Acad. Sci.*, 1961, **94:** 604–654.
41. Purpura, D. P. Relationship of seizure susceptibility to morphologic and physiologic properties of normal and abnormal immature cortex. In: *Neurological and Electroencephalographic Correlative Studies in Infancy.* (P. Kellaway and I. Petersen, Eds.). Grune & Stratton, New York, 1964: 117–157.
42. Purpura, D. P. Comparative physiology of dendrites. In: *The Neurosciences: A Study Program.* (G. C. Quarton, T. Melnechuk, and F. O. Schmitt, Eds.). Rockefeller Univ. Press, New York, 1967: 308–323.
43. Purpura, D. P. Stability and seizure susceptibility of immature brain. In: *Basic Mechanisms of the Epilepsies.* (H. H. Jasper, A. A. Ward, and A. Pope, Eds.). Little, Brown, Boston, Massachusetts, 1969: 481–505.
44. Purpura, D. P. Analysis of morphophysiological developmental processes in mammalian brain. *Res. Publ., Ass. Res. Nerv. Ment. Dis.*, 1973, **51:** 79–110.
45. Purpura, D. P., Carmichael, M. W., and Housepian, E. M., Physiological and anatomical studies of development of superficial axodendritic synaptic pathways in neocortex. *Exp. Neurol.*, 1960, **2:** 324–347.
46. Purpura, D. P., and Pappas, G. D. Structural characteristics of neurons in feline hippocampus during postnatal ontogenesis. *Exp. Neurol.*, 1968, **22:** 379–393.
47. Purpura, D. P., Prelevic, S., and Santini, M. Postsynaptic potentials and spike variations in the feline hippocampus during postnatal ontogenesis. *Exp. Neurol.*, 1968, **22:** 408–422.

48. Purpura, D. P., and Shofer, R. J. Excitatory action of dibutyryl cyclic adenosine monophosphate on immature cerebral cortex. *Brain Res.*, 1972, **38:** 179–181.
49. Purpura, D. P., Shofer, R. J., Housepian, E. M., and Noback, C. R. Comparative ontogenesis of structure-function relations in cerebral and cerebellar cortex. *Progr. Brain Res.*, 1964, **4:** 187–221.
50. Purpura, D. P., Shofer, R. J., and Scarff, T. Properties of synaptic activities and spike potentials of neurons in immature neocortex. *J. Neurophysiol.*, 1965, **28:** 925–942.
51. Rabinowicz, T. The cerebral cortex of the premature infant of the 8th month. *Progr. Brain Res.*, 1964, **4:** 39–86.
52. Rabinowicz, T. Quantitative appraisal of the cerebral cortex of the premature infant of 8 months. In: *Regional Development of the Brain in Early Life.* (A. Minkowski, Ed.). Davis, Philadelphia, Pennsylvania, 1967: 91–118.
53. Raisman, G., Cowan, W. M., and Powell, T. P. S. The extrinsic afferent, commissural and association fibres of the hippocampus. *Brain*, 1965, **88:** 963–966.
54. Scheibel, M. E., and Scheibel, A. B. Hippocampal pathology in temporal lobe epilepsy. A Golgi survey. In: *Epilepsy. Its Phenomena in Man.* (M. A. B. Brazier, Ed.). UCLA Forum in Medical Sciences, No. 17. Academic Press, New York, 1973: 311–337.
55. Schwartz, I. R., Pappas, G. D., and Purpura, D. P. Fine structure of neurons and synapses in the feline hippocampus during postnatal ontogenesis. *Exp. Neurol.*, 1968, **22:** 394–407.
56. Shofer, R. J., Pappas, G. D., and Purpura, D. P. Radiation-induced changes in morphological and physiological properties of immature cerebellar cortex. In: *Response of the Nervous System to Ionizing Radiations.* (T. J. Haley and R. S. Snider, Eds.). Academic Press, New York, 1964: 476–508.
57. Shofer, R. J., and Purpura, D. P. Spread of transcallosally evoked responses in immature association cortex. *Exp. Neurol.*, 1972, **37:** 431–445.
58. Sholl, D. A. *The Organization of the Cerebral Cortex.* Methuen, London, 1956.
59. Szentágothai, J. Synaptology of the visual cortex. In: *Handbook of Sensory Physiology.* Vol. 8, Part 3. (R. Jung, Ed.). Springer-Verlag, Berlin and New York, 1973: 269–324.
60. Thatcher, R. W.. and Purpura, D. P. Postnatal development of thalamic synaptic events underlying evoked recruiting responses and electrocortical activation. *Brain Res.*, 1973, **60:** 21–34.
61. Umezaki, H., and Morrell, F. Developmental study of photic evoked responses in premature infants. *Electroenceph. clin. Neurophysiol.*, 1970, **28:** 55–63.
62. Voeller, K., Pappas, G. D., and Purpura, D. P. Electron microscope study of development of cat superficial neocortex. *Exp. Neurol.*, 1963, **7:** 107–130.
63. Watanabe, K., Iwase, K., and Hara, K. Visual evoked responses during sleep and wakefulness in pre-term infants. *Electroenceph. clin. Neurophysiol.*, 1973, **34:** 571–577.
64. Weinzimer, S. H. A modification of the Bodian stain for neurofibrils. *Lab. Med.*, 1974, **5:** No. 4, April.
65. Westrum, L. E., White, L. E., and Ward, A. A. Morphology of the experimental epileptic focus. *J. Neurosurg.*, 1964, **21:** 1033–1046.
66. Zimmer, J. Ipsilateral afferents to the commissural zone of the facia dentata, demonstrated in decommissurated rats by silver impregnation. *J. Comp. Neurol.*, 1971, **142:** 393–416.

6A

Discussion: CNS Maturation and Behavorial Development

GUENTER ROSE
Mental Retardation Research Center,
University of California Los Angeles,
Los Angeles, California

As a psychologist, I have chosen to focus on problems which arise in relating *behavioral* events to indices of maturation obtained by other disciplines. The outstanding contributions of Drs. Purpura and Huttenlocher covering anatomical and physiological changes during neuronal development provide a basis for such comparisons. Furthermore, the delineation of distinctive patterns of emergent behaviors in neonates, which parallel the concomitant anatomical-physiological differentiation of neural substrates, as reported in these studies, will provide an important investigatory tool in understanding the maturation of normal as well as abnormal structural-functional relationships.

A crucial assumption underlying this type of research is that there are relatively abrupt changes in the nervous system which are reflected in the sudden emergence of the potential for new behavior. The difficulties in demonstrating these relationships experimentally have tended to erode the concept of critical stages in development. However, a few successes in such correlations lend some support to the concept of threshold age, and the elusiveness of many structural–functional correlations may be explained in terms of inadequate fundamental concepts and techniques. I would like to focus briefly on such problems by raising two major points.

First of all, while most studies of behavioral or central nervous system (CNS) maturation emphasize gradual, usually linear, increases in amount or proficiency of the phenomenon under investigation, there are, in contrast, other studies which indicate nonlinear increases, increases then decreases, or events unique to a particular growth period, such as pseudospines on the cell bodies of neurons. Typical age-unique alterations are especially seen in biochemical studies of maturation. With regard to behavior, gross activity levels in rat pups, for example (4), do not continue to increase with maturation, but peak at approximately 15–20 days of age, then decrease at later ages. Cortical spindles during slow wave sleep are present between 15–25 days of age in kittens. After the twenty-fifth day, the spindles disappear only to reappear at approximately 6 weeks of age (3). It is useful, I think, to recognize that there are events unique to a particular developmental period which may or may not be easily identified as the precursors of later behavioral or physiological responses but which have significance within a circumscribed age-period.

Of perhaps greater importance, is the fact that differential maturational rates within functional systems must be considered, especially when constructing neural models of immature behaviors. Dr. Dobbing has emphasized the different rate of development of the cerebellar as opposed to the cerebral cortex. Paralleling Dr. Dobbing's data on humans, Figure 1 illustrates the comparative growth rates of selected subcortical nuclei in the kitten brain, expressed as the percent of total volume seen in the adult. Note, for example, the high growth rate of the lateral geniculate body in contrast to the red nucleus during the first 30 days of life.

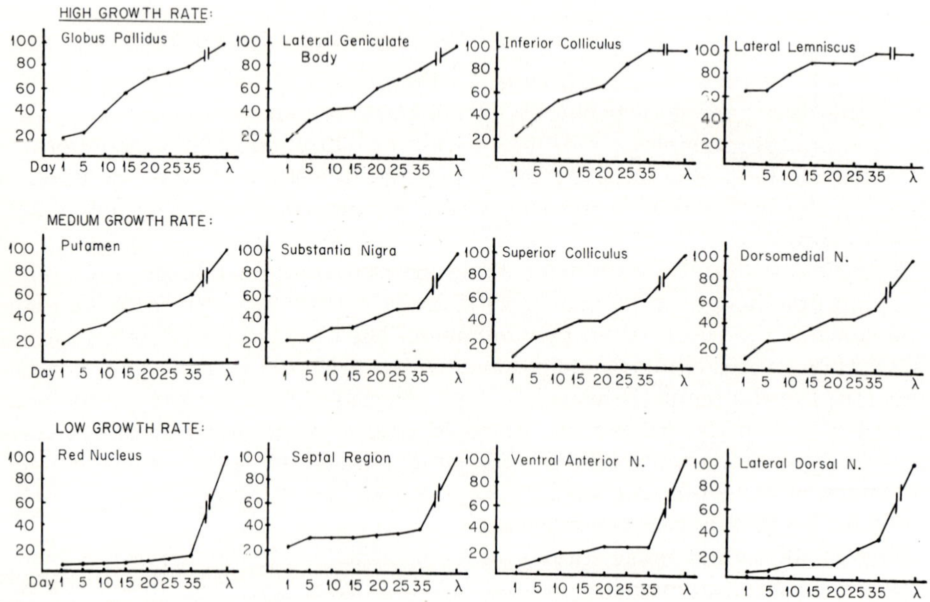

FIGURE 1. Comparative growth rates of selected brain nuclei in kittens, expressed as percentages of total volume in the adult.

If, as we expect, the electrophysiological data to be obtained support the anatomical data, it would indicate that adult neurological models of behavioral phenomena cannot be easily applied to developing behaviors since the functional capability of parts of the model varies with age. This fact should contribute to a focus on neurological models which complement behaviors unique to particular stages of development, deëmphasizing the noncritical reliance on established adult models.

The second major point that I wish to make relates to the difficulties in obtaining meaningful behavioral data per se from immature animals, i.e., data to be utilized for subsequent correlations with other indices of maturation. Our own research, for example, is primarily concerned with the relationship between emerging visual behavioral capabilities and electrophysiological indices of the developing visual system, as reflected by alterations in the cortical potential evoked by light input (6,9). In unanesthetized kittens, this consists of a characteristic sequence of waveform changes beginning with a single long-latency negative component at 0–4 days of age and ending with an adult-like complex W-shaped wave at 25–35 days of age. With the exception of a recent brief report (5), similar subcortical alterations have yet to be delineated.

In assessing visual maturation at the behavioral level, two approaches predominate: those which look at unlearned reflexive kinds of behavior, and those dealing with learned behavior. The former includes tests of eye opening, acuity utilizing optokinetic responses, depth perception via visual cliff techniques, extensive and guided placing, visual following, etc. To date, we can make only a rough approximation concerning neural relationships by stating that most of the more complex visual behaviors seem to emerge when the visual cortical response has attained a maturelike waveform at approximately 4 weeks of age. This ignores the most certain influence of subcortical events which to date remain unexplored.

In undertaking developmental studies such as the above, as well as those attempting an assessment of early learning-discriminative abilities, there are a number of unique conceptual and methodological problems one must consider (1): (a) both the sensory response to various stimuli as well as the motor expression of behavior varies with age; (b) motivational levels vary with age, as do the value of various reinforcers, e.g., younger animals with higher metabolic rates and general activity are likely to be hungrier after a given period of food deprivation; (c) unlearned preferences to certain stimuli used in learning studies, such as light versus dark, may vary with age; and (d) finally, early experiential factors can play a role in establishing learning ability, e.g., the previous experience of the animal may make that animal more or less emotional in a novel test situation which may impede or enhance learning depending on the task.

Because of all or some of these factors, few, if any, studies have established visual discrimination capabilities in kittens below 6 weeks of age. To overcome some of the response, motivation, and reinforcement problems, we devised a system of training the animals on a black-white discrimination utilizing a Y-water maze (7). The kittens are capable of swimming by 1 week of age, detest the water, and hence are motivated to escape. Two age groups were studied: one, beginning at 35 days of age when evoked potentials are mature-like, and the second beginning at about 3 weeks of age when evoked potentials are still immature. Both groups had 1 week of pretraining before actual testing. Figure 2 schematically summarizes the data which indicated that the age at which the kittens performed above chance level, regardless of when they started the initial training, seemed to be related to a time zone, between 25 and 35 days of age, when a mature-like visual evoked potential is achieved. Again, this is a very crude correlation; it may be very task-specific. Furthermore, it is very hard to show a one-to-one correspondence in these situations unless one is actually recording the electrophysiological responses during the acquisition of the task.

We have recently carried out a study of this latter type (8). Beginning at 10 days of age, kittens were in a Pavlovian conditioning paradigm with light as the conditioned stimulus and leg flexion as the conditioned response. Cortical evoked potential and GSR measures were taken during the training. Although the animals still did not show behavioral conditioning until about 6 weeks of age, a difference between control and experimental animals with regard to physiological measures was seen as early as 2 weeks of age. This study suggests that while the associative phase of learning may occur early in development, the overt motor expression of learning occurs later when neural–muscular systems are sufficiently mature.

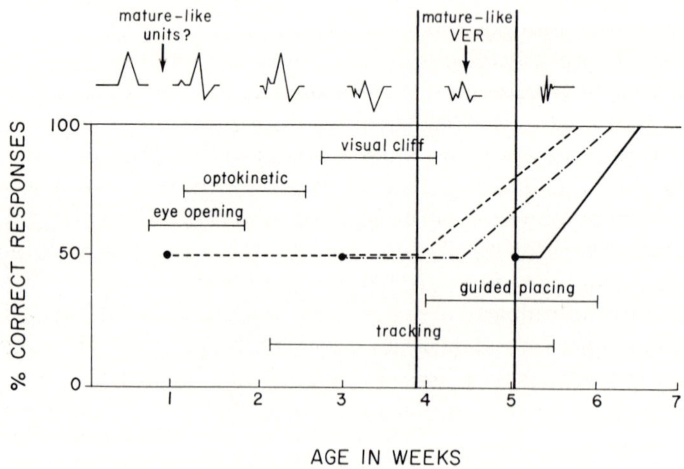

FIGURE 2. Schematic representation of black-white discrimination in Y-water maze (kittens). Learning curves beginning at 3 and 5 weeks of age based on actual data; hypothetical curve beginning at 1 week of age. Electrophysiological (9) and behavioral (2) data taken from previous studies.

Hence, we are now searching for unique ways of establishing the onset of learning abilities which take the inability of motor expression into account. I shall conclude this discussion with two examples.

In pilot studies on classic conditioning in our laboratory, Dr. Robert Norman selected the conditioned eyeblink as a model response system, because it is a relatively simple and highly stereotyped reflex, unencumbered by postural or gamma motor feedback mechanisms. Furthermore, extensive studies in adult animals have provided normative data on stimulus and response parameters for this paradigm. We have attempted to train kittens by pairing an auditory conditioned stimulus (CS) (1 kHz, 400 msec, 85 db) with a shock to the eye (40 V, 2 msec), as the unconditioned stimulus (US). Our initial studies indicated that, independent of when training was initiated, and independent of the number of training trials, conditioned responses could not be established until 30 days of age. However, it was noticed that often when conditioning did appear, responses were seen on the first trials of a session, implying that acquisition had begun initially in earlier sessions, but with an absence of motor expression. This idea was tested in a subsequent study by training experimental kittens for 7 days beginning at age 21 days while control littermates received random presentations of both CS and US. After 2 days' rest, both groups received conditioning trials. The animals which had previous pairings showed immediate conditioning, often on the first trials, while the control animal took 200–300 trials to condition (Figure 3). We tentatively concluded that the prior experience of paired presentation of the CS and US was facilitated at some earlier age (21–27 days) but could not be expressed because of some maturational block beyond the associative stage in neural processing.

A CNS feedback design provides another alternate technique to this dilemma. In pilot studies, Dr. Jerry Collins, Dr. Robert Norman, and I attempted to answer the following: Could we demonstrate learning in very immature systems by bypassing motor responses, treating the potential evoked by light flash as an independent variable, and reinforcing it directly to produce specified changes? The desired change in this case would be an increase or decrease of the whole visual electrocortical response (VEP) to establish learning ability per se. Additional payoff would occur if we could selectively condition particular components of the VEP.

To date, we have been able to train eight 1½–3-week-old kittens to increase or decrease, by as much as 500%, an immature long-latency negative VEP component (N_2) recorded from the visual cortex, using tone as a discriminative stimulus (S^D), light flash as the CS, and mild electrical shock as a negative reinforcer in a shock-avoidance paradigm (10). Amplitude alterations in yoked controls (e.g., light flash only; noncontingent shock) reached a maximum increase or decrease of 35% from baseline, depending on age. This occurs in both awake kittens with implanted electrodes and in Flaxedilized preparations. The results are not due to trivial factors such as orientation

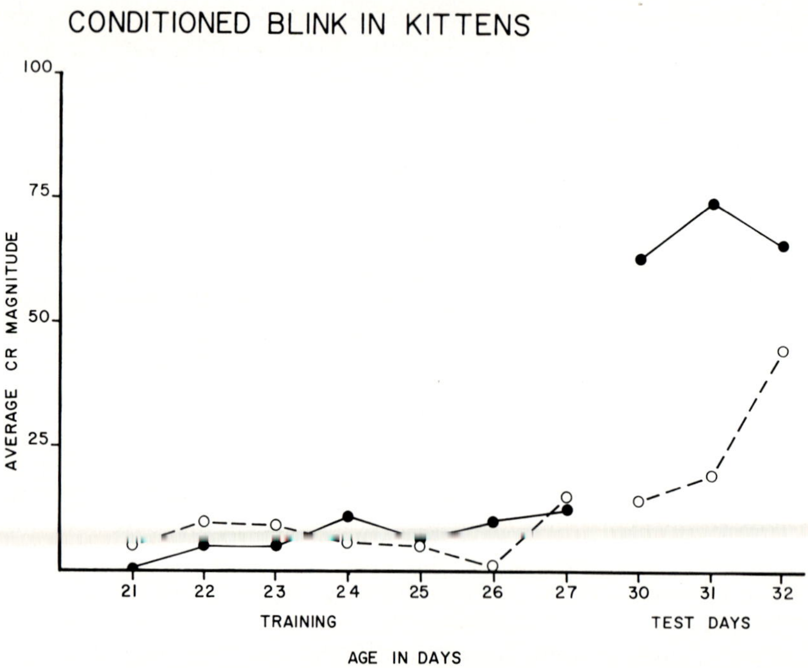

FIGURE 3. Conditioned eyeblink magnitude (integrated EMG from orbicularis oculi) in arbitrary units averaged over 100 trials per daily session. Conditioned (solid line) group received conditioning trials on all days, while the random (dashed line) group received random presentation of CS and US during days 21–27 and were switched to paired presentation on days 30–32. The immediate acquisition of the conditioned group on test days indicates that the response was "learned" during initial training in the absence of motor expression.

toward the light and pupillary changes. The evoked potential increases and decreases can, however, be interpreted as indicating that tonic state alterations, as opposed to discrete neural responses, have been conditioned.

An example of the data obtained in such studies is seen in Figure 4. A criterion specified by a time-amplitude "window" was set so as to require a 14-day-old kitten (awake, chronic implant) to lower the amplitude of a N_2 component recorded from the visual cortex. This animal showed good control through three cycles of acquisition and extinction. (The first extinction period was only partially completed.) The evoked potentials sampled during the same trials but from the midectosylvian cortex remained relatively stable, providing an additional control, suggesting that the changes seen in the visual cortex were not simply due to peripheral phenomena, such as pupillary dilation. It suggests, furthermore, that the mechanisms which modulated the changes are either contained within a specific cortical locus or that various pathways to the cortex can have separate gating mechanisms which can function independently of one another during the establishment of brain–behavior relationships.

The youngest animal successfully conditioned was 12 days of age, which, to our knowledge, is the earliest age at which learning involving the visual modality has been demonstrated. It reinforces our opinion that other studies using motor responses have failed to identify the earliest age of visual learning, due to the immaturity of response systems. As mentioned above, it would have been sufficient in these studies to have demonstrated any significant amplitude changes over controls. The fact that it can be confined to specified waves is an added advantage in kittens in view of hypotheses concerning the anatomical and functional basis of waveform changes during maturation. The technique, if sufficiently validated, becomes a potential experimental tool for further research in attempting to impede or accelerate electrophysiological maturation, accompanied by testing for behavioral effects or alteration or CNS modification. In addition, transfer studies involving evoked potentials or other electrophysiological activity can be undertaken. Sterman, for example, has operantly conditioned a substantial increase in the sensory motor rhythm recorded from the cortex of adult cats and then demonstrated specific transfer effects. Such conditioning produces a significant increase in

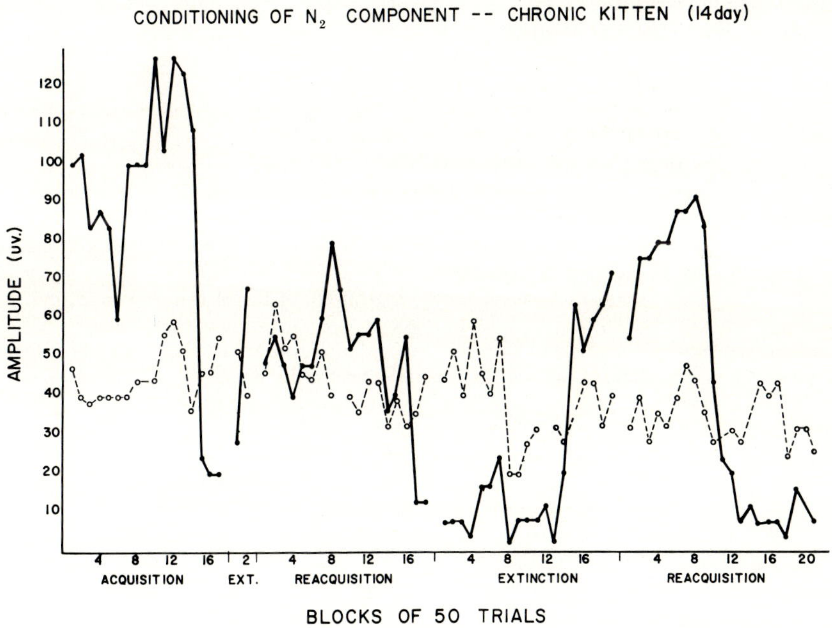

FIGURE 4. An example of feedback conditioning of an N_2 component evoked by light flash in the visual cortex (solid line). The criterion was set so as to require the kitten to lower the evoked potential amplitude at a prespecified latency. This animal showed good control through three cycles of acquisition and extinction. The evoked potentials sampled during the same trials but from the midectosylvian cortex (dotted line) remained relatively stable, suggesting that the changes in visual cortex were not simple peripheral phenomenon. Each data point represents the algebraic summation of 50 responses.

sleep spindles (12) and a significant increase in the threshold of seizures induced by hydrazine compounds (13). Finally, Sterman (11) demonstrated the effectiveness of SMR conditioning in reducing the incidence of grand mal seizures in one epileptic patient.

It is our opinion that these alternate techniques are particularly useful in dealing with developing animals and humans where one is faced with unique assessment problems, but also finds considerable potential for CNS plasticity. With regard to the present symposium, we would stress that any models of mental retardation, especially in early development, must take into account not only the possibility of CNS retardation in the higher centers, but peripheral sensorimotor deficiencies as well.

REFERENCES

1. Campbell, B. A. Developmental studies of learning and motivation in infra-primate mammals. In: *Early Behavior: Comparative and Developmental Approaches.* (H. W. Stevenson, E. W. Hess, and H. L. Reingold, Eds.). Wiley, New York, 1967: 43–71.
2. Fagen, L. Unpublished observations.
3. Jouvet-Mounier, D., Actic, L., and Lacote, D. Ontogenesis of the states of sleep in rat, cat, and guinea pig during the first postnatal month. *Dev. Psychobiol.,* 1969, **2:** 216–239.
4. Moorcroft, W. A., Lytle, L., and Campbell, B. A. Ontogeny of spontaneous locomotor activity in the rat. *J. Comp. Physiol. Psychol.,* 1971, **75:** 59–67.
5. Norman, J. L., and Wilson, P. P. Development of subcortical evoked potentials in kittens. *Brain Res.,* 1973, **55:** 446–450.
6. Rose, G. H. The relationship of electrophysiological and behavioral indices of visual development in mammals. In: *Neural Ontogeny and Behavior.* (M. B. Sterman, D. J. McGinty, and A. M. Adinolfi, Eds.). Academic Press, New York, 1971: 145–183.
7. Rose, G. H., and Collins, J. P. Light–dark discrimination and reversal learning in early postnatal kittens. *Develop. Psychobiol.,* in press.
8. Rose, G. H., and Dalhouse, A. Neurophysiological correlates of learning in young kittens. *Electroenceph. clin. Neurophysiol.,* 1974, **37:** 428.
9. Rose, G. H., Gruenau, S. P., and Spencer, J. W. Maturation of visual electrocortical responses in unanesthetized kittens: Effects of barbiturate anesthesia. *Electroenceph. clin. Neurophysiol.,* 1972, **33:** 141–158.
10. Rose, G. H., Norman, R. J., Naifeh, K., and Collins, J. P. Plasticity of visual evoked potentials in kittens demonstrated by operant conditioning. 9. *Physiol. Behav.* in press.
11. Sterman, M. B., and Friar, L. Suppression of seizures in an epileptic following sensorimotor EEG feedback training. *Electroenceph. clin. Neurophysiol.,* 1972, **33:** 89–95.
12. Sterman, M. B., Howe, R. C., and MacDonald, L. R. Facilitation of spindle-burst sleep by conditioning of the electroencephalographic activity while awake. *Science,* 1970, **167:** 1146–1148.
13. Sterman, M. B., LoPresti, R. W., and Fairchild, M. D. *Electroencephalographic and Behavioral Studies of Monomethyl Hydrazine Toxicity in the Cat.* Tech. Rep. AMRL-TR-69-3. Wright-Patterson Air Force Base, Air Systems Command, 1969.

6B

Discussion: Development of Postsynaptic Potentials Recorded from Immature Neurons in Kitten Visual Cortex

CHESTER D. HULL and D. R. G. FULLER
Mental Retardation Research Center,
University of California Los Angeles,
Los Angeles, California

This information on the changed morphology of neurons in the human cerebrum, gained from some of nature's unfortunate experiments, is interesting. It certainly strengthens the suggestion that, to a considerable degree, severe mental retardation results from the functioning of maldeveloped neurons which have fewer normal (and possibly more abnormal) synapses with each other. The case for the abnormally functioning neuron in mental retardation, rather than loss of neurons per se, is strengthened by Weinstein and Teuber's studies (7) of World War II victims of cranial penetrating wounds in whom little or no loss of measured intelligence occurred in spite of extensive cortical loss (7). However, the effects of impoverishment in neuronal growth and synaptic contacts on neuronal functions are not yet very clear. A frequently suggested model is the immature neuron in which the dendritic growth is still curtailed, as is the number of synaptic contacts. In this regard, we are reporting some results concerning the electrophysiological development of the immature neuron which we feel are generally supportive of Dr. Purpura's views (4) on synaptogenesis in the cerebral cortex.

Recently, we have been engaged in the assessment of age-related changes in postsynaptic potentials recorded from neurons in the visual cortex of the kitten. Recordings have been made from kittens ranging from 4–17 days of postnatal age. For kitten visual cortex, this age span brackets the onset of intense synaptic development and functional change as represented by alterations in light evoked potentials recorded with macroelectrodes from the cortical surface. Estimations by Cragg of the number of synapses per neuron in kitten cortex (2) indicate a low rate of synaptic development up to the post-partum age of 8 days (112 synapses per neuron), when a rapid growth sets in, which by age 18 days, has reached 7000 synapses/neuron.

While the rapid rate of synaptic growth continues until about 37 days of age, it is about 20 days of age when myelin first appears in this cortex. Thus, the effects of myelination of this part of the visual system are probably not responsible for the changes we are reporting here.

As Dr. Rose has indicated, and as has been reported elsewhere (3,6), the light evoked potentials recorded from the cortical surface undergo a series of progressive changes in waveform and latency of response. For the period of about 500 msec following the onset of a light flash, the predominant response at the earliest age is a relatively late negative wave followed, in turn, by a longer positive response. With increasing age, shorter latency components appear and the later components of the response tend to be attenuated until a relatively adult form is reached by about 35 days of age.

It should be made clear that we have confined our attention to the earlier more temporally reliable components of a complex response which, particularly in younger kittens, can have a quite long duration. This is illustrated in Figure 1. The bottom traces of Figure 1 show a slow recording from the visual cortex of a 4-day-old kitten, illustrating several cortical responses evoked by a 100-msec flash whose intensity is approximately 17 mL. Note the long series of

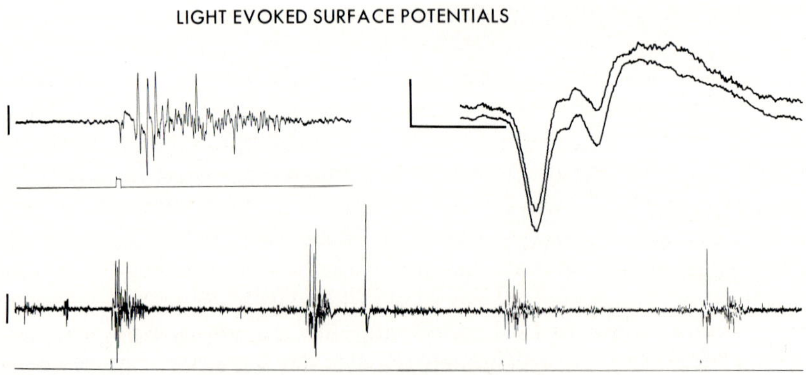

FIGURE 1. Example of a light evoked surface potential recorded from a 4-day kitten with a macroelectrode. Bottom of figure shows a slow recording of 4 consecutive responses evoked by a 100-msec flash (1 per 20 seconds). Note long afterdischarge. Upper right: expanded time scale. Vertical distance between these two traces represents one standard deviation. Calibration: vertical base at left of figures are 100 μV, positive upward. Horizontal line for average represents onset and duration of 100-msec flash. Vertical calibration is 50 μV.

high amplitude waves evoked by a single flash. The trace at the upper left shows one of these responses on an expanded time scale. At the upper right is an average of 10 consecutive responses on a still more expanded time scale and represents the part of the light evoked potential with which the remainder of this report will be concerned. The visual evoked potential in the young kitten is highly dependent on rate of stimulation. For this reason, low rates of stimulation (one per 10, or one per 20 seconds were employed).

As a further word on methodology, all kittens were prepared under either gas or short-acting barbiturate anesthesia, and were subsequently administered local anesthesia, paralyzed, and artificially ventilated. Eyelids were separated and retracted by means of a polyethylene cylinder with a flared base, which was inserted under the eyelids. Light was introduced into the retina by means of a Maxwellian view system and the entire retina was illuminated.

As we previously indicated, our goal is to examine the development of PSPs during the onset of rapid synaptic development. Technically, we have found the intracellular recording from these immature cortical neurons to be difficult and have not yet been able to vary the stimulation parameters to any significant degree. As other investigators have reported (5), we have found these neurons to be extremely fragile and difficult to impale for long periods of time. An example of one of our better recordings taken from an 8-day-old kitten is shown in Figure 2. As in Figure 1, the response is shown on different time bases. The bottom traces show responses of a slowly depolarizing cell to a series of stimulations. At this time scale, the only clearly identifiable response is an inhibitory one. A single response at an expanded time scale is

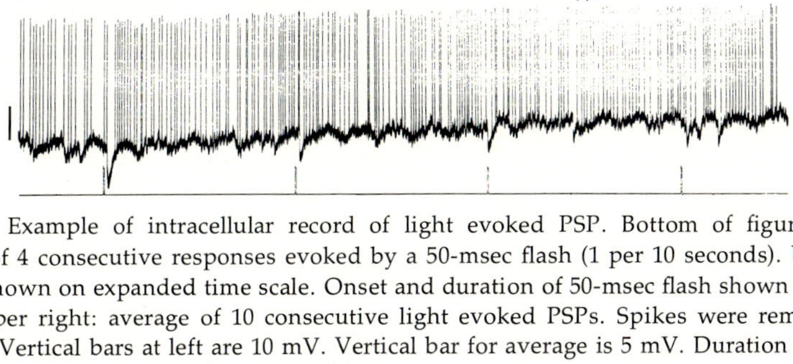

FIGURE 2. Example of intracellular record of light evoked PSP. Bottom of figure is a slow recording of 4 consecutive responses evoked by a 50-msec flash (1 per 10 seconds). Upper left: 1 response shown on expanded time scale. Onset and duration of 50-msec flash shown immediately below. Upper right: average of 10 consecutive light evoked PSPs. Spikes were removed before averaging. Vertical bars at left are 10 mV. Vertical bar for average is 5 mV. Duration and onset of 50-msec light flash is shown by horizontal line.

shown in the upper left of the figure in which an EPSP appears to be evoked prior to the inhibitory response. The spikes were "sliced off" by means of a computer program, and then ten consecutive responses were averaged to generate the tracing shown on the upper right, indicating the postsynaptic response to be a conventional excitatory–inhibitory sequence. Examples of these averaged PSPs were then grouped according to ages as shown in Figure 3, corresponding to age before intense synaptic development (first column), age at the beginning of rapid synaptic development (second column), and the age just before the onset of myelinization (third column). Tracings below the dashed line are averages of the average PSPs for the corresponding age groups. Considering these averages at the bottom as an indication of the contribution of the additional synapses per neuron, at least for this type of stimulation, the most prominent feature would appear to be an excitatory process growing out of a previously laid down inhibitory process, and probably corresponds to the surface-negative potential reported by Dr. Rose. As further synaptic development takes place, this excitatory response becomes sharper and decreases in latency.

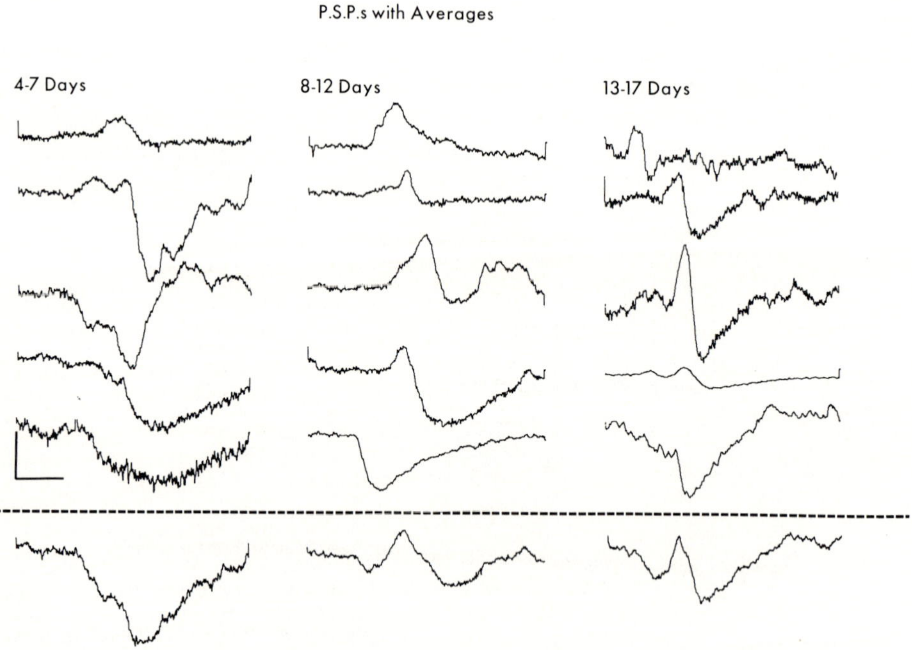

FIGURE 3. Averaged PSPs arranged according to age group. Each average is based on 4 to 10 separate responses. Traces below dashed line are average of the average PSPs and are based on different numbers of averaged PSPs. 4–7 days (N = 6), 8–12 days (N = 5), and 13–17 days (N = 15). Calibration: vertical line is 5 mV; horizontal line is 100 msec. Onset of light flash occurred at the beginning of the trace.

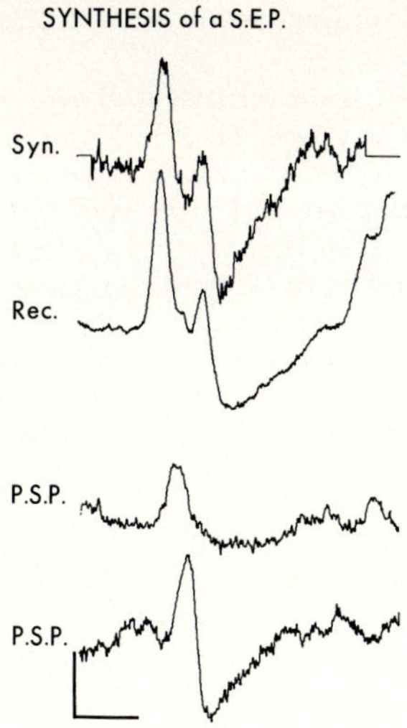

FIGURE 4. Synthesis of surface evoked potential. Top trace is weighted combination of the two PSPs shown at bottom. The latency of these PSPs were changed in the synthesis to achieve a better description of the actual surface evoked potential—second trace from top. In this case, negative is up for the surface evoked potential and down for the PSPs. Calibration for the PSPs is 5 mV (vertical bar) and 50 μV for the surface evoked potential. Horizontal is 100 msec.

One of the long-term purposes of making these recordings is to establish a computerized "bank" of averaged PSPs of individual neurons. Attempts will then be made to synthesize a given surface evoked potential, at a given age, from a weighted combination of PSPs from this bank as a potential index of individual differences in the rate of maturation of the visual system in individual animals. An example of this synthesis for the surface evoked potential of Figure 1 is shown in Figure 4. Note that the surface evoked potential has been inverted such that a negative deflection is now upward.

There is, of course, no necessity that any of the changes in these evoked potential changes are reflecting the concomitant addition of new synapses. Developmental alterations in individual synaptic contacts from "immature" to mature form is also possible (1). Contributions from maturation of the visual pathway from the retina onward also can and probably do contribute. The pattern of synaptogenesis shown by these recordings is consistent with Dr. Purpura's conclusions (4) that the earliest development in the cortex is a long inhibitory process on which subsequent synaptic development builds.

REFERENCES

1. Aghajanian, G. K., and Bloom, F. E. The formation of synaptic junctions in developing rat brain: A quantitative electron microscopic study. *Brain Res.*, 1967, **6:** 716–727.

2. Cragg, B. G. The development of synapses in cat visual cortex. *Invest. Ophthalmol.*, 1972, **11:** 377–385.
3. Ellingson, R. J., and Wilcott, R. C. Development of evoked responses in visual and auditory cortices of kittens. *J. Neurophysiol.*, 1960, **23:** 363–375.
4. Purpura, D. P. Intracellular studies of synaptic organizations in the mammalian brain. In: *Structure and Function of Synapses.* (G. D. Pappas and D. P. Purpura, Eds.). Raven Press, New York, 1972: 257–302.
5. Purpura, D. P., Shofer, R. J., and Scarff, T. Properties of synaptic activities and spike potentials of neurons in immature cortex. *J. Neurophysiol.*, 1965, **28:** 925–942.
6. Rose, G. H., and Lindsley, D. B. Development of visually evoked potentials in kittens: Specific and non-specific responses. *J. Neurophysiol.*, 1968, **31:** 607–623.
7. Weinstein, S., and Teuber, H. Effects of penetrating brain injury on intelligence test scores. *Science*, 1957, **125:** 1036–1037.

Role of the Basal Ganglia in Normal and Abnormal Development

7

Neurophysiological and Anatomical Interrelationships of the Basal Ganglia

N. A. BUCHWALD, C. D. HULL,
and M. S. LEVINE

Mental Retardation Research Center, Brain Research Institute, and Departments of Anatomy and Psychiatry, University of California Los Angeles, Los Angeles, California

The term "mental retardation" is used to describe many different cognitive dysfunctions. At one extreme are the catastrophic changes found in the assaults on the nervous system which result from inborn metabolic errors such as those occurring in Tay-Sachs disease and metachromatic leukodystrophy. At the other extreme are the undetermined subtle changes in the nervous system which are "programmed in" by developmentally early experiential factors and which impair an individual's ability to acquire knowledge. Intermediate between these extremes is a broad range of dysfunctions that involve complex interactions among localized brain pathology, the time of onset of the pathology, and experiential factors.

Many research strategies have been used to investigate these cognitive dysfunctions. One of these strategies is to abstract from the total nervous system, an anatomically well-defined set of interrelated structures, manipulate them experimentally during prenatal or early postnatal periods of development, and then to assess the outcomes of these manipulations in terms of alterations of brain function and behavior. A fruitful example of this strategy is exemplified by the research on the role of the cerebellum reported by Altman in this volume (2).

The system we have focused on is the basal ganglia, a group of telencephalic and diencephalic nuclei which include the caudate nucleus, the putamen, the globus pallidus, the substantia nigra, and the interconnections of these structures. To date, most of the research in our own laboratory has concerned studies in adult animals, but we have now begun to extend our work to the developmental sphere using the research strategy indicated above.

There are good reasons for considering developmental studies of the basal ganglia to be of importance in providing a model of the kind of cognitive brain deficits which might result in mental retardation. These reasons relate, on the one hand, to consideration of the important functions which the basal ganglia have during development, and on the other, to the attractiveness of the basal ganglia for experimental investigations because of the relative ease with which they can be studied and manipulated.

With regard to their functions during development, current evidence suggests that the basal ganglia, and particularly the striatum, play a significant role with respect to sparing of behavioral deficits subsequent to perinatal cortical damage. For example, in primates, experimental lesions in the head of the caudate nucleus made in infancy lead to persisting "cognitive" deficits in adulthood, as demonstrated by the animals' failure to perform delayed-response or similar tasks involving mnemonic abilities (33). Similar deficits in delayed-response performance occur in adult monkeys in which prefrontal cortical lesions have been made. However, these deficits do not appear if the cortical lesions are made in infancy (13). Presumably, the striatum in the developing animal is able to assume functions which the cortex controls at maturity. One might suppose, therefore, that the striatum in infancy is an important component of the brain mechanisms subserving the performance of complex behaviors, gradually relinquishing this role with development of the cortex. Goldman, in her chapter in this volume, discusses the data and the implications of the complex relationship between striatum and cortex during development (12). In addition to the experimental data, clinical evidence is also available suggesting that prenatal damage involving the basal ganglia frequently results in mental retardation. Much of this evidence comes from cases of severe mental disability in which abnormalities of the ventricular ependymal lining are accompanied by drastic distortions of the caudate nucleus (51). In this situation, and in most cases in which morphological changes in the brain have been correlated with existence of "mental retardation," the behavioral deficit is only part of a syndrome of abnormalities, many of which are apparently unrelated to the reduced level of cognition. The sufferer is the victim of what amounts to a catastrophic multiorgan disease process resulting in death, hence, the availability of the brain for study. Whether the cellular pathology discovered in these disease states can provide leads to understanding milder forms of retardation is unknown. However, brains from such catastrophies (with the exception of an occasional specimen made available by accidental death or by unrelated disease) are the only human material generally available for study [cf. chapters by Purpura (46) and Huttenlocher (24) in this volume].

Although our particular interest is focused on nonmotoric aspects of basal ganglionic function, dysfunctions of the basal ganglia are certainly related to "extrapyramidal" motor disorders, including Parkinson's and Huntington's diseases. The search for any single concept (i.e., motor function, sensory function, attention) to express the role of the basal ganglia in regulating behavior, however, may not be meaningful. While the internal structure of each of the nuclei composing the basal ganglia is relatively homogeneous, the topographical distribution of corticostriatal inputs (27) suggests that different regions of the striatum may serve different functions. Experimental damage or ablation of the caudate nucleus has now been shown to result in minimal motoric or metabolic deficiencies, even though more subtle cognitive and motoric abnormalities can be demonstrated. Villablanca and Marcus, in their chapter in this volume, discuss this subject and also detail experimental methods for caudate nuclear ablation, which do not result in gross cortical damage (52).

From a practical point of view, the basal ganglia, and particularly the striatum, are attractive for investigation because of their biochemical, anatomical, and electrophysiological properties. Biochemically they are rich in a number of putative neurotransmitters. These include dopamine, acetylcholine, and γ-aminobutyric acid (GABA), as well as their associated enzymes (7,8,14,19,38,44). The significance of the high striatal dopamine content has been the subject of considerable investigation. Its depletion with pharmacological agents and with lesions interrupting the nigrostriatal pathway are well known phenomena (18,40). Heller and Hoffman discuss these matters in their chapter (17). Striatal dopamine appears relatively late in the development of the nervous system. Tennyson *et al.* describe the course and nature of the development of the dopamine-containing fibers emanating from the substantia nigra in their chapter (50). The role played by dopamine in regulation of striatal neural activity, however, remains elusive, and in the present chapter, we will present some data on this subject. There is increasing evidence that GABA is present in a large fraction of striatal output fibers, and that the synaptic effects of gabaminergic fibers on their target cells is inhibitory (26,32,43–45). There is little doubt that the concentration of acetylcholine in the striatum is the highest in the brain, although exact *in vivo* quantitative estimates of the concentration of this substance have been difficult to make because of the rapid destruction of acetylcholine by cholinesterase. Lesions of brain sites which supply afferents to the striatum (intralaminar thalamus, cortex, or substantia nigra) produce little or no change in the striatal content of enzymes which are involved in metabolism of acetylcholine (37). The implication of these studies is that the striatopetal axons do not utilize acetylcholine as their synaptic transmitter. Recent work (25) in which striatal acetylcholine content was measured directly by biological assay, seems to indicate, however, that a cholinergic input does indeed emanate from certain nigral cells. This fact, of course, does not contradict the probability that the bulk of acetylcholine is located in axon terminals of interneurons. In contrast to acetylcholine, the striatal dopamine content is removed almost completely by the destruction of nigrostriatal afferents.

The remainder of this chapter will be addressed to reviewing our current knowlege of the relationships of the neurophysiology and anatomy of the basal ganglia in adult animals with the implications of this knowledge for studies in normal and abnormal aspects of the developmental process. We will begin with a brief description of the anatomy of the basal ganglia.

ANATOMY OF THE BASAL GANGLIA

For this discussion, the basal ganglia are defined to include the caudate nucleus and putamen (striatum), the two shells of the globus pallidus (the inner shell is called nucleus entopenduncularis in carnivores) and because of its close anatomical and functional relationship with the other basal ganglionic components, the substantia nigra. Some authors use the term neostriatum or corpus striatum as identical with striatum. Figure 1 is a schematic of these structures and includes some of the principal connections of the basal ganglia.

The striatum receives major inputs from cerebral cortex, intralaminar thalamus, and the substantia nigra.

All or nearly all parts of the cerebral cortex project upon the striatum in a topographical manner (27,53). Recent work by Heimer (15) even considers that the cortex of the rhinencephalon projecting on the nucleus accumbens represents a limbic extension of the basal ganglionic system. Projections from the contralateral cortex to the striatum have also been described (27).

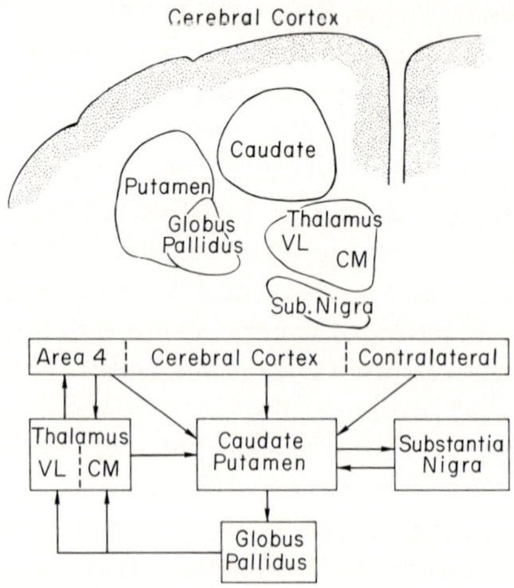

FIGURE 1. Schematic of the principal connections of the basal ganglia.

Thalamic afferents reach the striatum from the intralaminar thalamic nuclei, principally the central median and the parafascicular nuclei (39). There is no secure anatomical evidence concerning the topography of this distribution.

The remaining direct afferents to the striatum come from the midbrain, the bulk of which are nigrofugal. At least part of this projection is made up of dopamine-containing fibers (3,4,40). Striatal afferents not originating in the nigra include serotonin-containing fibers (16).

Extensive details of the neuronal make-up and synaptic contacts of striatal neurons have been provided recently by Kemp and Powell (28–31). More than 90% of the neurons of the caudate nucleus and putamen appear to be small to medium-sized interneurons with extensive dendritic fields. These neurons are distributed homogeneously throughout the striatum. Less than 5% of striatal neurons have long axons which project outside the nucleus.

Kemp and Powell's work (28–31) details the pattern of synaptic contacts on the short-axoned striatal interneurons. Dendrites of these neurons are densely covered with spines, except at their bases. The majority of synapses formed by input fibers are axodendritic. Incoming axons typically cross the dendrites of a number of these neurons at right angles, making synaptic contacts *en passant*. An individual striatal interneuron may receive inputs from cortical, thalamic, and nigral fibers. Cortical and thalamic inputs are equally distributed over the spiny regions of the dendrites. However, cortical afferents are more numerous at the dendritic base. Nigral inputs are sparser. Their exact terminations have not been ascertained.

The two principal structures receiving striatal efferents are the globus pallidus and the substantia nigra. In addition to the striatal projection, a major input to the pallidum (and nigra) comes from the subthalamic nucleus (9). A nigropallidal pathway has also been described (9).

In contrast to the striatum, most neurons in the globus pallidus are large and fusiform (1,10,30). Synaptic contacts on these neurons are usually made by axons running parallel to the dendrites. The majority of the neurons are long-axoned and terminate extranuclearly. Short-axoned interneurons are scarce. According to both Kemp and Powell (30) and Fox (10), the most common synaptic endings are terminals of striatal output cells which appear large and contain large vesicles. Small terminals may represent endings of subthalamic or nigral inputs to the pallidum, while rare large endings with few vesicles may be the termination of intrapallidal axonal branches.

The substantia nigra possesses a cellular appearance very similar to that of the globus pallidus. The major input to the nigra comes from the striatum. Apparently, striatofugal fibers make contact with dendrites of nigral cells in the reticular portion of the substantia nigra.

The major projections of the globus pallidus are to the ventral-anterior and ventral-lateral nuclei of the thalamus. Pallidal projections also occur to the subthalamic nucleus and to the midbrain tegmentum (42). The thalamic pathway (Figure 1) serves to close the loop between the basal ganglia and the cerebral cortex, although pallidal efferents also synapse on intralaminar thalamic neurons and are thus part of a more local basal ganglionic-thalamic-basal ganglionic circuit. Recently, Nauta (41) has provided anatomical evidence for the existence of an important pathway from the pallidum to the habenular nucleus.

Although the nigra, as well as the pallidum, possesses a thalamic afferent (9), more attention has been paid to the fine nigrostriatal fibers. The existence of this pathway, established by fluorescent microscopic techniques, has recently been confirmed by the Fink-Heimer method (40). Chapters by Heller and Hoffman (17) and Tennyson *et al.* (50) in this volume describe facets of the nigrostriatal pathway in detail.

ELECTROPHYSIOLOGY OF THE BASAL GANGLIA

We believe that it is now possible to understand the neurophysiology of the basal ganglia. Detailed information on the synaptic relationships of basal ganglionic nuclei has been provided by recent definitive studies using morphological (28–31) and electrophysiological (5,6,20–22,34) techniques. The account which follows is essentially a summary of our own work on basal ganglionic neurophysiology. Those details which we believe can be useful either now or in the near future in understanding basal ganglionic function in the developing organism are stressed. First, we will consider the intrinsic activity of caudate and pallidal neurons, and second, the responses which can be evoked in these neurons by stimulation of their afferents.

Intrinsic Activity

Neurons in the caudate nucleus and putamen fire more slowly than do neurons in many other brain sites (6,20,35,47,48). When systematic measurements are made under conditions in which the states of consciousness of the experimental subjects are taken into account, the mean firing rate of caudate neurons is found to be slower than that of neurons in the thalamus or of neurons in the neocortex (35). Table I expresses this result in terms of the mean interval between recorded neuronal spikes. Translated into spikes/second, caudate neurons fired 0.67/second, cortical neurons 1.36/second, and thalamic neurons (ventral anterior and ventral lateral nuclei) 1.96/second. In a separate study (34) of neurons in the globus pallidus and entopeduncular nucleus, it was found that cells in these structures generally fired at much higher rates (5.1/second). The slower overall mean firing rate of caudate neurons is due to a larger number of caudate cells with very long mean interspike intervals (greater than 2000 msec), and a relatively smaller number of fast

Table I Mean Interspike Intervals in Normal Cats[a]

	No. of Cats	*Number of Units*	*Mean Interspike Interval (msec)*
Caudate	7	234	1656
Cortex	4	110	738
VA-VL thalamus	4	151	510

[a] These values are derived from experiments performed on paralyzed, locally anesthetized cats.

firing caudate cells (mean interspike intervals less than 400 msec). In contrast, most cells in the cortex and thalamus have short mean interspike intervals (less than 400 msec) with relatively few cells with long mean interspike intervals (Figure 2, left panel).

The low firing rate of striatal neurons may result from their intrinsic anatom-

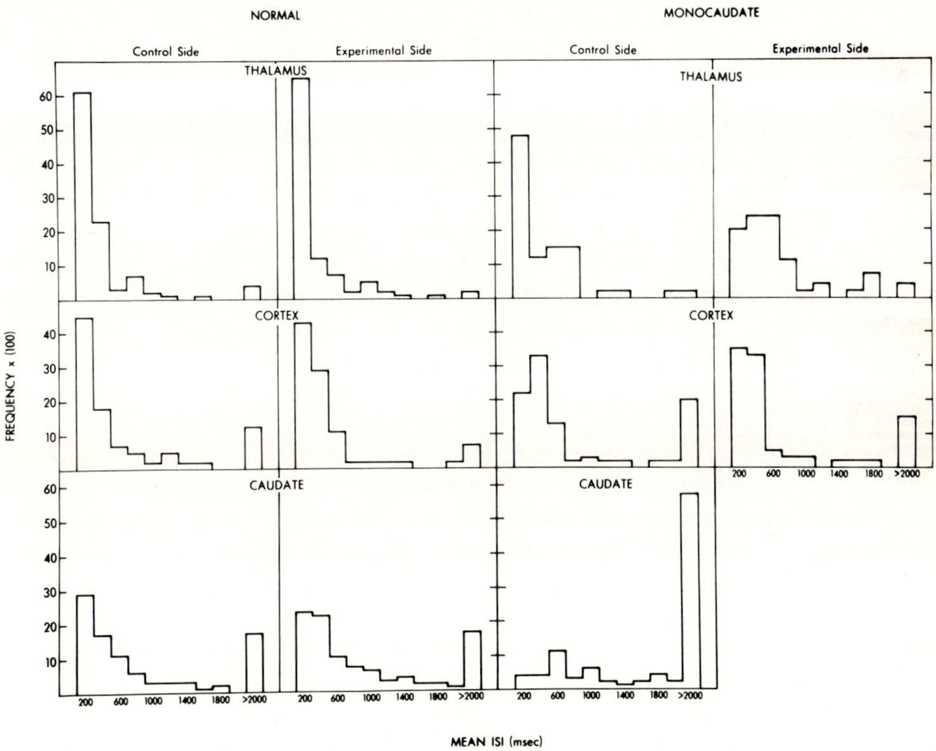

FIGURE 2. Distributions of mean interspike intervals (ISIs) for caudate, cortical, and thalamic units in intact cats (left panel) and in cats with one caudate nucleus removed (monocaudate) (right panel). Unilateral caudate ablation produced a slowing of unit firing in the contralateral caudate seen by the increase in the proportion of slowly firing caudate units in monocaudate cats. Bin widths = 200 msec. Frequency × 100 indicates percent of total number of units in each bin. Figure adapted from Levine *et al.* (35).

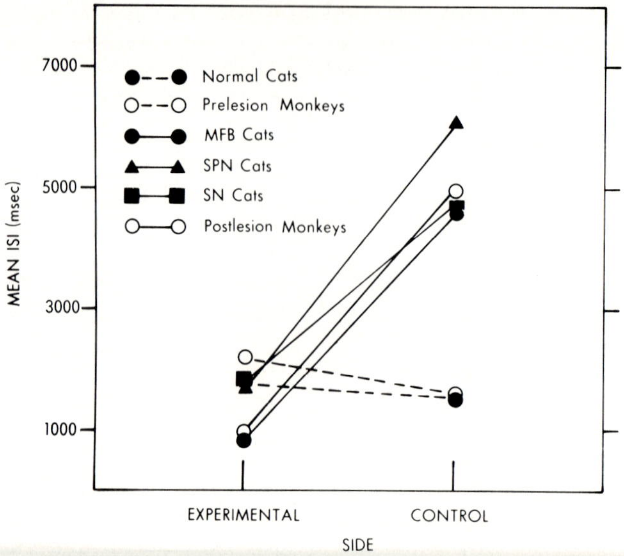

FIGURE 3. Overall group mean interspike intervals for intact cats and monkeys with unilateral lesions. Unilateral MFB and SN lesions in cats interrupted the nigrostriatal pathway and depleted dopamine and its biosynthetic enzymes from the ipsilateral caudate nucleus. SPN lesions in cats and unilateral lesions in monkeys did not produce depletion of dopamine in the ipsilateral caudate. (See text for further description.) Figure adapted from Hull *et al.* (23).

ical, physical, or chemical characteristics and/or from the nature of synaptic inputs to them from striatopetal axons. The latter possibility was investigated in an experiment designed to examine the consequences of interruption of the nigrostriatal pathway on spontaneous firing rates of caudate nucleus neurons (23). Unilateral lesions in the substantia nigra (SN), just dorsal to the nigra (SPN) or more rostrally, in the lateral hypothalamus along the course of the nigrostriatal pathway (MFB lesions), all produced an asymmetry in caudate nucleus firing represented mainly by a marked slowing of single unit firing rates in the caudate nucleus contralateral to the lesion (Figure 3). Interruption of the dopaminergic nigrostriatal pathway did not appear to be the prime cause of this postlesion asymmetry. The contralateral slowing occurred whether or not postlesion depletions in concentrations of ipsilateral striatal dopamine or alterations in the activity of its biosynthetic enzymes, tyrosine hydroxylase and DOPA decarboxylase occurred.

Postmortem examination of the brains of animals in this study indicated that the lesions probably interrupted striatal outputs as well as striatal inputs. We thought that the contralateral slowing might have been a consequence of interrupting striatal outputs which by multisynaptic pathways produced a tonic inhibition in the striatum on the opposite side of the brain. To test this hypothesis, we removed the caudate nucleus on one side using the surgical technique reported by Villablanca (52). Following this operation, a marked slowing of unit firing in the remaining caudate nucleus occurred (Figure 2, right panel) (35). This effect was quite similar to that produced by the unilateral lesions in the previous experiment (23) and provides positive evidence to suggest that interruption of striatofugal fibers had indeed been of importance.

The question as to how ipsilateral lesions produce contralateral neurophysiological effects still remains to be answered, although recent experiments have provided possible answers to this question. When the firing rates of cortical and thalamic units were examined in animals previously subjected to unilateral caudate ablation, a slight slowing was found in the thalamus ipsilateral to the lesion and in the cortex on both sides of the brain (35). This slowing was statistically insignificant for cortical neurons. For thalamic units, however, although overall mean firing rates did not appear to be significantly altered by the lesions, a significant decrease appeared in the occurrence of units with the shortest mean interspike intervals (fastest firing rates) (Figure 2, right panel). The fact that distributional differences in thalamic firing rates occurred postlesion, while overall mean rates were unchanged is probably related to the neuronal heterogeneity of the thalamus compared to the striatum. The possibility that the thalamus is involved in the alteration of neuronal firing rates of the contralateral striatum, which occurs after removal of striatofugal influences, seems reasonable in view of the fact that the target cells of the striatum in globus pallidus and substantia nigra project to both intralaminar and ventral anterior and ventrolateral thalamic nuclear groups (42). To provide a more direct test of thalamic involvement, we prepared animals with combined lesions in the area of the medial forebrain bundle (MFB) and in the ipsilateral intralaminar region (the parafascicular-central median nuclei (CM-PF) of the thalamus). Table II shows that in animals with combined lesions the side-to-side asymmetry in caudate firing rates produced by damaging striatal outputs alone no longer existed. Taken together, these results provide evidence that the low spontaneous firing rates of striatal neurons are at least partly due to the nature of the synaptic inputs to this nucleus from the thalamus. The data also provide a physiological clue to the events which might underlie the partial success of thalamic lesions in alleviating symptoms in certain extrapyramidal diseases.

Table II Mean Interspike Intervals (ISIs) for Caudate Neurons Recorded from Intact Cats, Cats with Unilateral MFB Lesions and Combined MFB and CM-PF Lesions

	Intact Cats		*Unilateral MFB Lesion*		*Combined MFB and CM-PF Lesions*	
	Left	*Right*	*Ipsilateral*	*Contralateral*	*Ipsilateral*	*Contralateral*
Mean ISI (msec)	1768	1544	955	4786	1238	1095

Synaptic Responses of Neurons in the Caudate Nucleus and the Globus Pallidus

Caudate Nucleus

In assessing the electrophysiological characteristics of caudate nuclear neurons, it is important to make intracellular recordings because even in response to stimulation of excitatory inputs, caudate neurons frequently remain polarized below their firing levels. In a series of experiments (5,6,20–22), we studied the responses of caudate neurons to excitation of known anatomical inputs (cortex, intralaminar thalamus, and substantia nigra) and to a number of peripheral inputs. Such stimulation almost always elicited initial excitation in caudate neurons, which was followed by a longer period of inhibition (an EPSP-IPSP sequence). The only major exception to the EPSP-IPSP sequence evoked in caudate cells occurred when the intralaminar thalamus (the central median-parafascicular region) was stimulated. This stimulation evoked relatively pure EPSPs in 30-40% of caudate neurons impaled (6).

We believe that the initial excitation evoked in caudate neurons by stimulation of striopetal axons is a consequence of activation of excitatory inputs on the dendrites of the ubiquitous short-axoned interneurons in the caudate nucleus. The succeeding IPSPs are generated internally and are mediated by these interneurons which project onto each other. In most instances, input axons to the striatum form contacts with a number of caudate interneurons. However, in those cases in which incoming excitatory axons terminate on a small number of caudate neurons, a "pure" EPSP would be generated.

Table III summarizes responses of caudate neurons to stimulation of cortex,

Table III Postsynaptic Response of Caudate Neurons

Brain Site Stimulated	*No. Tested*	*EPSP-IPSP*	*EPSP Only*	*IPSP Only*	*No Response*
Substantia nigra	18	14		3	1
Fields of Forel and subthalamus	8	3	1	1	3
Supranigral midbrain	9	7		2	
Caudate n.	7	7			
Suprageniculate n.	3	1	2		
Lat. posterior n.	13	5	4		4
Ventral lat. and ventral ant. nn	23	19	2	1	1
Ant. thalamic radiations	29	25	3		1
Medial dorsal n.	13	8	2		3
Central median and parafascicularis	32	18	10		4
Precruciate cortex	41	30		4	7
Peripheral stimulation	18	14			4
	214	151	24	11	28

thalamus, and substantia nigra and to a number of peripheral stimuli. Responses are classified according to the postsynaptic sequence recorded intracellularly.

During the course of the investigation of the synaptic responses of striatal neurons, we also studied the result of combinations of stimuli on the evoked postsynaptic responses. An important finding of these experiments (21) was the demonstration of the prepotency of cortical over thalamic or nigral activation. When stimuli to two different brain sites were paired, a preceding stimulus to the cortex prevented or attenuated the excitation produced by a thalamic or nigral stimulus (Figures 4 and 5). Conversely, a preceding thalamic or nigral stimulus failed to suppress cortically evoked excitation (Figures 4 and 5).

The corticostriatal functional relationships emphasized in these studies may be of importance with regard to the changing roles of cortex and striatum during development suggested by the lesion experiments mentioned earlier in this chapter. The results of those experiments imply that the striatum in the infant operates independently of the less mature cerebral cortex. Increasing "corticalization" as the organism develops may include synaptic "capture" of the striatum by the cortex, as indicated by our electrophysiological findings in mature animals. Electrophysiological experiments to investigate the time of onset of this synaptic "capture" are currently being carried out in our laboratory.

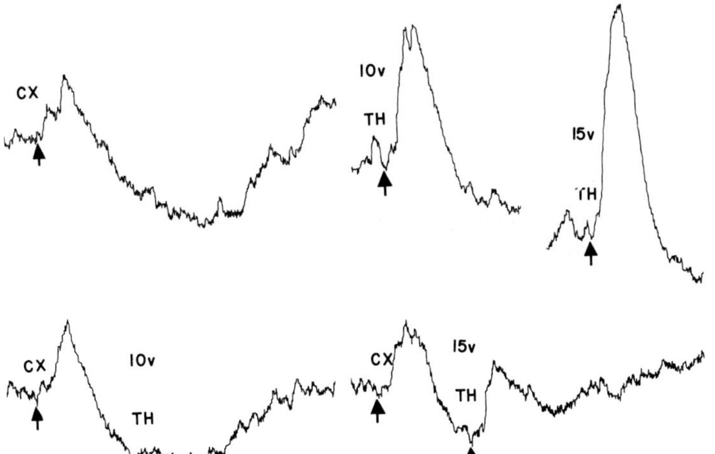

FIGURE 4. Suppression of a central median (TH) evoked EPSP in a caudate neuron by a cortically evoked IPSP. Shocks delivered to the cortex at 10 V, 0.5 msec duration, and 0.3 Hz. Pulse duration for thalamic shock was the same as for the cortex. Responses to 10 and 15 V intensity shocks to the TH alone are shown in middle and right, upper traces; responses to cortex alone (upper left trace). Paired cortex (CX) and 10-V TH response, lower left trace; paired cortex and 15-V TH response, lower right trace. All traces are averages of ten consecutive responses. Figure adapted from Hull *et al.* (21).

sensory, a single cell responding to a variety of sensory inputs (34,36,49). Although the pathways involved in the production of sensory-evoked responses in pallidal neurons are unknown, there is a strong possibility that these projections occur via the striatum. Both the consideration of the connections of the striatum to the pallidum and the fact that postsynaptic potential shapes and sequences evoked in pallidal neurons by activation of caudate and sensory inputs are similar (34), provide indirect evidence that sensory inputs to the pallidum are mediated by the striatum.

FUNCTIONAL INTERRELATIONSHIPS OF THE BASAL GANGLIA

From our knowledge of the anatomy and neurophysiology of the basal ganglia, we can make guesses as to their functional interrelationships. The "head end" of the system is the striatum, which processes neural information sent by other brain structures. The results of this processing is a modulated output to the globus pallidus and the substantia nigra. The guessed at function of these latter structures is to increase the "gain" in the system. Small changes in slowly firing striatal neurons are translated into much larger changes in faster firing pallidal cells. The outputs of the basal ganglia are relayed to the cortex from the pallidum and nigra via the thalamus, and on the basis of recent evidence, to the limbic system via the habenular nuclei. Feedback control of the striatum probably occurs by way of striatonigrostriatal paths and by indirect loops from the pallidum and nigra via the thalamus and/or cortex back to the striatum.

We believe that there is now enough knowledge of these interrelationships which, together with information available with regard to the process of maturation of the chemical constituency of the striatum, will allow the use of the basal ganglia as a model system to study development. Surgical or pharmacological insults can be inflicted upon the basal ganglia during infancy and the results of these insults can be determined as the animal matures.

ACKNOWLEDGMENT

This research was supported by USPHS Grant Nos. MH-07097, HD-05958, and HD-04612.

REFERENCES

1. Adinolfi, A. M. The fine structure of neurons and synapses in the entopeduncular nucleus of the cat. *J. Comp. Neurol.*, 1969, **135:** 225–248.
2. Altman, J. Effects of interference with cerebellar maturation on the development of locomotion. An experimental model of neurobehavioral retardation. Chapter 2, this volume.

3. Andén, N. E., Carlsson, A., Dahlström, A., Fuxe, K., Hillarp, N.-Å., and Larsson, K. Demonstration and mapping out of nigro-neostriatal dopamine neurons. *Life Sci.*, 1964, **3:** 523–530.
4. Andén, N. E., Dahlström, A., Fuxe, K., Larsson, K., Olson, L., and Ungerstedt, U. Ascending monoamine neurons to the telencephalon and diencephalon. *Acta Physiol. Scand.*, 1966, **67:** 313–326.
5. Buchwald, N. A., Hull, C. D., Vernon, L., and Bernardi, G. Physiological and psychological aspects of basal ganglia function. *U. S. Pub. Health Serv., Publ.* #1938, 1969: 82–91.
6. Buchwald, N. A., Price, D. D., Vernon, L., and Hull, C. D. Caudate intracellular responses to thalamic and cortical inputs. *Exp. Neurol.*, 1973, **38:** 311–323.
7. Burgen, A. S. W., and Chipman, L. M. The location of cholinesterase in the central nervous system. *Q. J. Exp. Physiol. Cog. Med. Sci.*, 1952, **37:** 61–74.
8. Campbell, L. B., and Jenden, D. J. Gas chromatographic evaluation of the influence of oxatremorine upon the regional distribution of acetylcholine in rat. *J. Neurochem.*, 1970, **17:** 1697–1699.
9. Carpenter, M. B., and Strominger, N. L. Efferent fibers of the subthalamic nucleus in the monkey. A comparison of efferent projections of subthalamic nucleus, substantia nigra and globus pallidus. *Am. J. Anat.*, 1967, **121:** 41–72.
10. Fox, C. A., Andrade, A. M., Luqui, J. J., and Rafols, J. A. The primate globus pallidus: A Golgi and electron microscopic study. *J. Hirnforsch.*, 1974, **15:** 75–93.
11. Fuller, D. R. G., Hull, C. D., and Buchwald, N. A. Caudate neurons antidromically activated from nucleus entopeduncularis and substantia nigra. (Manuscript in preparation.)
12. Goldman, P. Age, sex, and experience as related to the neural basis of cognitive development. Chapter 13, this volume.
13. Harlow, H. F., Blomquist, A. J., Thompson, C. I., Schlitz, K. A., and Harlow, M. K. Effects of induction age and size of frontal lobe lesions on learning in rhesus monkeys. In: *The Neuropsychology of Development.* (R. Isaacson, Ed.). Wiley, New York, 1968: 79–120.
14. Hebb, C., and Silver, A. Choline acetylase in the central nervous system of man and some other mammals. *J. Physiol. (Lond.)*, 1956, **134:** 718–728.
15. Heimer, L. and Wilson, R. D. The allocortical projections to the basal ganglia in the rat—similarities in the neural associations of the hippocampus, the piriform cortex and the neocortex. *Golgi Centennial Symposium.* (Santini, Ed.). Raven Press, Hewlett, 1974.
16. Heller, A. Neuronal control of brain serotonin. *Fed. Proc.*, 1972, **31:** 81–90.
17. Heller, A., and Hoffman, P. C. Neuronal control of neurochemical processes in the basal ganglia. Chapter 8, this volume.
18. Heller, A., and Moore, R. Y. Control of brain serotonin and norepinephrine by specific neural systems. *Adv. Pharmacol.*, 1968, **6:** 191–206.
19. Heller, A., and Moore, R. Y. Localization and neural control of brain monoamines. In: *Biochemistry, Schizophrenia and Affective Illnesses.* (H. E. Himwich, Ed.). Williams & Wilkins, Baltimore, Maryland, 1970: 431–469.
20. Hull, C. D., Bernardi, G., and Buchwald, N. A. Intracellular responses of caudate neurons to brain stem stimulation. *Brain Res.*, 1970, **22:** 163–179.
21. Hull, C. D., Bernardi, G., Price, D. D., and Buchwald, N. A. Intracellular responses of caudate neurons to temporally and spatially combined stimuli. *Exp. Neurol.*, 1973, **38:** 324–336.
22. Hull, C. D., Buchwald, N. A., and Vernon, L. Intracellular responses in caudate and cortical neurons. *U. S. Pub. Health Serv., Publ.* #1938, 1969: 92–97.
23. Hull, C. D., Levine, M. S., Buchwald, N. A., Heller, A., and Browning, R. A. The spontaneous firing pattern of forebrain neurons. I. The effects of dopamine and non-dopamine depleting lesions on caudate unit firing patterns. *Brain Res.*, 1974, **73:** 241–262.
24. Huttenlocher, P. R. Dendritic and synaptic development and mental defect. Chapter 5, this volume.
25. Jones, B. E., Guyenet, P., Cheramy, A., Gauchy, C., and Glowinski, J. The *in vivo* release of

acetylcholine from cat caudate nucleus after pharmacological and surgical manipulation of dopaminergic nigrostriatal neurons. *Brain Res.*, 1973, **64:** 355–369.

26. Kataoka, K., Bak, I. J., Hassler, R., Kim, J. S., and Wagner, A. L-Glutamate decarboxylase and choline acetyltransferase activity in substantia nigra and striatum after surgical interruption of the strio-nigral fibres of the baboon. *Expl. Brain Res.*, 1974, **19:** 217–227.
27. Kemp, J. M., and Powell, T. P. S. The cortico-striate projection in the monkey. *Brain*, 1970, **93:** 525–546.
28. Kemp, J. M., and Powell, T. P. S. The structure of the caudate nucleus of the cat: Light and electron microscopy. *Philos. Trans. R. Soc. Lond. [Biol. Sci.]*, 1971, **262:** 383–401.
29. Kemp, J. M., and Powell, T. P. S. The synaptic organization of caudate nucleus. *Philos. Trans. R. Soc. Lond. [Biol. Sci.]*, 1971, **262:** 403–412.
30. Kemp, J. M., and Powell, T. P. S. Site of termination of fibers in the caudate nucleus. *Philos. Trans. R. Soc. Lond. [Biol. Sci.]*, 1971, **262:** 413–427.
31. Kemp, J. M., and Powell, T. P. S. Termination of fibers from cerebral cortex and thalamus upon dendritic spines in the caudate nucleus: A study with the Golgi method. *Philos. Trans. R. Soc. Lond. [Biol. Sci.]*, 1971, **262:** 429–439.
32. Kim, J. S., Bak, I. J., Okada, Y., and Hassler, R. Role of γ-aminobutyric acid in extrapyramidal motor system. II. Some evidence for existence of a type of GABA-rich strionigral neurons. *Expl. Brain Res.*, 1971, **14:** 95–104.
33. Kling, A., and Tucker, T. J. Effects of combined lesions of frontal granular cortex and caudate nucleus in neonatal monkey. *Brain Res.*, 1967, **6:** 428–439.
34. Levine, M. S., Hull, C. D., and Buchwald, N. A. Pallidal and entopeduncular intracellular responses to striatal, cortical thalamic and sensory inputs. *Exp. Neurol.*, 1974, **44:** 448–460.
35. Levine, M. S., Hull, C. D., Buchwald, N. A., and Villablanca, J. The spontaneous firing patterns of forebrain neurons. II. Effects of unilateral caudate nuclear ablation. *Brain Res.*, 1974, **78:** 411–424.
36. Lidsky, T. I., Buchwald, N. A., and Hull, C. D. Pallidal and entopeduncular single unit activity in cats during drinking. *Soc. Neurosci.*, 1974, **4:** 308.
37. Lynch, G. S., Lucao, P. A., and Deadwyler, S. A. Demonstration of acetylcholinesterase containing neurons in caudate nucleus of rat. *Brain Res.*, 1972, **45:** 617–621.
38. McCaman, R. E., and Hunt, J. M. Microdetermination of cholineacetylase in nervous tissue. *J. Neurochem.*, 1965, **12:** 253–259.
39. Mehler, W. R. Further notes on the center median nucleus of Luys. In: *The Thalamus*. (D. Purpura and M. Yahr, Eds.). Columbia Univ. Press, New York, 1966: 109–122.
40. Moore, R. Y., Bhatnagar, R. K., and Heller, A. Anatomical and chemical studies of a nigroneostriatal projection in the cat. *Brain Res.*, 1971, **30:** 119–135.
41. Nauta, H. W. J. Evidence of a pallidohabenular pathway in the cat. *J. Comp. Neurol.*, 1974, **56:** 19–28.
42. Nauta, W. J. H., and Mehler, W. R. Fiber connections of the basal ganglia. *U. S. Pub. Health Serv., Publ.* #1938, 1969: 67–72.
43. Obata, K., and Yoshida, M. Caudate evoked inhibition and actions of GABA and other substances on cat pallidal neurons. *Brain Res.*, 1973, **64:** 455–459.
44. Okada, Y., Nitsch-Hassler, C., Kim, J. S., Bak, I. J., and Hassler, R. Role of γ-aminobutyric acid (GABA) in the extrapyramidal motor system. I. Regional distribution of GABA in rabbit, rat, guinea pig and baboon CNS. *Expl. Brain Res.*, 1971, **13:** 514–518.
45. Precht, W., and Yoshida, M. Blockage of caudate-evoked inhibition of neurons in the substantia nigra by picrotoxin. *Brain Res.*, 1971, **32:** 229–233.
46. Purpura, D. P. Normal and aberrant neuronal development in the cerebral cortex of human fetus and young infant. Chapter 6, this volume.
47. Purpura, D. P., and Malliani, A. Intracellular studies of the corpus striatum. I. Synaptic potentials and discharge characteristics of caudate neurons activated by thalamic stimulation. *Brain Res.*, 1967, **6:** 325–340.

48. Rocha-Miranda, C. E. Single unit analysis of cortex-caudate connection. *Electroenceph. clin. Neurophysiol.*, 1965, **19:** 237–247.
49. Soltysik, S., Hull, C. D., and Buchwald, N. A. Caudate and pallidal unit activity during delayed instrumental response performance in monkey. *Soc. Neurosci.*, 1974, **4:** 431.
50. Tennyson, V. M., Mytilineou, C., Heikkila, R., Barrett, R. E., Cohen, G., Côté, L., Duffy, P. E., and Marco, L. Dopamine-containing neurons of the substantia nigra and their terminals in the neostriatum. Chapter 9, this volume.
51. Tobin, A. Mental retardation due to germinal matrix infarction. *Science.*, 1969, **164:** 156–158.
52. Villablanca, J. R., and Marcus, R. Effects of caudate nuclei removal in cats. Comparison with effects of frontal cortex ablation. Chapter 10, this volume.
53. Webster, K. E. The cortico-striatal projection in the cat. *J. Anat.*, 1965, **99:** 329–337.

8

Neuronal Control of Neurochemical Processes in the Basal Ganglia

ALFRED HELLER and PHILIP C. HOFFMANN
Department of Pharmacological and Physiological Sciences,
The University of Chicago,
Chicago, Illinois

The neurochemistry of the caudate nucleus and the associated basal ganglia is as complex and intriguing a subject as is the examination of its anatomical organization and physiological function. This division of the telencephalon has a neuronal population capable of synthesizing and storing a number of biologically active substances including acetylcholine, γ-aminobutyric acid, norepinephrine, serotonin, and dopamine. The presence of such substances, all of which may act as chemical transmitters, in a brain area which subserves motor as well as behavioral functions, provides an attractive model for the study of the role of specific neurochemical substances in physiological functions. Analyses of this type, however, require direct information as to the association of particular neurochemical substances with specific neuronal elements. One approach to this problem, which has proved particularly useful in the case of the monoaminergic systems, is the selective destruction of specific central pathways by lesions followed by examination of the neurochemical or histochemical changes produced by such neuronal destruction.

The lesion technique was initially applied to the identification of the medial forebrain bundle, a tract whose presence is essential for the biosynthesis and storage of brain serotonin and norepinephrine (for review, see 24,25,27,28,30,47). The lesion method combined with the use of the Falck-Hillarp histochemical method (12,13) has, in addition, led to an extensive mapping of central monoaminergic pathways (8,17,63). The medial forebrain bundle is a complex tract interconnecting the hypothalamus, the basal telencephalon, and the midbrain (21,39,53), and its destruction leads to a profound and permanent loss in serotonin and norepinephrine in all areas of the telencephalon (30,31,50,52). The primary biochemical deficit which accounts for the reduction of brain monoamines is a loss of enzymatic activities essential for their biosynthesis, including tyrosine hydroxylase, 5-HTP/dopa decarboxylase, and dopamine β-hydroxylase (26,32,33,48,59). Telencephalic norepinephrine or serotonin can be selectively reduced by lateral versus medial placement of lesions in tegmental areas projecting to the medial forebrain bundle (28) (Table I).

In the basal ganglia, primary interest has been focused on the presence of dopamine. In mammals, the high concentration of dopamine in the basal ganglia is quite striking as compared to other areas of brain (6,37) and there is now abundant evidence that the presence of this monoamine in the basal ganglia is a function of the existence of a direct projection of dopamine-producing axons to the neostriatum from cell bodies in the substantia nigra. Evidence for such a pathway is available from a variety of sources: (a) The dopamine content of the basal ganglia is markedly reduced in the neostriatum of parkinsonian patients in association with cell loss in the substantia nigra (10,20,36); (b) application of the Falck-Hillarp fluorescence histochemical method (12,13) has demonstrated the presence of dopamine-containing cell bodies in the pars compacta of the substantia nigra and adjacent areas and dopamine-containing terminals in the neostriatum (4,7,8,18); and (c) a variety of lesions involving destruction of the substantia nigra, the ventral midbrain tegmentum, or rostrally along the course of the internal capsule all result in a marked reduction in striatal dopamine (1–3,5,14,22,49,51,56,57).

Despite a good deal of suggestive evidence for a direct nigrostriatal system, it had not been possible until recently to demonstrate such a projection by conventional anatomical techniques. By application of the Fink and Heimer modification of the Nauta method for silver impregnation of degenerating axons and terminals (16) it has recently been possible to study the course and distribution of axon degeneration following lesions of the substantia nigra (46,49). Following lesions of the substantia nigra and ventral tegmentum in

Table I Effects of Central Nervous System Lesions Involving Components of the Medial Forebrain Bundle on Telencephalic Serotonin and Norepinephrine in the Rat[a]

Experimental Lesion	*% Serotonin*[b]	*% Norepinephrine*[c]
Lateral hypothalamus	−82	−82
Medial tegmentum	−78	ns[d]
Ventrolateral tegmentum	ns[d]	−73

[a] Reprinted with permission from Heller (25).
[b] Control telencephalic serotonin = 0.68 μg/gm wet weight of tissue.
[c] Control telencephalic norepinephrine = 0.26 μg/gm wet weight of tissue.
[d] ns refers to differences between control and lesion levels not statistically significant, $P > 0.05$.

the cat it can be shown that axons of the nigrostriatal projection pass through the ventral tegmentum and ascend via the internal capsule and lateral hypothalamus to innervate the putamen and caudate nucleus. The distribution of degenerating terminals is homogeneous in the putamen whereas in the caudate more terminals are evident laterally than medially. Of particular interest is the distribution of degenerating nigrostriatal axons within the hypothalamus. At the rostral tuberal level of the hypothalamus, the fibers run entirely in the medial internal capsule and the adjacent lateral hypthalamus. Thus, lesions transecting the lateral hypothalamic area and extending into the medial part of the internal capsule produce profound effects on caudate nucleus dopamine, tyrosine hydroxylase, and dopa decarboxylase restricted to the side of the brain containing the lesion (49). The magnitude of the effect is dependent upon the size and exact location of the combined lesion and some well-placed lesions cause a nearly total loss of amines and enzymes. Lesions involving only the medial internal capsule, but sparing the lateral hypothalamic area result in decreases in caudate nucleus dopamine, tyrosine hydroxylase, and dopa decarboxylase in the range of 40–50%. Lesions involving both the medial internal capsule and the lateral hypothalamic area have a more marked effect on dopamine and the enzymes producing a 70–90% loss of each.

The rate of loss of caudate dopamine following lesions of the nigrostriatal pathway has been studied in some detail in the rat (25). Dopamine is lost more rapidly following transection of this central monosynaptic catecholamine pathway than are serotonin and norepinephrine following certain central lesions (24,25). The loss of serotonin and norepinephrine following such lesions may involve transsynaptic mechanisms (for review, see 25,29,30,47). Following transection of the nigrostriatal projection either within the diencephalon or at the mesencephalic level by destruction of the substantia nigra, there is a rapid fall in dopamine with a 50% reduction by 2 days and a 70–80% reduction in 4 to 6 days (25). This time course is quite similar to that observed in peripheral tissues following direct sympathetic denervation and therefore consistent with a direct central denervation phenomenon.

At 1 day following lesion placement, dopamine is elevated to 30% above normal (25). This observation is of interest in view of the recent finding that after lesions of the nigrostriatal pathway at the level of the rostral end of the supramammillary decussation, there is a very rapid increase in dopamine. By 18 minutes after the lesion, dopamine levels are increased by 64% and this effect is sustained for at least 20 hours. It has been suggested that the increase in dopamine caused by axotomy results from an initial inhibition of impulse flow in the nigroneostriatal pathway and a reduction in dopamine release (64).

The ontogenic development of dopamine and its biosynthetic enzymes in the rat provides additional evidence for a direct nigrostriatal projection. The rat is a useful animal for such studies since the increase of monoamine and enzyme activity takes place almost entirely postnatally and in addition, the brain is of sufficient size, even at a young age, to permit reliable dissection and analysis (58). The caudate shows a more or less steady increase in dopamine from about 15% of adult values at 4 days of age to about 50–65% of the adult levels at 45 days. The increase in the biosynthetic enzymes, tyrosine hydroxylase and dopa decarboxylase, is quite similar to that of dopamine. Thus, there is a concurrent development of amines and biosynthetic enzymes in this area. This differs from the sequential development of the enzymes and norepinephrine in the mesencephalon, pons–medulla, and diencephalon (58). The concurrent appearance of enzymes and amines in the caudate may represent the arrival at nerve terminals of enzymes synthesized in the cell bodies and transported by axoplasmic flow to the caudate in a unicellular system (15).

Recently it has been shown that the placement of lesions in the diencephalon of the neonatal rat prevents the postnatal increase of telencephalic catecholamines with development (11). Animals with unilateral lesions placed at 4 days of age have markedly lower levels of norepinephrine (−74%) and dopamine (−84%) in the ipsilateral telencephalon at 6–12 weeks, a time at which catecholamines have reached adult values on the control side. No significant side-to-side differences in either norepinephrine or dopamine were seen in animals with lesions restricted to the medial hypothalamus (Table II). The correlation between anatomical placement of the lesion and the monoamine reduction is identical to that seen in the adult. The fibers involved are presumably the same as those implicated in maintenance of adult levels of catecholamines, i.e., the medial forebrain bundle for norepinephrine and the nigrostriatal projection for dopamine. Nonterminal dopamine-containing axons have been visualized in newborn rats [(42,43,45,55), Tennyson *et al.*, Chapter 9, this volume] and it is likely that lesions in the neonatal rat are at least partially transecting immature monoaminergic fibers. The lesions may also be blocking the ingrowth of neurons into the telencephalon. The placement of lesions in the neonate which prevent catecholamine development in the caudate nucleus makes possible the study of metabolic and behavioral

Table II Effect of Neonatal Unilateral Lesions on Telencephalic Catecholamine Development in the Rat[a]

Lesion Group	*Norepinephrine*[b] *% Change*	*Dopamine*[c] *% Change*
Lateral hypothalamus and medial internal capsule	−74	−84
Medial hypothalamus	−9	+1

[a] The lesions were placed at 4 days of age and the animals killed 6–12 weeks later.
[b] Norepinephrine control side value = 0.23 μg/gm.
[c] Dopamine control side value = 0.99 μg/gm.

phenomena in animals which have matured in the absence of normal levels of dopamine in this structure.

There is little doubt that the nigrostriatal projection is a direct dopaminergic input to the neostriatum and that its destruction results in the loss of dopamine-containing nerve endings in this structure. The functional consequences of the loss of dopaminergic innervation for the postsynaptic cellular elements of the caudate have not yet been elucidated. Neurophysiological studies of the effects of lesions removing the dopaminergic input in the cat and monkey have cast doubt on the concept that there is a simple relation between dopamine and the regulation of caudate neuronal activity [(38), Buchwald *et al.*, Chapter 7, this volume]. We have been studying the possible role of dopamine in the caudate nucleus as a regulator of metabolic events, particularly with respect to carbohydrate metabolism. In many peripheral tissues, both epinephrine and norepinephrine have been shown to influence basic reaction sequences involved in intracellular metabolism such as glycogenolysis. The classic work of Cori and Sutherland has established the enzymatic basis for epinephrine's accelerating effect on glycogenolysis in liver and skeletal muscle. More recently, these neurohumors have also been shown to affect glycogen synthesis (35). Sutherland and his co-workers have developed the hypothesis of the "second messenger" in which many diverse humoral agents produce their effects by activating the enzyme, adenylate cyclase (60). This, in turn, results in an increase in the intracellular 3′,5′-adenosine monophosphate (cyclic AMP) level which acts as a regulator for particular metabolic processes such as glycogenolysis and glycogen synthesis.

The glycogenolytic response to catecholamines is of particular interest since stimulation of parasympathetic and sympathetic nerves to the liver can markedly alter the rates of glycogenolysis and glycogen synthesis through a demonstrated effect on the activities of the enzymes controlling these processes, namely, glycogen synthetase and phosphorylase (61,62). This response to sympathetic stimulation is presumably mediated by norepinephrine released at the neuro-effector junction which in turn activates adenylate cyclase producing increased phosphorylase and glucose-6-phosphatase activity. In accordance with the view that peripheral autonomic nerves can regulate metabolic events in innervated tissues are the findings that sympathectomy or total denervation of the heart results in accumulation of glycogen in this tissue (40,65). Presumably, the loss of norepinephrine from the heart following degeneration of adrenergic neurons slows the rate of glycogen breakdown and stimulates glycogen synthesis in the myocardium until a new and higher steady-state glycogen level is achieved. The loss of norepinephrine would decrease adenylate cyclase activity resulting in lowered intracellular cyclic AMP, which in turn would appropriately change the activities of phosphorylase and glycogen synthetase. This model does not, however, take into account additional metabolic modulators which regulate glycogen metabolism in-

some of the terminals having symmetrical junctions originate from intrinsic neurons of the neostriatum, since they degenerate after lesions of the caudate nucleus and putamen (42,57). Since AChE is present in the striatonigral fibers (69), these boutons may be cholinergic (43). A much smaller percentage of boutons (about 10%) contain some large dense core vesicles (also called large dense core granules in this manuscript) among the clear vesicles. This type of bouton forms asymmetric junctions (43,78). Gulley and Smithberg (43) postulated in their studies of the rat that the latter type of bouton might contain norepinephrine, and that another type of asymmetrical synapse, which has small clear vesicles and some large dense core vesicles, may contain serotonin. Since boutons having elongated vesicles are assumed to be inhibitory, terminals with this type of ending on the axon hillock are presumed to contain the inhibitory transmitter GABA (43). The large 700- to 1200-Å dense core vesicle discussed in the latter two types of boutons in the rat appears to be even more ubiquitous in other species. Rinvik and Grofová (78) reported that all types of synaptic boutons in the substantia nigra of the cat could contain the large dense core vesicle. They are found frequently in the rabbit as well. The attempt by Gulley and Smithberg (43) to correlate morphology with the transmitter is provocative, but it should be pointed out that definitive experiments proving these assumptions have not been accomplished without question as yet.

ADULT NEOSTRIATUM

The fluorescent preterminal axons and boutons of neurons of the substantia nigra, pars compacta, terminate in the neuropil of the neostriatum (Figure 1B). The tiny axons and terminals are numerous and so widely distributed that the neuropil appears diffusely and intensely fluorescent, in contrast to the nonfluorescent fibers of the internal capsule and the neuronal cell bodies of the neostriatum (arrow). The size and shape of neostriatal neurons, as well as the extent of the dendritic arborization and the length of their axons, have been the subject of studies using the Golgi impregnation method (30–32,54,55,58). Over 96% of the cells in the caudate nucleus are medium-sized Golgi type II neurons, about 12 to 18 μm in diameter, and have five or six dendrites which are studded with spines on their branches. These cells are intrinsic to the caudate nucleus; their axons ramify within the limits of the spread of the dendrites of the parent cell and form a dense plexus with the dendrites of neighboring intrinsic cells. Less than 1% of the neurons are large fusiform cells, about 22 to 30 μm in size, and have large straight dendrites with few spines and long axons. Unlike the short axons of the Golgi type II neurons, the long axons of the large neurons become lightly myelinated and probably give rise to the thinly myelinated radial fibers that enter the globus pallidus

(31,59). Collaterals of these fibers may lose their myelin when they reach the "comb system" through which they travel to reach the substantia nigra (31).

Electron microscopic studies have also been done on the adult neostriatum in the cat (1,2,55–57,87), monkey (30–32,75), rat (35,66), mouse (7), and rabbit (83,84). The most common neuron, the medium-sized Golgi type II cell, has a spherical nucleus and a moderate amount of clear cytoplasm with few inclusions and scattered elements of the endoplasmic reticulum that do not form Nissl bodies. Their dendrites have a large number of spines. The pale dendritic cytoplasm contains dilated smooth-surfaced cisternae and poorly developed microtubules. The largest cells have an indented nucleus and a large amount of cytoplasm with many stacks of granular endoplasmic reticulum forming Nissl bodies. The mitochondria of these cells are large and pale with few cristae. The presence of this type of mitochondrion in dendrites having conspicuous microtubules and few spines aids in identifying these dendrites as originating from the large neurons (55).

Most of the synaptic terminals in the neostriatum are small axodendritic spine synapses with round clear vesicles in the axonal bouton and asymmetrical membrane thickenings (Figure 3A, crossed arrow). A much smaller number of the terminals have symmetrical junctional contacts. The axonal bouton in this case may have either rounded vesicles or pleomorphic vesicles. Although many of the isolated synapses may be the terminal boutons of axons, at least some of them are sections through boutons "en passage," i.e., synaptic varicosities occurring along the course of the axon proper (Figures 3A and B). Boutons "en passage" can be demonstrated after silver impregnation (30,54,55) and have previously been seen by electron microscopy (1,2,30,56,57,83,84,87). Unlike axons in most areas of the central nervous system, clear vesicles are frequently found all along their course, particularly in those that form synapses "en passage."

Axons forming synapses "en passage" can originate from the cortex, thalamus, or midbrain, since they are found in various stages of degeneration after lesions of fiber tracts from these respective areas (57). In addition, some synapses "en passage" are present along the axons of neurons intrinsic to the caudate nucleus, since a large number of them remain after a combined cortical and thalamic lesion (54). This conclusion is confirmed by the varicosities "en passage" in Figure 3B which was found in the caudate nucleus after section of all of its afferent connections (87).

Kemp and Powell (57) studied the characteristics of degenerating terminals after lesions in the cortex, thalamus, or midbrain in an attempt to describe the various afferent boutons in the caudate nucleus. A large number of the terminals having clear vesicles and asymmetrical membrane thickenings degenerate after lesions in the cortex or thalamus, up to 40 and 25%, respectively (57). These terminals contain small clear vesicles (30,31,53) and end predominantly on dendritic spines of the Golgi type II neurons (31). Large lesions in the

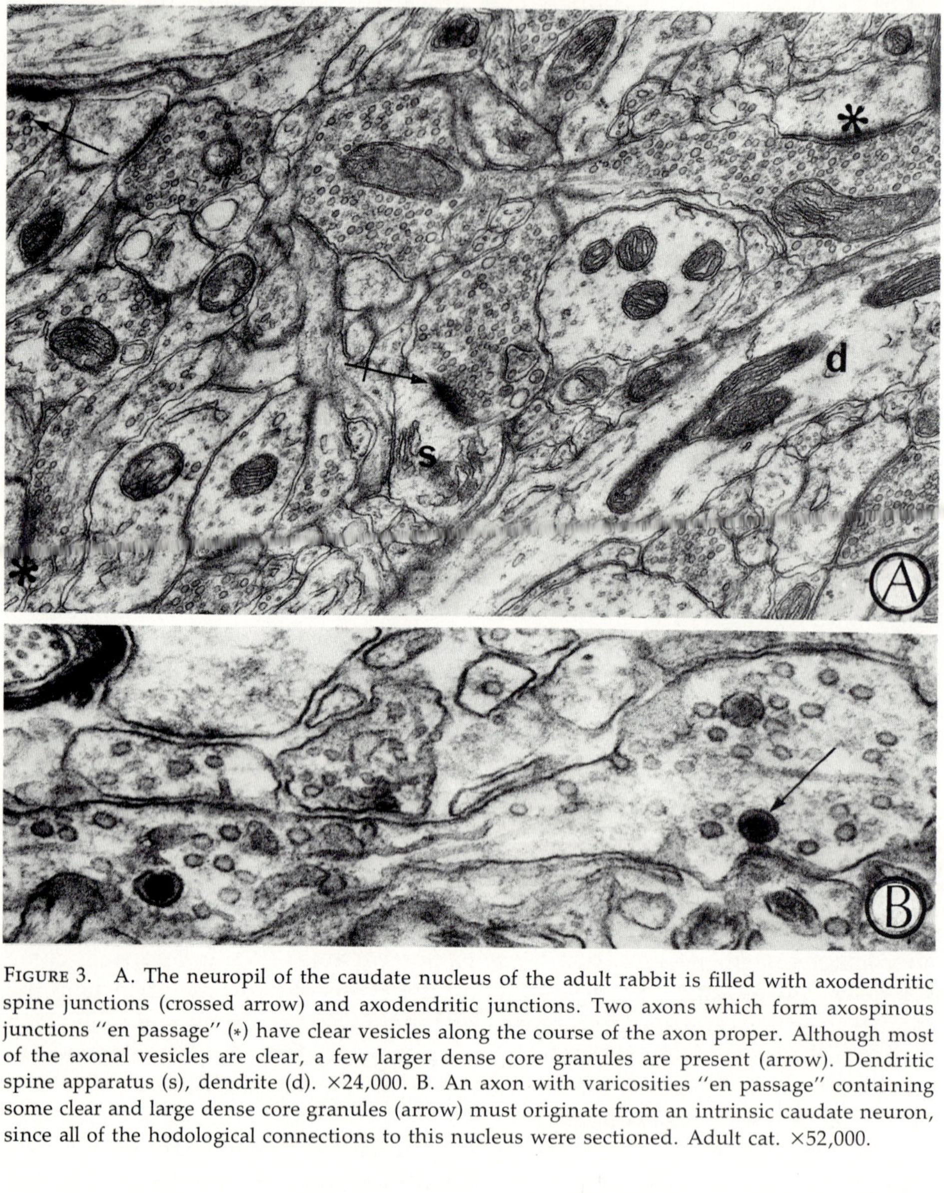

FIGURE 3. A. The neuropil of the caudate nucleus of the adult rabbit is filled with axodendritic spine junctions (crossed arrow) and axodendritic junctions. Two axons which form axospinous junctions "en passage" (*) have clear vesicles along the course of the axon proper. Although most of the axonal vesicles are clear, a few larger dense core granules are present (arrow). Dendritic spine apparatus (s), dendrite (d). ×24,000. B. An axon with varicosities "en passage" containing some clear and large dense core granules (arrow) must originate from an intrinsic caudate neuron, since all of the hodological connections to this nucleus were sectioned. Adult cat. ×52,000.

midbrain produce very sparse, though widespread, degeneration of synaptic terminals in the caudate nucleus (57). The degenerating terminals observed had asymmetrical membrane thickenings. Most were found in contact with dendritic spines.

FETAL DEVELOPMENT

Substantia Nigra, Pars Compacta

As early as day 14 of gestation in the rabbit, the anlage of the substantia nigra, zona compacta, and the area ventralis tegmenti can be recognized in the midventral region of the caudal midbrain (Figure 4A, arrow). There are a few faintly fluorescent cell bodies (Figure 4B, arrow) and processes in the mantle layer. By day 16 of gestation (Figure 4C), the fluorescent cells have become more numerous (Figure 4D); and they extend almost to the pial surface dorsoventrally forming an inverted V-shaped fluorescent zone. They are present throughout the caudal third of the midbrain. This confirms earlier studies using other techniques which show that the midventral proliferation of the midbrain is the site in which the neurons of the substantia nigra (18) and of the area ventralis tegmenti originate (45). Our fluorescent data cannot provide information on the origin of the pars reticulata. Hanaway *et al.* (45) recognized that some nigral neurons might arise from the midline anlage, but they state that the primary site of origin of neurons of the substantia nigra is from the middle third of the basal neuroepithelium. Since we did not see any fluorescent cells in that location, the cells studied by Hanaway *et al.* (45) may have been destined only for the pars reticulata. This suggests a less close embryological relationship between the cells of the pars compacta and pars reticulata of the substantia nigra than between neurons of the pars compacta and the area ventralis tegmenti.

When one compares the ultraviolet photomicrograph of the midventral proliferation of the 16-day gestation rabbit with the same section seen in darkfield using white light to reveal the nuclei and cellular packing in the tissue, one sees that the fluorescent profiles appear immediately ventral to the ependymal zone (Figure 4D, ep). We examined by electron microscopy the region corresponding to the fluorescent inverted V-shaped area in littermate embryos. Elongated spindle-shaped bipolar neuroblasts (Figure 5A) are oriented dorsoventrally immediately beneath the ependymal zone. They are aligned in tandem with the cell body of one adjacent to a trailing process of another as if the preceding cell were directing the course of migration of the following cell. The nuclei of the neuroblasts are elongated and often indented. Numerous ribosomes (r) fill the cytoplasm, but there are only a few channels of granular endoplasmic reticulum (er). The Golgi complex (g) is small and may be located near the nucleus or close to the base of a process. A moderate number of mitochondria (m) are scattered throughout the cell body and its process. The earliest processes (p) consist of perikaryal cytoplasm. More mature processes in the neuropil (n) have developed microtubules and neurofilaments. Neuroblasts closer to the pial surface appear more mature than the spindle-shaped

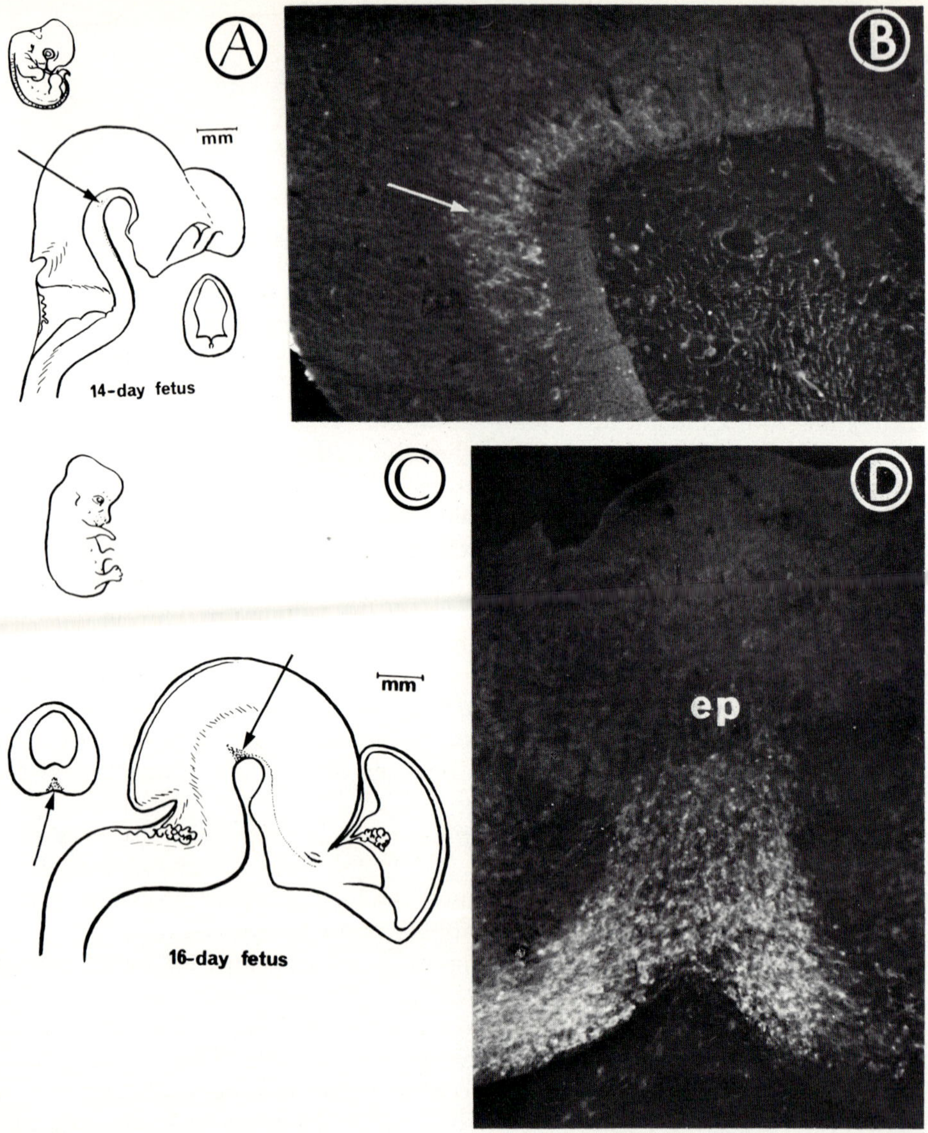

FIGURE 4. A. A diagram of a transverse section of the midbrain, a parasagittal section of the brain, and of the stage of development of a 14-day fetus. The arrow points to the location of the cells in Figure 4B. Reproduced by permission of *J. Comp. Neurol.*, 1973, **149:** 233. B. A fluorescence micrograph showing some fluorescent cells (arrow) and processes in the mantle layer of the basal plate of the caudal mesencephalon of a 14-day fetus. See Figure 4A for orientation. ×152. C. A diagram of a transverse section of the midbrain, an oblique parasagittal section of the brain, and of the stage of development of a 16-day fetus. The arrows indicate the location of the fluorescent zones in Figure 4D. The dotted line indicates the course of the fluorescent axons in Figure 6A. Reproduced by permission of *J. Comp. Neurol.*, 1973, **149:** 233. D. A fluorescent inverted V-shaped zone is apparent immediately ventral to the stratified ependymal zone (ep). Most of the fluorescence appears as dots or linear processes, but occasionally fluorescent perikarya can be recognized. See Figure 4C transverse section, arrow, for orientation. 16-day fetus. ×155. Reproduced by permission of *J. Comp. Neurol.*, 1973, **149:** 233.

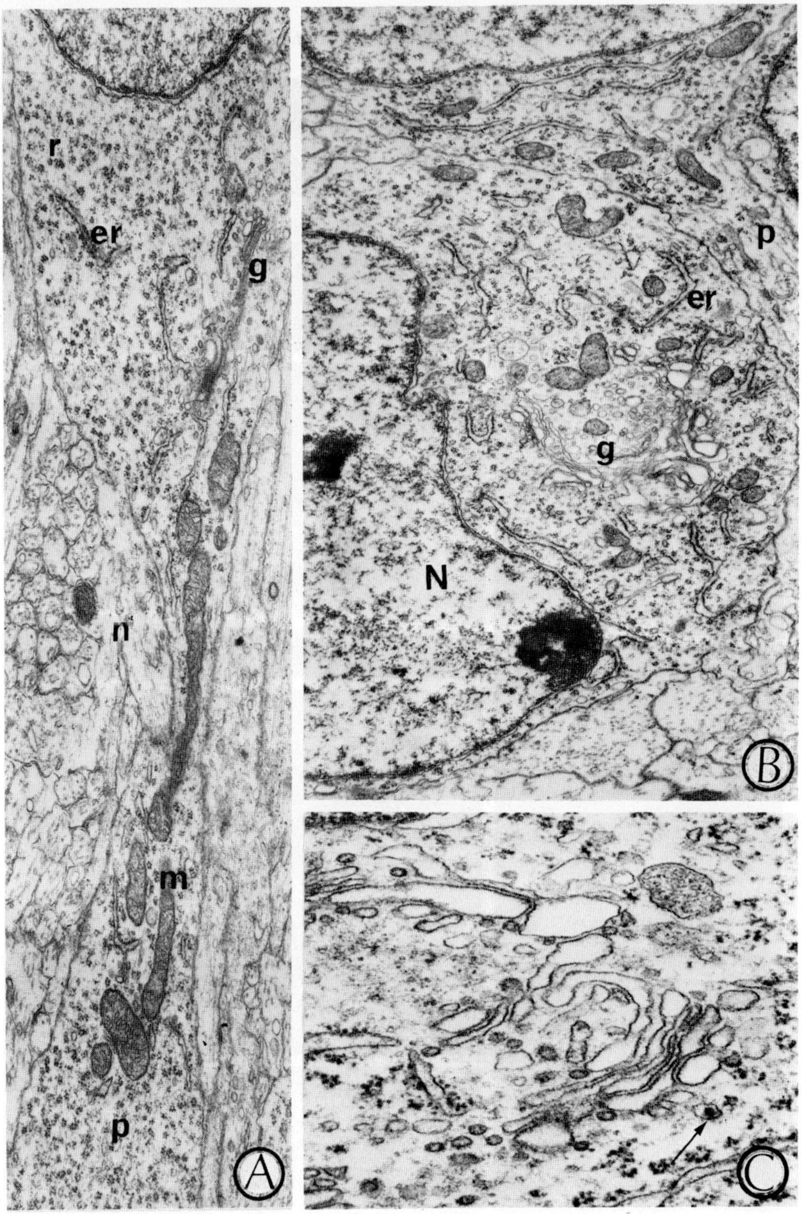

FIGURE 5. A. A bipolar neuroblast courses ventrally from the ependymal zone. Scattered mitochondria (m), polyribosomes (r), and a few cisternae of granular endoplasmic reticulum (er) fill the cytoplasm and immature process (p) of the neuroblast. A Golgi complex (g) is present in the cytoplasm. The other processes in the neuropil (n), which are more mature, have microtubules and a few neurofilaments. 16-Day fetus. ×13,600. B. The globular neuroblasts in the ventral mantle layer are directly adjacent to one another. Their nuclei (N) are eccentric and indented toward the cell center which contains the Golgi complex (g). There is more granular endoplasmic reticulum (er) than previously. The process (p) contains neurofilaments and microtubules. 16-Day fetus. ×13,600. C. A vesicle containing a dense core (arrow) is present close to the Golgi complex. 16-Day fetus. ×14,800.

axons, since they have not yet established their ultimate connections. Is it possible that dopamine acts as a chemotactic agent serving to establish communication with distally placed cells? For instance, dopamine might be released into the neuropil, where it can signal the dopamine-sensitive neuroblasts in the neostriatum to respond with the release of an appropriate substance. The latter substance, in turn, might form a diffusion gradient to attract the dopaminergic axons. The release of dopamine from these relatively undifferentiated neuroblasts, therefore, may serve as an important link in a feedback mechanism which directs the catecholaminergic axons to their target in the neostriatum.

The fluorescent anlage extends rostrally to include the upper midbrain by days 17 and 18 of gestation. By this time, the fluorescent cells have migrated laterally from the midline (Figure 6B, *) and their cell bodies are more discrete (arrow). Their fluorescent axons (Figure 6C, arrow) run parallel to the pial surface in the midbrain and course through the hypothalamus to enter the putamen at day 18 of gestation (Figures 6D and E, arrows). The neuroblasts continue to migrate laterally and by day 20 of gestation the mature topography is established, i.e., a fluorescent area ventralis tegmenti (Figure 7A, *) lies medial to the substantia nigra, which consists of a thin semicircular pars compacta (arrow) dorsal to a nonfluorescent pars reticulata (r). Fluorescent axons from the midbrain can be traced to the tuberculum olfactorium, putamen, nucleus accumbens, and septum, but the caudate nucleus still lacks fluorescence at this time.

A second wave of migration of neuroblasts takes place in the substantia nigra at day 23 of gestation (Figure 7B). The cells seem to be concentrated in a fluorescent wedge-shaped zone (inset, arrow) in the rostral portion of the midbrain. Medially only wispy fluorescent profiles (crossed arrow) indicate the site of these cells which appear as immature as those at earlier stages of development in the caudal region of the midbrain (Figure 4D). Those cells close to the junction with the zona reticulata (Figure 7B, r), however, are more mature (arrow). A thin rim of fluorescent cytoplasm surrounds the nucleus (Figure 7C, arrow) and short processes can be distinguished. By day 27 of gestation, the pars compacta is a fairly compact semicircular zone of fluorescent neurons (Figure 7D, arrow) dorsal to the zona reticulata (r). They have a greater volume of cytoplasm than previously and are more mature. The neurons of the substantia nigra, pars compacta, appear to reach their final development in the early postnatal period. By the ninth postnatal day (Figure 7E), the fluorescent neurons are as large and as fluorescent as in the adult (compare Figure 7E with Figure 1A). The perikarya of neonatal nigral neurons (Figure 7E, arrow) are ovoid or angular, and elongated fluorescent processes can frequently be seen. The nucleus may be either centrally located or eccentric.

Electron microscopic examination of the cells of the substantia nigra from days 18 to 20 of gestation shows that many of them have matured into mul-

tipolar neurons. The cell bodies
dendritic processes, some of w
organelles have increased greatly
tions of granular endoplasmic r
have more randomly disposed
filopodia of growth cones contai
numerous in the neuropil. The
microfilaments, which may be
(10,96). It is uncertain whether
dendritic, since both types cont
until they become more mature (
are present in the neuropil, bu
have also been seen, but they
synapses (88). Many of the term
somewhat bulbous, have few ve
rial seen in the growth cone. Al
we seem to find asymmetrical j
frequently than symmetrical junc
clear vesicles in the axonal bout
shape may be spherical, ovoid,
are found (crossed arrow).

The neurons at day 25 of ge
viously, and they usually exhi
complex (g) is well developed
number consistent with the inc
more numerous, but they are sp
still immature in appearance, wh
of the types of synaptic terminals
stage.

Examination of the neurons o
period by phase microscopy rev
phology, as compared to adult n
more obvious in adult neurons

seen in the neuron. 20-Day fetus. ×20,00
149: 233. B. Two axonal boutons, contain
ture dendrite. One junction is cut obliqu
dense core granule (crossed arrow) is pr
agranular reticulum, and a filamentous m
of *J. Comp. Neurol.*, 1973, **149:** 233. C. A
nucleus (N), clumps of endoplasmic re
tochondria, and dense bodies. Two axon
basal portion of a process (arrow) as it
developed at time, axonal processes (ax)
25-Day fetus. ×16,200.

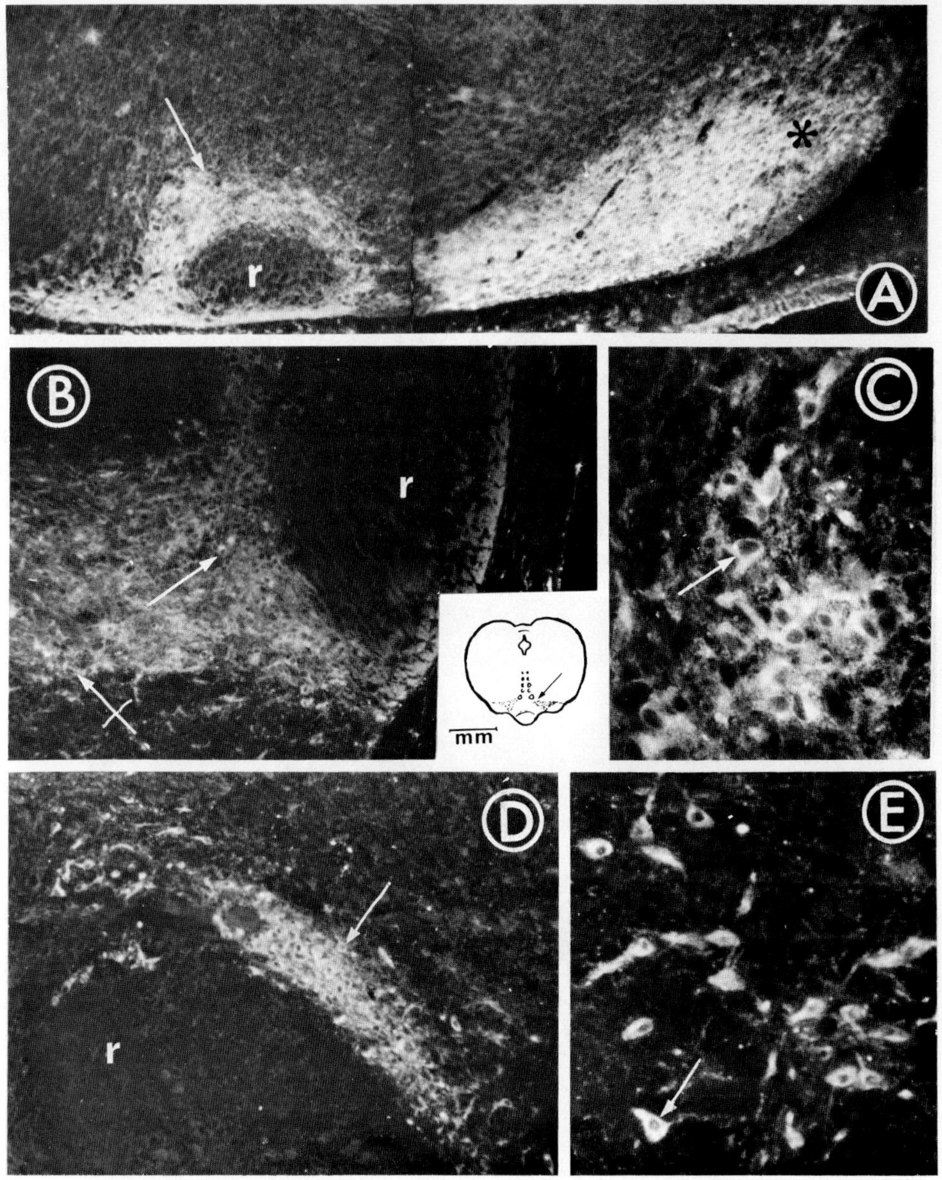

FIGURE 7. A. The fluorescent area ventralis tegmenti (*) is separated laterally from the substantia nigra, which now has a fluorescent pars compacta (arrow) distinct from the nonfluorescent pars reticulata (r). 20-Day fetus. Montage. ×125. B. A wedge-shaped zone of fluorescent neurons is present in the rostral midbrain at day 23 of gestation. The outlines of cell bodies (arrow) close to the zona reticulata (r) are easier to distinguish than those located more medially (crossed arrow). ×125. (Inset) A diagram of the location of the wedge-shaped zone of migrating cells (arrow). C. The fluorescent cell bodies and proximal processes (arrow) of the more developed cells adjacent to the zona reticulata. 23-Day fetus. ×300. D. The pars compacta forms a semicircular zone of relatively mature fluorescent cells (arrow) dorsal to the zona reticulata (r) at day 27 of gestation. ×125. E. A large number of the fluorescent neurons of the pars compacta (arrow) in the 9-day postnatal rabbit appear to be as large and as mature as those of the adult. ×325.

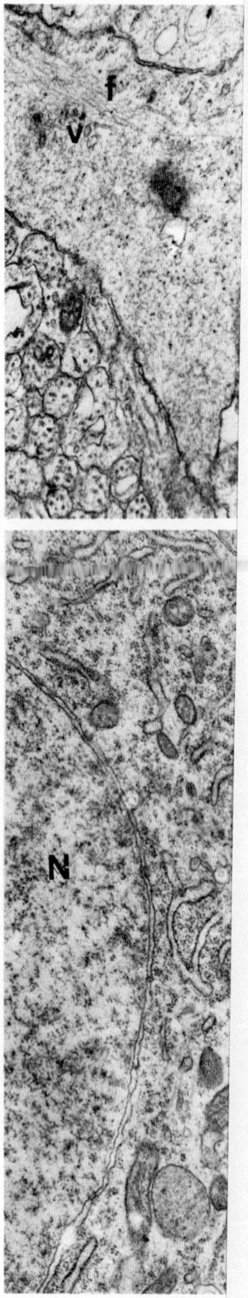

FIGURE 8. A. An electron mic
ments (f), microtubules, and sca
portion of a perikaryon (N). Mit

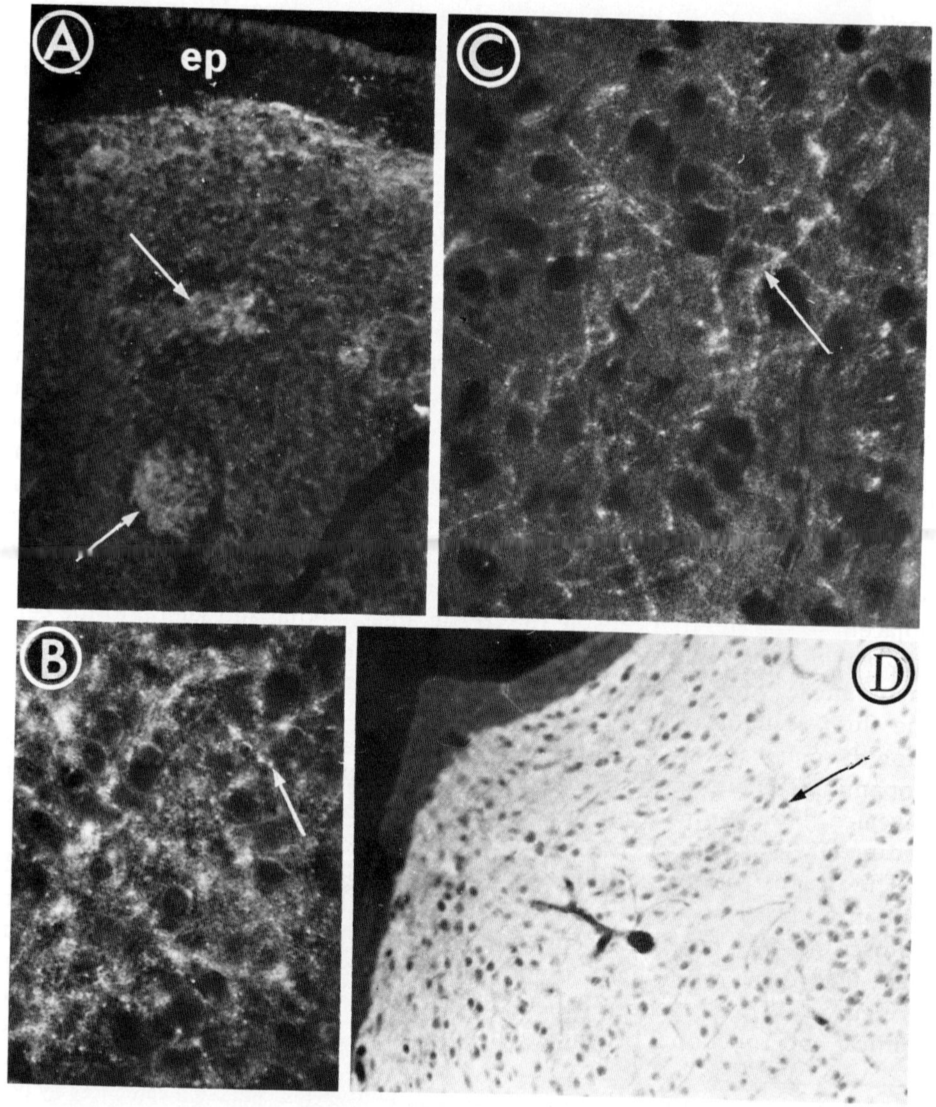

FIGURE 11. A. Scattered punctate fluorescence fills the neuropil of the caudate nucleus below the subependymal zone (ep) at the tenth postnatal day. Fluorescent islands in the caudate nucleus show fine punctate and linear fluorescence surrounded by a nonfluorescent zone (arrows). ×145. B. Small discrete fluorescent dots (arrow) are evident. Irregular twiglike profiles of a lower intensity fluorescence are numerous. Caudate nucleus, postnatal day 9. ×420. C. Punctate dots and extremely thin linear fluorescence (arrow) are present in the putamen at the ninth postnatal day. ×365. D. The neuropil of the caudate nucleus beneath the narrow nonfluorescent subependymal zone appears intensely and homogeneously fluorescent at the twenty-fifth postnatal day. The cell bodies (arrow) are rather closely packed. ×145.

with the usual histological preparations, nor by histofluorescence in the mature stage, when the entire neuropil has become filled with fluorescent axons. The circumscribed islands, which appear to be a cluster of neurons enclosing a core of dopamine-containing axons, create a glomerular-like pattern in which a localized axonal input could effect a synchronous modulation on the dendrites of the cluster of neurons. We have not identified these islands by electron microscopy as yet, but we hope to do so, since they may be of interest to neurophysiologists.

The remainder of the neuropil of the caudate nucleus is filled with tiny fluorescent varicosities (Figure 11B, arrow), which are particularly numerous beneath the subependymal region (Figure 11A). Fluorescent varicosities are present in the putamen, as well, and their presence along the course of axons (Figure 11C, arrow) is additional evidence that these dopamine-containing axons form synapses "en passage." Thereafter, there is a rapid ingrowth of dopamine-containing terminals and from days 16 to 25 of postnatal life the entire neostriatum becomes diffusely and intensely fluorescent (Figure 11D). It would be difficult to recognize this specimen from one of an adult animal. The majority of the synapses in the neuropil appear mature ultrastructurally, except for the fact that the nonfluorescent cell bodies are closer together in the 25-day-old rabbit.

Biochemical Studies

The endogenous levels of dopamine present in the caudate nucleus and putamen (Figure 12) were correlated with the fluorescence microscopic studies. Dopamine was assayed by the method of Anton and Sayre (6). As expected, endogenous dopamine concentrations are very low in the early fetal period (days 20 to 22) and increase gradually during the prenatal and early postnatal period. By the twenty-fifth postnatal day, however, when the caudate nucleus appears to be as fluorescent as that of the adult when examined microscopically, the endogenous dopamine concentrations are only about half that found in the adult. This phenomenon of a concentration-dependent quenching has been studied by Jonsson (52), who showed that above a certain level the eye cannot appreciate a further rise in fluorescence intensity. Our biochemical studies indicate that the neostriatum of the rabbit does not reach adult levels even by the forty-fifth postnatal day, although the neuropil is intensely fluorescent.

Studies have also been done on the relative uptake and accumulation of ^{3}H-dopamine by fresh tissue slices of the neostriatum in an effort to assess the degree of maturity of the dopamine-containing axons at each stage of development (Figure 13). The uptake of ^{3}H-dopamine was measured by a modification of the method of Shaskan and Snyder (80). The accumulation of ^{3}H-dopamine from days 19 to 28 of gestation rises to a value of 20 (tissue-to-medium ratio),

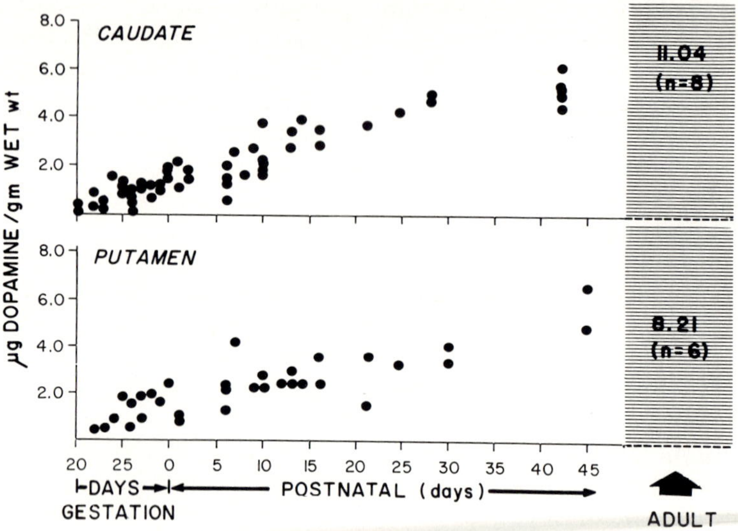

FIGURE 12. Endogenous dopamine levels in the rabbit caudate nucleus and putamen. Reproduced by permission of *Brain Res.*, 1972, **46:** 251.

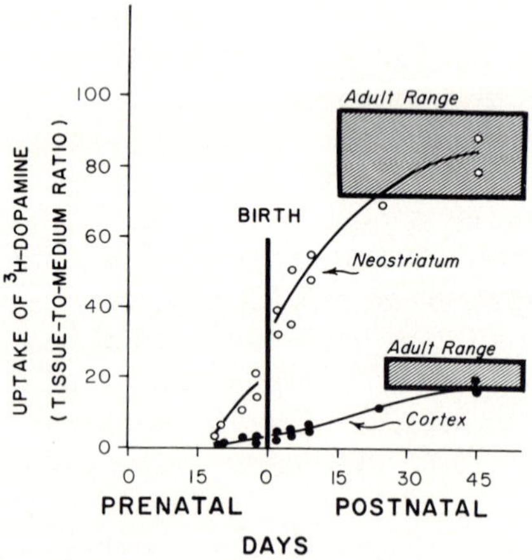

FIGURE 13. The uptake of ^{3}H-dopamine into tissue slices of rabbit neostriatum. The data are expressed as the ^{3}H-dopamine (disintegrations/minute, dpm) per gram of tissue divided by the ^{3}H-dopamine (dpm) per ml of medium (tissue to medium ratio, T/M) after 15 min at 37°C. A T/M greater than 1.0 is generally considered to reflect an active uptake process. Reproduced by permission of *Brain Res.* 1972, **46:** 251.

then there is a rapid increase shortly after birth. By the twenty-fifth postnatal day, the uptake and accumulation of dopamine in the neostriatum approach that found in the adult. As mentioned, this is long before endogenous dopamine levels approach maximum values. The uptake of ^{3}H-dopamine, therefore, achieves adult values much earlier than the endogenous dopamine content. The development of the uptake mechanism in the neostriatum correlates well with the morphological signs of synaptic terminal maturation by electron microscopy.

STORAGE SITES OF DOPAMINE

Neuronal Cell Body

It is well established by fluorescence microscopy that dopamine is present in neuronal perikarya of the substantia nigra compacta, but the localization of the amine at the ultrastructural level is a controversial issue. Van Orden *et al.* (93) have discussed the evidence that norepinephrine in the peripheral sympathetic nervous system is correlated with small dense core vesicles, which were first described by Richardson (77) and Grillo and Palay (41). Similar catecholamine storage vesicles have been sought in the substantia nigra. Lenn (61) failed to find a significant number of granular or agranular vesicles in catecholamine neurons to explain the hypothesis of a perikaryal vesicular pool of monoamines. Fuxe *et al.* (36) concluded that a vesicular pool of monoamines exists, but that it is represented by agranular vesicles found in the perinuclear area of the neuron near the Golgi complex. Bak (7), on the other hand, assumed that dopamine was present in large dense core granules in the perikarya and in axonal boutons, because he found a decrease in these granules after treatment of mice with reserpine, which depletes catecholamines and indolamines. It should be pointed out that it is a formidable task to document such a decrease in granules without question by electron microscopy, because the granules are relatively sparse in the cell bodies, even in untreated animals. Gulley and Wood (44), moreover, noted that there are fewer dense core vesicles in the perikarya of the zona compacta (the fluorescent neurons) than in the cell bodies of the zona reticulata (mostly nonfluorescent neurons). Grofová and Rinvik (42) attempted a systematic quantitative analysis of the effects of reserpine treatment on the axonal boutons in the neuropil of the substantia nigra reticulata. The clear and dense core vesicles were counted in 100 boutons from 16 cats. They reported a significant reduction of dense core vesicles compared to normal animals from 5 to 49 hours after reserpine treatment, with a minimum at 24 hours. As discussed later, it is possible that the dense cores depleted in their study are the storage sites of serotonin.

Electron microscopic autoradiographic studies after the intraventricular injection of catecholamines have been done in an attempt to elucidate the problem. Silver grains due to uptake of tritiated norepinephrine were ubiquitously distributed throughout the neuronal perikarya and dendrites in the substantia nigra (24,72,81). Descarries and Droz (24) suggested that exogenous catecholamines are bound to a macromolecular complex in the perikarya rather than to preformed synaptic-like vesicles. Sotelo (81) supported this hypothesis and showed that the large dense core vesicles in nigral neurons have a high acid phosphatase activity, and thus, those near the Golgi complex are related to primary lysosomes, not to storage sites of monoamines. The axonal boutons in the neuropil of the substantia nigra seem to have less affinity for exogenous catecholamines than the neuronal perikarya. In two studies, in which ^{3}H-norepinephrine was used, there was no concentration of label over axonal boutons (24,81), but in another investigation, some ^{3}H-dopamine- and ^{3}H-norepinephrine-labeled nerve terminals were observed in axodendritic synapses (72). More conspicuous, however, was the labeling of axodendritic terminals in the substantia nigra after injections of radioactive serotonin and its precursors (72). Silver grains were found over boutons containing clear vesicles and large dense core vesicles. It is possible that the large dense core granules in axonal boutons that were depleted by reserpine (7,42) may be storage sites of serotonin rather than dopamine. This would be in accord with fluorescence microscopic findings (33) that the zona compacta of the substantia nigra has a very sparse population of catecholamine terminals, but there is a mass of densely packed, very fine serotonin terminals in the zona reticulata.

Axons in the Neostriatum

The neuropil of the neostriatum contains a wide variety of terminals from various sources. Although attempts have been made to identify the dopamine-containing axons, their characteristics have not been fully demonstrated with certainty by electron microscopy as yet. Our fluorescence microscopy studies of the developing neostriatum lead us to conclude that the mature dopamine-containing axon is thin and has small varicosities which form synapses "en passage." After a lesion in the midbrain, Kemp and Powell (57) illustrated degenerating axons forming synapses "en passage," but this type of terminal originates in other parts of the brain as well. All of the junctional contacts of degenerating extrinsic terminals in the caudate nucleus which they observed were asymmetrical. In an autoradiographic study, Hattori *et al.* (46) presented other evidence suggesting that nigrostriatal terminals in the neostriatum end predominantly in asymmetrical synapses. Several days after the stereotaxic injection of ^{3}H-leucine into the zona compacta of the substantia nigra of the rat, 75% of the silver grains in the neostriatum were located over synapses with moderately pleomorphic vesicles and asymmetrical junctions, whereas only

25% were over terminals with highly pleomorphic vesicles and symmetrical junctions. Since intraventricular injection of 6-hydroxydopamine caused degeneration of only the former type of nerve ending, it was assumed that dopaminergic nigrostriatal boutons in the neostriatum contain moderately pleomorphic vesicles and make asymmetrical synaptic contacts (46).

The ultrastructural localization in the neostriatum of the various putative neurotransmitters, dopamine, acetylcholine, γ-aminobutyric acid, serotonin, and norepinephrine, has not been established. Biochemical studies have indicated that at least a portion of the dopamine may be stored in vesicles (94). Although some investigators have suggested that the large dense core granules may be dopamine storage sites (7,66), others (1,2,9,30,35,55,83,84) have pointed out that the clear vesicles are by far the most abundant type of vesicle in the neostriatum. The large dense core vesicles, moreover, can be found in postsynaptic dendrites (83), which are not thought to contain dopamine. The dense core vesicles remain in axons in the neuropil (Figure 3B) after all of the hodological connections to the caudate nucleus, including nigrostriatal fibers, have been sectioned and dopamine fluorescence is absent (87). Further evidence which suggests that dopamine may be present in some clear vesicles is the finding that silver grains due to intraventricular injections of labeled norepinephrine are localized over nerve endings containing primarily the agranular type of vesicle (3).

Uptake Studies in Tissue Slices

The incubation of fresh tissue in the presence of "false transmitters," such as α-methylnorepinephrine, 5-hydroxydopamine (5-OH-DA), 6-OH-DA, and 6,7-dihydroxytetrahydroisoquinoline (6,7-diOHTIQ), forms dense cores in vesicles of catecholaminergic boutons of the peripheral nervous system (48,85,90) and central nervous system (48,76). Since 6-OH-DA results in destruction of terminals after a period of time (91), the incubation period with this substance should be kept as short as possible. 6,7-diOHTIQ, which is a condensation product of dopamine with methyl or ethyl aldehyde, may be relevant to the biological effects of alcohol ingestion (16,17,85). The technique of incubating fresh tissue in the presence of false transmitters has also been employed to give additional data concerning the morphological characteristics of the dopamine-containing axons in the neostriatum (48,50,84). Although there is considerable damage to most of the brain tissue, the axonal boutons are relatively well preserved. After incubation, some boutons can be visualized owing to the uptake and storage of the exogenous transmitter by small vesicles. There is formation of a dense precipitate in the vesicles due to the reaction of $NaMnO_4$ (the fixative) with the transmitter (49). This is a convenient method to "tag" the vesicles for electron microscopy. The amount of reaction product in the vesicles, therefore, is dependent not only on the ability of the vesicles to store

dures. We suggest that the low K_m PDE activity can be correlated, in part, with monoamine content. However, the heterogeneity of possible neurotransmitters acting at cortical synapses makes exceedingly difficult the correlation of PDE activity with postsynaptic sites belonging to any single group of axonal endings.

Perhaps a better model to test this hypothesis can be found in the caudate nucleus. There, projections from the substantia nigra and adjacent midbrain on to dendritic spines and dendrites represent the sole source of dopamine. Manipulation of this system during its development which results in a significant alteration in the striatal levels of cyclic AMP and related enzymes should provide strong evidence for the existence of the "dopamine receptor." For the neuroanatomist, cytochemical localization of phosphodiesterase and, better still, of adenylate cyclase will then afford a ready means of seeing these receptors within the neostriatum.

REFERENCES

1. Adinolfi, A. M. The organization of synaptic junctions in cat putamen. *Brain Res.*, 1971, **32:** 53–67.
2. Adinolfi, A. M., and Pappas, G. D. The fine structure of caudate nucleus of the cat. *J. Comp. Neurol.*, 1968, **133:** 167–184.
3. Adinolfi, A. M., and Schmidt, S. Y. Cytochemical localization of cyclic nucleotide phosphodiesterase activity at developing synapses. *Brain Res.*, 1974, **76:** 21–31.
4. Andén, N. E., Carlsson, A., Dahlström, A., Fuxe, K., Hillarp, N.-Å., and Larsson, K. Demonstration and mapping out of nigro-neostriatal dopamine neurons. *Life Sci.*, 1964, **3:** 523–530.
5. Andén, N. E., Dahlström, A., Fuxe, K., Larsson, K., Olson, L., and Ungerstedt, U. Ascending monoamine neurons to the telencephalon and diencephalon. *Acta Physiol. Scand.*, 1966, **67:** 313–326.
6. Appleman, M. M., Thompson, W. J., and Russell, T. R. Cyclic nucleotide phosphodiesterases. In *Advances in Cyclic Nucleotide Research*. Vol. 3. (P. Greengard and G. A. Robison, Eds.). Raven, New York, 1973: 65–98.
7. Breckenridge, B., and Johnston, R. E. Cyclic 3′,5′-nucleotide phosphodiesterase in brain. *J. Histochem. Cytochem.*, 1969, **17:** 505–511.
8. Brown, J. H., and Makman, M. H. Stimulation by dopamine of adenylate cyclase in retinal homogenates and of adenosine-3′,5′-cyclic monophosphate formation in intact retina. *Proc. Natl. Acad. Sci. USA*, 1972, **69:** 539–543.
9. Connor, J. D. The nigro-neostriatal pathway: The effects produced by iontophoretic dopamine. *Res. Publ. Assoc. Res. Nerv. Ment. Dis.*, 1972, **50:** 193–206.
10. De Robertis, E., Arnaiz, G. R., and Alberici, M. Subcellular distribution of adenyl cyclase and cyclic phosphodiesterase in rat brain cortex. *J. Biol. Chem.*, 1967, **242:** 3487–3493.
11. Florendo, N. T., Barrnett, R. J., and Greengard, P. Cyclic 3′,5′-nucleotide phosphodiesterase: Cytochemical localization in cerebral cortex. *Science*, 1971, **173:** 745–747.
12. Gaballah, S., and Popoff, C. Cyclic 3′,5′-nucleotide phosphodiesterase in nerve endings of developing rat brain. *Brain Res.*, 1971, **25:** 220–222.
13. Greengard, P., McAfee, D. A., and Kebabian, J. W. On the mechanism of action of cyclic AMP and its role in synaptic transmission. In *Advances in Cyclic Nucleotide Research*. Vol. 1. (P. Greengard and G. A. Robison, Eds.). Raven, New York, 1972: 337–355.

14. Hökfelt, T. G. M. *In vitro* studies on central and peripheral monoamine neurons at the ultrastructural level. *Z. Zellforsch. Mikrosk. Anat.* 1968, **91:** 1–74.
15. Hornykiewicz, O. Dopamine and extrapyramidal motor function and dysfunction. *Res. Publ. Assoc. Res. Nerv. Ment. Dis.*, 1972, **50:** 390–415.
16. Hull, C. D., Bernardi, G., and Buchwald, N. A. Intracellular responses of caudate neurons to brain stem stimulation. *Brain Res.*, 1970, **22:** 163–179.
17. Kebabian, J. W., and Greengard, P. Dopamine-sensitive adenyl cyclase: Possible role in synaptic transmission. *Science*, 1971, **174:** 1346–1349.
18. Kebabian, J. W., Petzold, G. L., and Greengard, P. Dopamine-sensitive adenylate cyclase in caudate nucleus of rat brain, and its similarity to the "dopamine receptor." *Proc. Natl. Acad. Sci. USA*, 1972, **69:** 2145–2149.
19. Kemp. J., and Powell, T. P. S. The structure of the caudate nucleus of the cat: Light and electron microscopy. *Philos. Trans. R. Soc. Lond.* [*Biol. Sci.*], 1971, **262:** 383–401.
20. Kemp, J., and Powell, T. P. S. The synaptic organization of the caudate nucleus. *Philos. Trans. R. Soc. Lond.* [*Biol. Sci.*], 1971, **262:** 403–412.
21. Kemp, J., and Powell, T. P. S. The site of termination of afferent fibres in the caudate nucleus. *Philos. Trans. R. Soc. Lond.* [*Biol. Sci.*], 1971, **262:** 413–427.
22. Rall, T. W., and Gilman, A. G. The role of cyclic AMP in the nervous system. *Neurosci. Res. Program, Bull.*, 1970, **8:** 221–323.
23. Tennyson, V. M., Barrett, R. E., Cohen, G., Cote, L. J., Heikkila, R., and Mytilineou, C. The developing neostriatum of the rabbit: Correlation of fluorescence histochemistry, electron microscopy, endogenous dopamine levels and (3H) dopamine uptake. *Brain Res.*, 1972, **46:** 251–285.
24. Tennyson, V. M., and Marco, L. A. Intrinsic connections of caudate neurons. II. Fluorescence and electron microscopy following chronic isolation. *Brain Res.*, 1973, **53:** 307–317.
25. Thompson, W. J., and Appleman, W. J. Multiple cyclic nucleotide phosphodiesterase activities from rat brain. *Biochemistry*, 1971, **10:** 311–316.

10

Effects of Caudate Nuclei Removal in Cats. Comparison with Effects of Frontal Cortex Ablation

JAIME R. VILLABLANCA and ROBERT J. MARCUS
Mental Retardation Research Center and Department of Psychiatry, University of California Los Angeles, Los Angeles, California

INTRODUCTION

There are several important conditions which should be met in any experimental study of the neurological and gross behavioral effects of caudate nuclei ablation: First, most of the caudate tissue must be removed. Second, damage to adjacent structures, particularly the dorsolateral frontal cortex, should be kept to a minimum. Finally, the ablation should be done in one surgical stage. The main reasons for meeting these criteria are respectively: (a) there are indications that the caudate tissue may have a large functional compensatory capability (2,51,74); (b) it has been repeatedly suggested that the frontal cortex may have some functions in common with the caudate nuclei (5,16,23); and (c) it has been shown that multistaged lesions of a given brain area may induce processes masking the effects which are seen following a one-stage, total lesion (1,19,62). Furthermore, the animals should be maintained in good health for a long enough period in order to be sure that any transitory effects which usually follow extensive brain surgery (1,27,75) have been attenuated or are no longer present. Finally, an adequate histological report of the lesions should be provided.

Since it appears that the above conditions have been only partially fulfilled in the caudate ablation studies performed to date in adult animals—which we know of (2,15,21,24,32,33,37,42,51,53,56,61,72–74)—we think that the full potential of the lesion method has not been used in studying the functions of the caudate nuclei. The present experiments are an attempt toward achieving this goal.

A method is described for performing a virtually complete, one-stage removal of the caudate nuclei (avoiding dorsolateral cortical damage) and for maintaining the animals in good health indefinitely. Three other experimental groups were studied concomitantly. Cats with unilateral removal of the caudate nucleus were studied for the purpose of disclosing any marked lateralized neurological function and for assessing the magnitude of the functional compensation by caudate tissue. Animals with bilateral ablation of the frontal cortical areas were studied so as to evaluate any frontal cortical contribution to the effects of the caudatal removal since many reports on similar ablations (28,40,47,70,85) either vaguely indicate that the caudate nuclei might also have been damaged or altogether fail to clarify this important point. Finally, a group of sham-operated cats was studied.

The neurological, gross behavioral, and EEG-polygraphic effects of these lesions are presented here and discussed comparatively. Several other studies of similar experimental adult cats or kittens have been or are being performed either in our own laboratory (48,49,77,79–81) or in collaboration with other laboratories of the UCLA Mental Retardation Center (44,57). It is expected that a coherent picture will emerge of the basic defect(s) resulting from the absence of whatever the caudate nuclei contribute to central nervous function.

METHODS

The experiments were performed in 37 adult male (unless otherwise stated) cats: twelve (two females) with bilateral removal of the caudate nuclei (BAc), eleven (one female) with unilateral removal of the caudate nucleus (UAc), ten (two females) with bilateral removal of the frontal cortical areas (BFr), and four sham-operated (ShO) cats.

Surgical Procedures

All surgery was performed under rigid aseptic technique using pentobarbital anesthesia with moderate hypothermia. The steps to ablate the caudate nucleus were as follows: The bone of the midline of the calvarium was removed (an area of about 40 mm anterior–posteriorly and about 13 mm on each side of the midsagittal plane) sparing the sagittal sinus. The dura was opened bilaterally. The sagittal sinus was ligated and cut just in front of the coronal suture; the underlying falx was cut at this level and the two ends were gently displaced away from the section. A spatula was stereotaxically positioned between the hemispheres and was used both to indicate the anterior margin of the underlying head of the caudate nucleus and to retract gently the hemisphere. Under visual control and using a thin glass pipette for aspiration, a small opening was made in the gyrus cinguli (area 24) just below the midline prolongation of the cruciate sulcus (Figure 1). The corpus callosum was penetrated at this site thereby gaining access to the lateral ventricle and exposing the dorsomedial aspects of the caudate. At this point, the softer consistency of the caudate tissue enabled the suction strength to be reduced to a level which was sufficient to aspirate the caudate without affecting neighboring fiber structures, particularly the internal capsule. A similar procedure was repeated on the contralateral side for bilateral ablation. In the ShO cats, all the above procedures were performed except for the actual aspiration of the caudate tissue.

For ablation of the frontal cortical areas, a more anterior bone flap was removed and most of the brain tissue in front of the head of the caudate nuclei—indicated by a needle stereotaxically positioned at A 22 on top of the brain—was removed by aspiration (Figure 5). In all animals, the cranial bone defect was covered with cranioplastic material.

In 30 cats (11 BAc, nine UAc, six BFr, and four ShO) recording electrodes were implanted during the same surgical session as follows: bilateral epidural screws (uni- or bipolar) in frontal, parietal, and occipital cortical areas; tripolar electrodes (twisted, 0.01-in. stainless-steel wires, insulated except for the tips), unilaterally in the ventral hippocampus (A 7.5, L 10.4, H-5.0,) and pontine re-

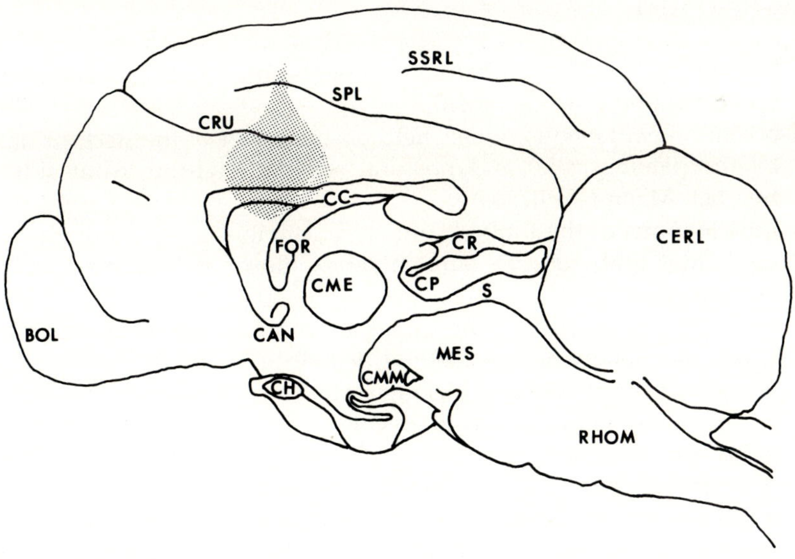

FIGURE 1. Schematic view of the medial surface of the cat brain showing the extent of the penetration lesion (stippled area) in order to expose the caudate nucleus.

ticular formation (P 5, L 2.0, H-6.0). The stereotaxic coordinates of Snider and Niemer (69) were used for all placements. In addition, bipolar silver wires were implanted in the nuchal muscles for EMG recording and a unipolar screw lead was affixed in the roof of each orbit for monitoring eye movements. Finally, one screw was affixed in the midline of the frontal bone and another in the bone overlying the cerebellum as reference and ground leads, respectively. The electrodes were affixed to the top of the cranioplastic bone cover with an amphenol strip connector and dental cement.

Postoperative Care

All cats were closely monitored during the acute postoperative period. The BAc cats were kept for 1 to 4 days in special cages (75) in order to monitor and control the rectal temperature and to collect urine (to assess the hydration state). Tube feeding was instituted when an animal was aphagic for more than 1 day; this was supplemented with parenteral fluids depending on the state of hydration.

Testing and Recording Procedures

Neurological Testing

A battery of neurological tests was applied periodically to all cats; the main items assessed were

a. locomotion (circling, obstinate progression, gait coordination and speed, stepping up or down)
b. posture (spontaneous, when held by the scruff of the neck or hanging by the pelvic girdle) and postural reflexes (righting from side or in free fall, Magnus reflexes)
c. muscle tonus of the limbs (rigidity, spasticity)
d. segmental limb reflexes (stretch reflex, flexor withdrawal, limb supporting reactions)
e. limb placing reactions: the tactile or contact placing reaction (CPR), was tested following the method described by Bard (4) as well as the visual and proprioceptive placing responses; in addition, the cat's ability to walk on a plank was assessed
f. gross somatic sensibility
g. presence of abnormal "involuntary" movements
h. pupillary and ocular activities, in particular, the orienting of the eyes toward the sources of visual and/or acoustic stimulation and the persistence of tracking objects in a horizontal or vertical pendular motion

Recordings

Recordings were done with the animals in a sound-attenuated chamber with a one-way observation window and under dim, although uninterrupted, illumination. The freely moving animals were connected to the polygraph (type B Dynograph recorder, Beckman Instruments) through a counter-weighted cable system and slip-ring assembly. The cats had unlimited access to water and food.

Overt motor activity and sleep-wakefulness were evaluated by means of 24-hour recording sessions conducted on or around the fifth postoperative day, every 10–15 days during the first 3 months, and every 10–30 days thereafter for up to 6 months. Shorter recording sessions were conducted during the first postoperative days to evaluate early EEG changes. The polygraphic criteria used to identify motor activity during wakefulness were a desynchronized EEG, a highly active EMG, as well as movement artifacts in the records. Moreover, the cats were frequently observed, not only during the day, but also during parts of the night. The time spent in quiet wakefulness (ocular movements and a less active EMG) was not considered as motor activity. The criteria used to score the sleep-wakefulness states and the corresponding results of this part of the study have been reported elsewhere (49,80); however, part of that information will be used to complement certain aspects of the present report.

Behavioral Observations

The animals were observed moving freely in the laboratory, where the spontaneous or the "motivated" behavior could be assessed, and in the restricted environment of the recording chamber as described above. Particular emphasis was devoted to the evaluation of the following items:

a. level of behavioral arousal and general motor activity; three criteria were used for assessment: (1) the amount of motor activity displayed by the animal in the recording cage; this, identified as described above, was expressed as a percentage of the 24-hour recording session for each animal; an average of the percentages for all animals in each recording session was calculated and shown, independently for each experimental group, by means of the bars in Figure 9. Finally, an average of the percentages for all sessions, or average cumulative percentage, was also calculated for each experimental group (Figure 8). (2) percentages of the sleep-wakefulness states for each group of animals; (3) an estimate of the animals' activity while free in the laboratory or in their open-view home cages (considered as a "reactivity" estimate)

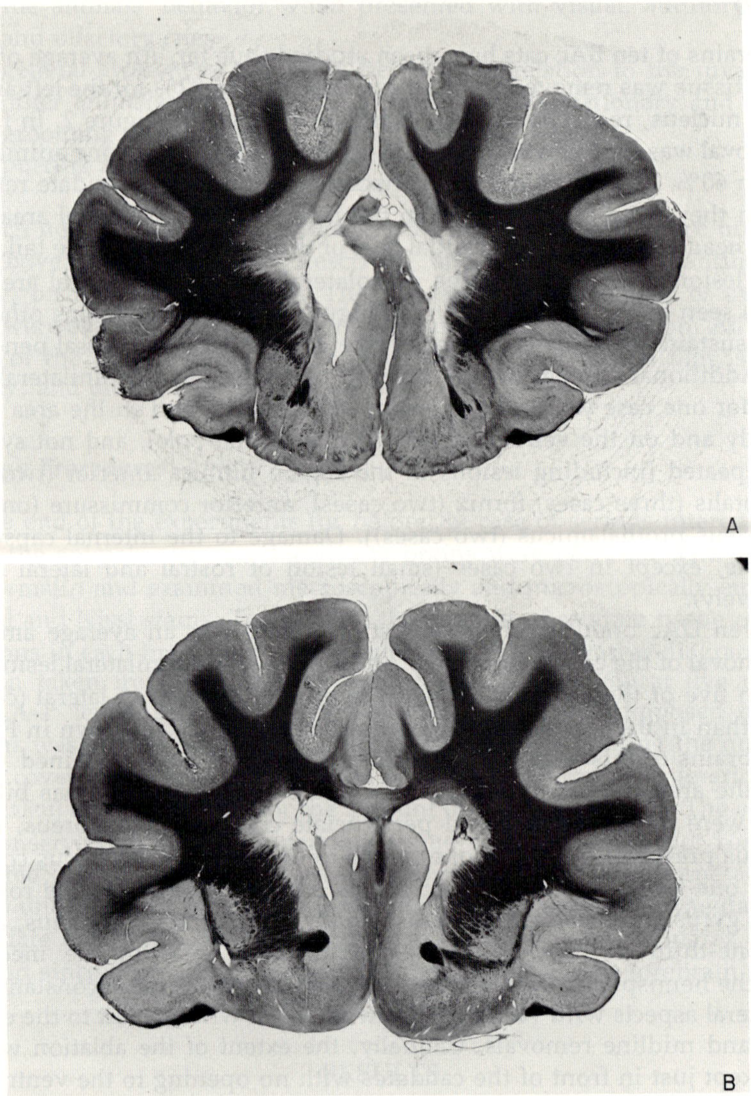

FIGURE 2. Histological sections of the brain of a cat with bilateral removal of the caudate nuclei. Weil-stained sections at approximately: A, A 18.0 (Snider and Niemer's atlas, 69); B, A 15.0; C, A 13.0; and D, A 8.0.

"COMPULSORY
we call "comp
other descript
all BAc cats. V
the cat emerge
tracking persi
visual field. T
yielded counts
to 10 postoper
sistence, but i
disappeared
tracking, howe

As soon as t
manifested, a
person, cat, o
typed in the s
usually with
changes of sp
sisting almost
onstrated its s
under unusual
from the inves
times as he w
pletely recover
by another cat
actually come
proach; this v
vocalization or
ject or person;
he was preven
jects or climbir
approaching b
animal sudden
would not retr
until the threa
flexibility and
tact cat which

Although vis
and tactile stin
change in dire
sound emanati
ing behavior. T
cat touching o

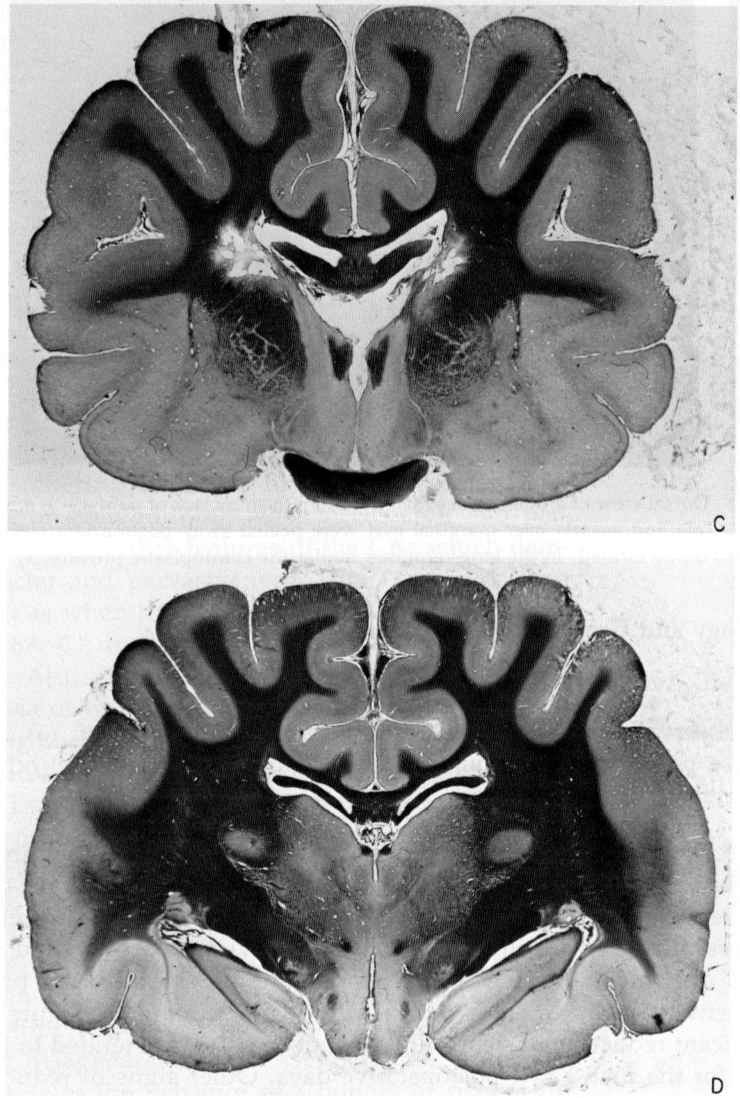

FIGURES 2 C and D.

BEHAVIOR. None of the UAc cats ever exhibited the CAs. Six animals showed very transitorily (up to the third postoperative day), weak visual tracking more markedly toward the side of the lesion. Thereafter, these animals behaved like ShO cats. They exhibited a slight, inconstant hyperactivity (see BAc cats and Figure 9) but no sleep reduction (80). By the third postoperative day they began to eat efficiently.

CATS WITH FRONTAL CORTICAL ABLATION

NEUROLOGY. All the cats exhibited moderate paresis of all four limbs and hypesthesia lasting from 6 to 12 days and declining slowly thereafter. Most of the animals exhibited an exaggerated extensor tonus of the limbs, particularly in the forelimbs, such that their hyperextended forelimbs would tightly adhere to the thorax when the cat was held by the scruff of the neck. This decreased or disappeared over a period of about 1 month. The CPR was abolished initially in all four limbs; its apparent recovery after 3 to 4 months is presently being further studied and documented.

BEHAVIOR. Eight cats did not exhibit any of the elements of the CAs except for the presence, in four animals, of the visual tracking described above for the BAc cats; however, this behavior was less marked and lasted for a shorter period (an average of 15 days) than in the BAc cats. Indeed, these animals were timid and tended to run away and hide as soon as placed upon the floor or counters in the lab. The brains for which the extent of the ablation has been verified and described above belonged to animals in this group.

Two cats, which are currently alive, transitorily exhibited some of the features of the CAs; however, these coexisted with aggression as described below. Both cats approached the investigator, but not objects, for 13 and 30 days, respectively, but displayed little of the stereotyped activity seen in BAc cats. The cat exhibiting the visual approaching for 30 days did not show any other form of approach or any tendency toward exaggerated treading or purring. The other animal tended later, when the visual following had disappeared, to develop marked purring and tactile approach. These two cats hissed and attacked when handled and particularly when touched, even gently, on the back; three investigators have been bitten several times by one of them.

The BFr animals started eating and were eating efficiently by 4 and 7 days after surgery, respectively. They exhibited motor hyperactivity although less marked than BAc cats (see BAc cats and Figure 9) and a moderate, sustained, reduction in the amount of sleep (49).

SHAM-OPERATED CATS

No permanent neurological or behavioral abnormalities were found in these animals. The CPR was altered, coarse, or absent in one or more limbs for a few days immediately after surgery but was fully recovered in all animals by the tenth day.

Electroencephalogram

The EEG was essentially normal in all the cats. In some BAc cats, during the first week, isolated bursts of high voltage slow waves occasionally interrupted the desynchronized cortical EEG during arousal, particularly over frontoparietal areas. No such abnormal bursts were observed in UAc or BFr cats. Thereafter, both the cortical and subcortical EEG appeared to be normal in all BAc cats as shown by an adequate display of all the EEG events characteristic of the EEG sleep-waking states and a good EEG reactivity to barbiturates and amphetamines (marked sustained desynchrony of the ECoG).

DISCUSSION

General Effects of Caudate Nuclei Ablation

Survival

To our knowledge, there have not been any publications reporting results in chronically maintained cats following bilateral, simultaneous removal of the caudate nuclei in the absence of dorsolateral cortical damage. Mettler and collaborators (24,51,53,54) did perform caudate nuclei ablation in cats in which cortical areas had been previously removed. However, their animals died within 3 to 5 days of the caudatal lesions. Ill-defined metabolic disturbances in which the striatum was thought to be specifically involved (54) were blamed for the deaths. Satisfactory, chronic survival was obtained later (73,74) in cats with subtotal ablation of the caudates after removal of aspects of the dorsolateral cortex in a preparatory stage. Fox *et al.* (21) also reported an "extremely high mortality" in an unsuccessful attempt to perform, one-stage, bilateral, caudate lesions, and recently Harik and Morris (26) found that cats with large caudate lesions could not be maintained beyond 3 days.

The present results support neither the above findings nor the concept of caudate nuclei participation in vital metabolic processes since our BAc cats could be kept alive indefinitely by using the routine techniques which we have previously developed for the care of cats with brain lesions (75). In fact, the acaudate cats were not any more difficult to maintain than the BFr cats.

Cognitive Deficit

The present results also failed to duplicate the observations by Mettler and collaborators (24,51,53,54) that bilateral removal of the caudates produces such a profound deficit in the cat as to warrant describing them as "real vegetables, completely out of contact, wandering aimlessly" (Heath, in 54). In the acute postoperative period, there were manifestations of lack of awareness and faulty relationship with the environment; but, since the signs disappeared soon afterward, it is difficult to conceive of them as being specific effects of caudate function deficit. Rather, they might be considered as unspecific manifestations of transitory processes (edema, neurological shock, irritation) concomitant with any extensive brain surgery. Thompson and Mettler's cats (73,74) did not exhibit the deficit of Mettler's earlier animals; however, they still showed "total and prolonged failure to learn" rather simple tasks. Preliminary results in our BAc cats (81) do not support the latter findings but suggest a perseverative defect in performance in line with the behavioral rigidity manifested in the CAs. More subtle defects in the cognitive sphere have been repeatedly demonstrated in cats (16,17,21), rats (57,66,88), and monkeys (5,14,23,63) with restricted caudatal lesions.

Behavioral Arousal and Motor Activity (Including UAc and BFr cats)

Enhanced behavioral arousal and hyperactivity have long been considered a result of caudate lesions. Although there are quantitative reports demonstrating hyperactivity in monkeys (13,60) and rats (35,87) following caudate lesions, the reports of hyperactivity in the cat have been based on nonquantified visual observations (53). Thus, the present study appears to be the first to quantify the presence of motor hyperactivity in the cat following large caudate lesions.

The literature is less clear regarding possible participation of lesions restricted to the frontal cortical areas in producing motor hyperactivity in cats. As far as we are aware, the only quantitative study is that of Langworthy and Richter (40); these authors reported a large increase in motor activity in cats with frontal lesions (in which some damage to the striatum was also inflicted). Other studies dealing with frontal lesioned cats either did not demonstrate any hyperactivity (43) or reported its presence in frontal cats in which, most probably, the caudate nuclei were also involved in the lesion (47,85). Thus, Brutkowski concludes in his review (8) that hyperactivity has not been reported in cats with frontal lesions. The present data demonstrate the participation of frontal cortical areas in the control of the level of motor activity in the cat. Therefore, the cats with frontal lesions appear to be similar in this respect to the rhesus monkey (33,60,64).

Since the increased motor activity in our animals was demonstrated in the monotonous environment of the recording cage, it indicates that hyperactivity existed independently of the amount of environmental stimulation. Whether the cats also manifested increased motor responsiveness vis-à-vis environmental stimulation (hyperreactivity), has not been demonstrated quantitatively by the present experiments. However, the behavioral observations strongly suggested that this was the case for the BAc cats only. The problem of hyperreactivity versus hyperactivity in animals with caudate lesions has been previously discussed by others (35,53). Kirkby (35) demonstrated a further increase in motor activity in his caudate lesioned rats and Mettler and Mettler (53) observed enhanced hyperactivity in their caudate lesioned cats following environmental darkening for the rats or blindfolding of the cats, respectively. Since both are nocturnal species, the authors interpreted the change as a hyperreaction to the decrease in illumination.

The results of our sleep-wakefulness studies (49,80), used as an additional criterion to assess the level of arousal in the present cats, fit well with our data on motor activity. Thus, the reduction in sleep was also greater during the first postoperative month in the BAc cats; it was less in the cats with frontal lesions during the same period, but in the latter animals it became more sustained thereafter. The sleep reduction in the UAc cats was not statistically significant.

Therefore, when all three criteria to assess behavioral arousal and motor activity (see Methods) are taken together, our results suggest that both caudate and frontal areas (although the caudate nuclei in a more marked manner) are involved in the control of the arousal-activity levels in the cat, with hyperreactivity probably being another factor in the acaudate animals. We have previously postulated (78) a forebrain system exerting an important control over a powerful arousal-activity mechanism located probably at ventral diencephalic level. The present experiment suggests that the caudate nuclei and frontal cortical areas may be a part of such a system.

Caudate Ablation in Monkeys

Attempts to ablate the caudate in the monkey have met with relatively more success than in the cat. Even though Teuber *et al.* (72) reported that their attempt to ablate the caudate bilaterally in the monkey was a "disaster" (since all their animals died shortly after surgery), two other authors were, apparently, more successful. Kennard (32,33) lesioned the caudate in a number of monkeys, either penetrating frontal areas 6 or 8 or using a transcallosal approach. The neurological and behavioral changes observed in the monkeys with destruction of areas 6 or 8 were interpreted as being due to the cortical lesion, whereas the absence of symptoms in the animals with the midline penetration was considered as evidence that caudate nuclei ablations do not produce any effects. Such a conclusion does not seem fully justified since in Kennard's monkeys:

a. There was not any clear statement regarding the extent of the caudatal ablation, except for mentioning that "only the head was lesioned in all of them" and that in one of them the caudate lesions "were small."

b. The lesions were performed in two stages.
c. No clear information was provided regarding the time of survival and the method used in studying the animals.
d. Some of the monkeys developed epilepsy.

Thus we think, the important conclusion quoted above lacks experimental evidence.

Denny-Brown (15) reported a remarkable change in behavior in the monkey after bilateral destruction of the caudate nucleus produced via a penetration in the prefrontal cortex. The main effects were the display of a "compulsive behavioral promenade" which "was related entirely to the presence of others" and of a number of visual compulsions "of which visual challenge (the leaping automatism), visual avoiding (facing the wall), and compulsive visual investigation" were the most obvious. He concluded that "in some manner bilateral lesion of the head of the caudate nucleus releases visually determined cortical automatisms" and that "the caudate nucleus must normally be concerned in the integrative balance of cortical responses to environmental contact stimuli with those of visual context." Unfortunately, there were not any histological reports on the brains of these animals. Recently, Watkins (83) interpreted these results as indicative that the caudate "is concerned with the control of automatic motor patterns and visually determined responses."

Subtotal Caudate Lesions

Numerous other caudate lesion studies in the cat (2,17,21,25) and in other species (5,14,23,63,66) have been reported (see also Ref. 42). In most of these studies, the lesion has been either relatively small or purposely localized to only parts of the caudate. The results of those studies, which are pertinent to the present observations, are discussed below. We would like to stress, however, the need for performing extensive or total lesions in order to evaluate caudate function. This need was recognized early by Mettler and collaborators after their observation that lesions destroying less than 50% of the caudate and putamen failed to produce readily observable changes (51). This is further emphasized by the present findings that complete unilateral removal of the caudate produces no long-lasting gross neurological or behavioral changes and that in cats with less than 80% of the caudate removed, the CAs was both less marked and shorter in duration than in the animals with larger ablations.

"Compulsory Approaching" Syndrome

CAs versus Obstinate Progression

A discussion of the main neurological behavioral change observed in BAc cats necessitates first that a clear differentiation be made between the CAs and the obstinate progression phenomenon. According to the original description by Bailey and Davis (3) and our own experience with diencephalic cats (78), the main features characterizing obstinate progression are

a. a pervasive tendency to walk incessantly; if the cat encounters an obstacle, he continues pushing against it until either the obstacle gives way, the animal accidentally gets started in another direction, or, if the propulsive effort is too strong, possibly inflicts serious damage (3,78) to his forehead
b. a lack of awareness to cliff—hence the animal can easily walk out of an open cage or walk over the edge of a counter or table
c. absence of any tendency to follow the observer or to attend to other environmental stimuli.

Furthermore, obstinate progression is usually a transient phenomenon, lasting at most a few weeks. Finally, while some of the reports (40,47,53) suggest a tendency for the lesions producing it to cluster in rostral areas of the brain, findings by other investigators indicate that lesions of many other areas (3,50,76,78) can also produce the syndrome; in fact, the most marked and lasting obstinate progression has been observed in animals following extensive neodecortication or complete removal of the cerebral hemispheres (see Ref. 78).

Because of the above reasons we consider obstinate progression to be an unspecific consequence of the removal of widespread inhibitory telencephalic influences acting upon a basic activity mechanism, probably located at a lower diencephalic level (78).

We did not observe obstinate progression in our BAc cats.

In contradistinction, the following features are essential to the CAs:

a. the displacement of the cat elicited by external stimuli and subsequent movement being stimulus bound; even with this qualification, walking is only one of the components of the CAs
b. stereotyped friendliness (compulsory stimulus attachment, rubbing, purring, vocalization, and treading)
c. monotonous, long-lasting syndrome present in animals virtually free of other neurological deficits

Specificity of the Caudate Ablation in Producing the CAs

Several observations in the present experiments as well as by others (2,13,15,51,53) suggest that large caudate lesions may play a central role in determining the CAs.

In the present study:

a. The CAs was observed in all the BAc cats.
b. It was a long-lasting or permanent change, thereby indicating that it

THE NATURE OF THE CAs

Two hypotheses, one neurological, the other behavioral, may explain the CAs in BAc cats.

Neurologically, the CAs could conceivably be thought of as resulting from the release of the basic drive to walk—providing it is accepted that the caudate nucleus is one of the forebrain structures involved in the inhibitory control of such a drive. A pure manifestation of such a release is seen in obstinate progression; however, obstinate progression, as pointed out earlier, is a non-guided walking activity which can occur even in the absence of the telencephalon [as in the "diencephalic" cat (78)], whereas the CAs is a stimulus-bound event. The stimulus-bound nature of the CAs could conceivably result from the fact that all sensory cortical areas are intact in the BAc cats and therefore can subserve the role of "guiding" the released walking activity. The CAs could thus be understood as a released walking mechanism "guided" by any of the sensory modalities. Moreover, one could even propose an enhanced effectiveness of sensory stimuli conducive to hyperactivity of the orienting reaction in BAc cats as proposed by Zernicki (89), for frontal cats. In this context, there are electrophysiological data (22,38) linking the caudate nuclei to the processing of sensory information which could provide the basis for understanding the increased effectiveness of sensory cues in caudate-ablated cats. This possibility would make it even more likely that a double release, that of the walking mechanism and of the orienting reaction, could account for CAs. In this context, the presence of hyperreactivity in the BAc cats could also be understood.

The main argument against the above hypothesis is that it does not account for other components of the CAs, e.g., the general friendliness of the BAc cats as manifested by their constant purring, treading, and peculiar mewing, the tactile or "bodily contact" component, the apparent preference for the animals to approach animate versus inanimate objects, and, finally, the possible, although not as yet well-documented, change in sexual behavior. Taken as a whole, the CAs appears to be a great change in the behavior of the cat. Indeed, this feline, which is usually considered to be independent and voluble (45), is suddenly changed into a stereotyped, persistent follower, and this might well be the central feature of the CAs.

Another alternative for understanding the CAs would be to conceive of it as an affective change, or at least as a change in the approach-withdrawal behavioral balance (67). In such a case the exaggerated purring-treading-rubbing, at a maximum when the animal reaches its target, could be conceived as being part of the "consummatory" aspect of the behavior, whereas the distress signs which the BAc cats display when attempts are made to prevent their approaching could be thought of as manifestations of a strong "motivational" component. Although most of the testing to prove or disprove this hypothesis remains to be done, it is interesting to note that several papers have reported impairments in avoidance and escape as a consequence of a striatal damage in rats (36,56,88), dogs, rabbits (61), and cats (24,41,74).

Unilateral Acaudate Cats

The major finding in the UAc cats was the virtual absence of neurological and behavioral changes. This result is in agreement with observations by Mettler (51) and by Anderson and Akert (2) in cats with large and small unilateral caudate lesions, respectively. This finding has at least two important implications. Thus, except for its probable participation in the contralateral CPR, the caudate nuclei appear not to have any lateralized gross neurobehavioral function, and it is strong evidence for a large functional reserve of this structure. This should not be considered as evidence that removing one caudate nucleus has no neurophysiological effect whatsoever; in fact, after such ablation there are changes in the firing patterns of neurons in the contralateral caudate (44), and our ongoing research (81) suggests slowing of bar pressing with the paw contralateral to the caudatal removal.

Other authors have reported a marked and long-lasting, compulsory, ipsiversive circling in animals with unilateral caudate damage (12,51,86). In some of these experiments (51,86) in which the caudate was approached through the dorsolateral cortex, the lesion of the latter might explain the postural and walking asymetry. A similar mechanism might explain the ipsiversive turning found in the rat after a unilateral caudate lesion (12) since abundant cortical-subcortical fibers cross through the caudate in this species, and these are bound to be destroyed by any caudate lesion.

Electroencephalogram

The EEG findings in the present study are markedly different from those of Kennard who is, as far as we are aware, the only other author having examined the effects of bilateral caudate lesions upon the EEG (31). Kennard reported a marked, persistent change in the electrocorticogram in monkeys with combined ablations of the head of the caudates and cortical areas 4 and 6; these consisted of intermittent high amplitude bursts, marked showing, "unevenness" and "diminution of amplitude" of the EEG patterns. However, epilepsy was a common postoperative occurrence in these animals. Moreover, a histological account of the extent of the lesions was not provided. The cortical involvement plus the epileptic nature of the lesions may explain the EEG effects in Kennard's experiments. Our results suggest, on the contrary, that the caudate nuclei are not grossly involved in the control of the EEG events; it has been demonstrated, however (10), that EEG spindle waves can be triggered by means of caudate stimulation. In general, the normality of polygraphic patterns in our caudate-lesioned cats is further proof of the relative intactness of noncaudate structures.

SUMMARY

A method is described for performing one-stage ablation of the caudate nuclei through a midline approach in cats. Ten bilateral acaudate cats (BAc), with an average of 84% of caudate tissue removed, were studied for an average of over 6 months (three, for over 1 year). In addition, 11 cats with unilateral caudectomy (UAc), with an average of 95% of the nucleus removed, 10 cats with bilateral removal of the frontal-cortical areas (BFr), and four sham-operated cats (ShO) were also studied. Most cats were implanted with recording electrodes in neocortical areas, the hippocampus, the pontine reticular formation, neck muscles, and orbits. The results of the gross behavioral, neurological, and polygraphic observations are reported.

1. A long-lasting, behavioral change labeled "compulsory approaching syndrome" (CAs) was observed following surgery in all BAc cats. This syndrome was characterized by stereotyped, "compulsory," and prolonged approaching or following of persons, cats, or objects apparently aimed at a physical contact with the approached target and persisting under unusual conditions. Visual cues (visual tracking was a transitory, early component of the CAs) were most effective in eliciting the CAs; acoustic and tactile stimuli were also adequate. Other components of the CAs were marked passivity, markedly exaggerated forelimb kneading or treading, marked purring, and hyperreactivity. The magnitude and duration of the CAs appeared to be related to the extent of the ablation, although some of its basic features persisted for over a year. The CAs was never observed in the ShO cats.

2. BAc cats were remarkably free of neurological and gross behavioral deficits. Except for some short-lasting deficits, probably nonspecific, during the early postoperative period (motor weakness, absence of contact placing reaction, faulty awareness, defective eating and drinking, and hyposomnia), only a moderate hyperactivity with a tendency toward hyposomnia, along with the CAs, persisted in the chronic state.

3. In all UAc cats, there was an absence of any permanent gross neurological or behavioral changes including the CAs. This finding suggests that the caudate nuclei do not have any gross lateralized behavioral or neurological function and indicates an ample compensatory functional reserve.

4. The BFr cats exhibited early, short-lasting visual tracking, but none of the characteristics of the CAs were present except in two animals in which there was a combination of aggressiveness and elements of the CAs. Other defects of the frontal cats were a consequence of the ablation of the sensory-motor areas (paresis, hypesthesia, and absence of contact placing reactions).

5. The cortical and subcortical EEG was normal in all cats including the BAc animals.

The CAs is discussed in terms of the specificity of the caudate nuclei ablation in its production. It is tentatively explained as resulting from a simultaneous release (from caudate nuclear inhibition) of a basic walking or activity mechanism coupled with the hyperactivity of the orienting reaction. Other possibilities are also considered.

It is concluded that total ablation of the caudate nuclei in the cat produces a characteristic behavioral change which is basically manifested as an exaggerated, stereotyped, approaching behavior, the exact nature of which remains to be elucidated. The caudate nuclei do not appear to have an essential role in the control of basic metabolic processes, elementary sensory-motor functions, elementary cognitive functions, and the EEG as previously postulated.

ACKNOWLEDGMENTS

This research was supported by USPHS Grant Nos. MH-07097, HD-05958, and HD-04612. We wish to thank Dr. C.E. Olmstead for his assistance in parts of the work and the UCLA Mental Retardation and Child Psychiatry Media Unit for making the 16-mm movies and video tapes.

REFERENCES

1. Adametz, J. H. Rate of recovery of functioning in cats with rostral reticular lesions. *J. Neurosurg.*, 1959, **16:** 85–97.
2. Akert, K., and Anderson, B. Experimentaller beitrag zur Physiologie des Nucleus caudatus. *Acta Physiol. Scand.*, 1951, **22:** 281–298.
3. Bailey, P., and Davis, E. W. The syndrome of obstinate progression in the cat. *Proc. Soc. Exp. Biol. Med.*, 1942, **51:** 1841.
4. Bard, P. Studies on the cerebral cortex. I. Localized control of hopping and placing reactions in the cat and their normal management by small cortical remnants. *Arch. Neurol. Psychiat.*, 1933, **30:** 40–74.
5. Battig, K., Rosvold, H. E., and Mishkin, M. Comparison of the effects of frontal and caudate lesions on discrimination learning in monkeys. *J. Comp. Physiol. Psychol.*, 1962, **55:** 458–463.
6. Bond, D. D., Randt, C. T., Bidder, T. G., and Rowland, V. Posterior septal, fornical, and anterior thalamic lesions in the cat. *Arch. Neurol. Psychiat.*, 1957, **78:** 143–162.
7. Brady, J. V., and Nauta, W. J. H. Subcortical mechanisms in emotional behavior: Affective changes following septal forebrain lesions in the albino rat. *J. Comp. Physiol. Psychol.*, 1953, **46:** 339–346.
8. Brutkowski, S. Functions of prefrontal cortex in animals. *Physiol. Rev.*, 1965, **45:** 721–746.
9. Brutkowski, S., Fonberg, E., and Mempel, E. Angry behavior in dogs following bilateral lesions in the genual portion of the rostral cingulate gyrus. *Acta Biol. Exp.* (*Warsaw*), 1961, **21:** 199–205.
10. Buchwald, N. A., Wyers, E. J., Okuma, T., and Heuser, G. The "caudate" spindle." I. Electrophysiological properties. *Electroenceph. Clin. Neurophysiol.*, 1961. **13:** 509–518.
11. Carman, J. B., Cowan, W. M., and Powell, T. P. S. The organization of corticostriate connections in the rabbit. *Brain*, 1963, **86:** 525–562.
12. Cools, A. R. *The Caudate Nucleus and Neurochemical Control of Behavior.* Drukkerif Brakkenstein, Nijmegen, The Netherlands, 1973.

13. Davis, G. Caudate lesions and spontaneous locomotion in the monkey. *Neurology,* 1958, **8:** 135–139.
14. Dean, W. H., and Davis, G. D. Behavior changes following caudate lesions in rhesus monkey, *J. Neurophysiol.,* 1959, **22:** 524–537.
15. Denny-Brown, D. Experimental lesions of the basal ganglia in the monkey In: *The Basal Ganglia and Their Relation to Disorders of Movement.* Oxford Univ. Press, London, and New York, 1962: 103–121. By permission of The Clarendon Press, Oxford.
16. Divac, I. Functions of the caudate nucleus. *Acta Biol. Exp.,* 1968, **28:** 107–120.
17. Divac, I. Delayed alternation in cats with lesions of the prefrontal cortex and the caudate nucleus. *Physiol. Behav.,* 1972, **8:** 519–522.
18. Ermolenko, S. F. Cortical projections of the caudal part of the head and body of the caudate nucleus in cats. *Arkh. Anat. Gist. Embriol.,* 1971, **61:** 24–32.
19. Finger, S., Walbran, B., and Stein, D. G. Brain damage and behavioral recovery: Serial lesion phenomena. *Brain Res.,* 1973, **63:** 1–18.
20. Fox, M. W. Reflex development and behavioral organization. In: *Developmental Neurobiology.* (W. A. Himwich, Ed.). Thomas, Springfield, Illinois, 1970: 553–580.
21. Fox, S. S., Kimble, D. P., and Lickey, M. E. Comparison of caudate nucleus and septal area lesions on two types of avoidance behavior. *J. Comp. Physiol. Psychol.,* 1964, **58:** 380–386.
22. Fox, S. S., and O'Brien, J. H. Inhibition and facilitation of afferent information by the caudate nucleus. *Science,* 1962, 423–425.
23. Goldman, P. S., and Rosvold, H. E. The effects of selective caudate lesions in infant and juvenile rhesus monkeys. *Brain Res.,* 1972, **43:** 53–66.
24. Gomez, J. A., Thompson, R. L., and Mettler, F. A. Effect of striatal damage on conditioned and unlearned behavior. *Trans. Am. Neurol. Ass.,* 1958, **83:** 88–91.
25. Gybels, J., Meulders, M., Callens, M., and Colle, J. Disturbances of visuo-motor integration in cats with small lesions of the caudate nucleus. *Arch. Int. Physiol. Biochim.,* 1967, **75:** 283–302.
26. Harik, S. I., and Morris, P. L. The effects of lesions in the head of the caudate nucleus on spontaneous and L-dopa induced activity in the cat. *Brain Res.,* 1973, **62:** 279–285.
27. Irwin, D. A., Criswell, H. E., and Kakolewski, J. W. Spontaneous whole brain slow potential changes during recovery from experimental neurosurgery. *Science,* 1973, **181:** 1176–1178.
28. Jeannerod, M., Kiyono, S., and Mouret, J. Effets des lésions frontales bilatérales sur le comportement oculo-moteur chez le chat. *Vision Res.,* 1968, **8:** 575–583.
29. Johnson, T. N., Rosvold, H. E., and Mishkin, M. Projections from behaviorally-defined sectors of the prefrontal cortex to the basal ganglia, septum, and diencephalon of the monkey. *Exp. Neurol.,* 1968, **21:** 20–34.
30. Kemp, J. M., and Powell, T. P. S. The connexions of the striatum and globus pallidus: Synthesis and speculation. *Philos. Trans. R. Soc. London.* [*Biol. Sci.*] 1971, **262:** 441–457.
31. Kennard, M. A. Effects on EEG of chronic lesions of basal ganglia, thalamus, and hypothalamus of monkeys. *J. Neurophysiol.,* 1943, **6:** 405–416.
32. Kennard, M. A. Experimental analysis of the functions of the basal ganglia in monkeys and chimpanzees. *J. Neurophysiol.,* 1944, **7:** 127–149.
33. Kennard, M. A., and Fulton, J. F. Corticostriatal interrelations in monkey and chimpanzee. *Res. Publ., Assoc. Res. Nerv. Ment. Dis.,* 1942, **21:** 228–245.
34. Kennard, M. A., Spence, S., and Fountain, G., Jr. Hyperactivity in monkeys following lesions of the frontal lobes. *J. Neurophysiol.,* 1941, **4:** 512–524.
35. Kirkby, R. J. Caudate nucleus and arousal in the rat. *J. Comp. Physiol. Psychol.,* 1973, **85:** 82–96.
36. Kirkby, R. J., and Kimble, D. P. Avoidance and escape behavior following striatal lesions in the rat. *Exp. Neurol.,* 1968, **20:** 215–227.
37. Klosovskii, B. N., and Bolzhina, N. S. Physical and behavioral development of puppies with removed subcortical nuclei (caudate nuclei) and spared cerebral cortex. *Arkh. Patol.,* 1956, **18:** 35–42.

38. Krauthamer, G. M., and Albe-Fessard, D. Electrophysiologic studies of the basal ganglia and striatopallidal inhibition of non-specific afferent activity. *Neuropsychologia,* 1964, **2:** 73–83.
39. Langworthy, O. R., and Kolb, L. C. The experimental production in the cat of a condition simulating pseudo-bulbar palsy. *Am. J. Physiol.,* 1935, **111:** 571–577.
40. Langworthy, O. R., and Richter, C. P. Increased spontaneous activity produced by frontal lobe lesions in cats. *Am. J. Physiol.,* 1939, **126:** 158–161.
41. Laursen, A. M. Conditioned avoidance behavior of cats with lesions in globus pallidus. *Acta Physiol. Scand.,* 1963, **57:** 81–89.
42. Laursen, A. M. Corpus striatum. *Acta Physiol. Scand.,* 1963, **59:** Suppl. 211, 1–106.
43. Lawicka, W., and Konorski, J. The effects of prefrontal lobotomies on the delayed responses in cats. *Acta Biol. Exp.,* 1961, **21:** 141–156.
44. Levine, M. S., Hull, C. D., Buchwald, N. A., and Villablanca, J. The spontaneous firing patterns of forebrain neurons. II. Effects of unilateral caudate nuclear ablation. *Brain Res.,* 1974, **78:** 411–424.
45. Leyhausen, P. *Verhaltensstudien an Katzen.* Parey, Berlin, 1973.
46. Liles, S. L., and Davis, G. D. Permanent athetoid and choreiform movements after small caudate lesions in the cat. *U.S., Pub. Health Serv., Publ.,* 1969, **1938:** 98–109.
47. Magoun, H. W., and Ranson, S. W. The behavior of cats following bilateral removal of the rostral portion of the cerebral hemisperes. *J. Neurophysiol.,* 1938, **1:** 39–44.
48. Marcus, R. J., and Villablanca, J. Is the striatum needed for amphetamine-induced stereotyped behavior? *Proc. West. Pharmacol. Soc.,* 1974, **17:** 219–222.
49. Marcus, R. J., and Villablanca, J. Long-term sleep reduction in frontal cats. *Physiologist,* 1974, **17:** 280.
50. McGinty, D. J., and Sterman, M. B. Sleep suppression after basal forebrain lesions in the cat. *Science,* 1968, **160:** 1253–1255.
51. Mettler, F. A. Relation between pyramidal and extrapyramidal function. *Res. Publ., Ass. Res. Nerv. Ment. Dis.,* 1942, **21:** 150–227.
52. Mettler, F. A. Perceptual capacity, functions of the corpus striatum and schizophrenia. *Psychiatry Q.,* 1955, **29:** 89–111.
53. Mettler, F. A., and Mettler, C. C. The effects of striatal injury. *Brain,* 1942, **65:** 242–255.
54. Mettler, F. A., Thompson, R. L., Hovde, C. A., Gomez, J., and Dupree, A. L. The striatal syndrome. *Trans. Am. Neurol. Ass.,* 1957, **82:** 24–31.
55. Meyer, P. M., Dalby, D. A., Glendenning, K. K., Lauber, S. M., and Meyer, D. R. Behavior of cats with lesions of the septal forebrain or anterior sigmoid neocortex. *J. Comp. Physiol. Psychol.,* 1973, **85:** 491–501.
56. Mitcham, J. C., and Thomas, R. K., Jr. Effects of substantia nigra and caudate nucleus lesions on avoidance learning in rats. *J. Comp. Physiol. Psychol.,* 1972, **81:** 101–107.
57. Norman, R. J., Villablanca, J. R., Brown, K. A., Schwafel, J. A., and Buchwald, J. S. Classical eyeblink conditioning in the bilaterally hemispherectomized cat. *Exp. Neurol.,* 1974, **44:** 363–380.
58. Parmeggiani, P. L., and Zanocco, G. A study on the bioelectrical rhythms of cortical and subcortical structures during activated sleep. *Arch. Ital. Biol.,* 1963, **101:** 385–412.
59. Reinoso-Suárez, F. *Topographischer Hirnatlas der Katze.* E. Merck A. G., Darmstadt, 1961.
60. Richter, C. P., and Hines, M. Increased spontaneous activity produced in monkeys by brain lesions. *Brain,* 1938, **61:** 1–16.
61. Romanovskaya, E. A. Certain consequences of destroying the caudate nuclei in rabbits and dogs. *Bull. Exp. Biol. Med. (USSR)* 1957, **44:** 1066–1069.
62. Rosen, J., Stein, D., and Butters, N. Recovery of function after serial ablation of prefrontal cortex in the rhesus monkey. *Science,* 1971, **173:** 353–356.
63. Rosvold, H. E., and Delgado, J. M. R. The effect on delayed-alternation test performance of stimulating or destroying electrically structures within the frontal lobes of the monkey's brain. *J. Comp. Physiol. Psychol.,* 1956, **49:** 365–372.

Behavioral Plasticity during Development

11

Brainstem Substrates of Sensory Information Processing and Adaptive Behavior

JENNIFER S. BUCHWALD
Mental Retardation Research Center and
Department of Physiology, School of Medicine,
University of California Los Angeles,
Los Angeles, California

Under the umbrella of mental retardation, the diversity of clinical entities clearly indicates a potential multitude of causal mechanisms. Two statistics, however, provide a point of departure for the present discussion: (a) the incidence of premature births, with anoxia as a common perinatal complication, is significantly elevated in mentally retarded populations (13,29); and (b) partial deafness is significantly more common among the mentally retarded (18,19).

While premature birth can potentially implicate any part of the central nervous system (CNS), several studies suggest that the sensory (especially auditory) relay nuclei of the brainstem are particularly vulnerable to the anoxia which often accompanies this birth complication. In an extremely detailed quantitative study employing cell counts and areal measurements, the CNS histopathology of 39 neonates (7–9 months gestational age) who died of perinatal asphyxia was studied by Hall (14,15), using, as controls, nine infants who suffered accidental deaths without CNS damage. The asphyxiated group showed periodic postnatal attacks of apnea, which failed to stabilize even with oxygen therapy, and death occurred within a period of 4 hours to 22 days after birth. On the basis of the detailed histories which accompanied these cases intrauterine anoxia and cerebral hemorrhage were ruled out as important prenatal complications and acute perinatal asphyxia per se was considered the most important etiology of observed brain pathology. The brains were perfused intraarterially within 2 hours after death with formalin and Heidenhain-Sousa solutions and subsequently prepared with thionine stain for histological examination. Temporal bones were additionally removed and decalcified so that cochlear histology could also be studied. After examination of the asphyxiated and control tissue a normal histological and cytological picture for both groups was found in the cortex (e.g., auditory cortex), the thalamus (e.g., medial geniculate body), in the motor nuclei of the brainstem, as well as in the cochlea. However, the asphyxiated brain series showed other specific loci of pathology, the most dramatic of which was in the cochlear nucleus, where a 20–45% cell loss consistently occurred (estimated by a sample cell count procedure). The subdivision of the dorsal cochlear nucleus showed the greatest amount of damage, which was reflected by cell losses of 36–66%. Additional areas of cell destruction or damage were consistently present in the superior olivary complex and inferior colliculus so that the brainstem auditory pathway appeared to be particularly vulnerable to anoxic stress, i.e., to have the least safety margin, in the neonatal brain. This unique susceptibility to anoxia may be explained by the high capillarity which has been quantitated for the cochlear nucleus (9).

The susceptibility of the neonatal auditory pathway to anoxia is also emphasized in the experimental studies of Windle and his colleagues (30–32). In these experiments on monkeys, birth anoxia was imposed for varying periods of time, ranging from 5 to 20 minutes. The animals were subsequently terminated at intervals of months, with a maximum follow-up time of 9 years, and both behavioral and anatomical observations were made. Because the duration of the anoxic episode was controlled by the experimenter, those brain areas most susceptible to this stress could be determined by relating observed pathology to degree of anoxia. In the monkey the inferior colliculus was consistently the most sensitive brain region to anoxic effects with clearly observed central regions of cell destruction or damage. Other brainstem components of the acoustic pathway likewise showed marked anoxic sensitivity with pathological changes in the superior olivary nucleus, nucleus of the lateral lemniscus, and cochlear nucleus. Brainstem nuclei of other sensory systems, e.g., vestibular and somatic, also showed pathology, in contrast to the more rostral visual system which consistently appeared normal throughout its entire extent. Additional loci in the basal ganglia also showed pathology, whereas other brain areas, including cerebral cortex, appeared normal up to 10 months. In monkeys ranging in age from 10 months to 9 years, however, transneuronal degeneration began to appear as secondary consequence of the primary anoxic pathology (11). Thus, in sensory areas of the reticular formation, in the thalamic relay nuclei, and in those cortical areas to which the ascending sensory systems normally project, transneuronal degeneration was observed. Other cortical areas, e.g., the frontal cortex, continued to appear histologically normal.

The behavioral consequences of such anoxic brain pathology have not yet been extensively investigated. Infant monkeys with severely anoxic births initially showed a variety of neurological signs but, as the animals matured, their behavior became increasingly normal (24,25,30–32); as adults, these animals showed no gross motor deficits and their performance in a visual discrimination task was normal (17). Auditory thresholds, however, were found to be elevated when quantitated in a behavioral test situation (1). A similar auditory finding has been reported for human subjects who sustained birth complications of anoxia; audiometric testing showed that these individuals had marked elevations of acoustic thresholds including high frequency deafness (12). Although sophisticated behavioral screening is only beginning to be carried out on anoxic subjects, studies of memory deficits (26), which have been replicated (17), showed that monkeys with anoxic births were unable to perform a 5-second delayed response task, although they scored at control levels when the "delay" aspect of the test was removed. As noted above, the brain histology on such animals has shown normal frontal cortex but extensive primary brainstem and secondary thalamic and cortical pathology in the ascending sensory systems, with the exception of the visual pathway. A relevant clinical study on 3-year-old children with anoxic perinatal histories showed that these subjects were significantly poorer than controls in tests of vocabulary skill and cognitive ability, although, in most of the psychological tests given, the two groups performed equally well (10).

Taken together, these clinical and experimental studies indicate a high degree of vulnerability of the brainstem sensory nuclei, particularly those of the auditory system, to the pathological effects of perinatal anoxia. In the monkey, control studies employing true anoxia (oxygen-free air), rather than asphyxia (air deprivation), did not result in brain pathology; thus, local increases in carbonic acid rather than oxygen lack per se appeared to be the more important causal element for the observed pathology (30–32). The extent to which these vulnerable brainstem loci might be selectively susceptible to other perinatal stresses has not been studied, but their high capillary density suggests that any nutritional disturbance might be severely registered by the cells within such richly vascularized beds.

Histopathology of the brainstem sensory nuclei could significantly disturb the normal encoding of stimuli into appropriate neuronal firing patterns, whereby higher centers receive information about the sensory environment. The form and degree of any resultant behavioral pathology would surely depend upon the extent of the primary lesions and subsequent secondary degeneration. Unfortunately, there are few data in the experimental literature which extensively examine behavior after disturbance of sensory information processing at the brainstem level. One of the few studies specifically directed to this problem was that of Sprague *et al.* (27,28) which indicated that dramatic behavioral aberrations emerged after surgical interruption of the somatic and acoustic sensory pathways in their ascent through the lateral brainstem. The adult cats subjected to this sensory interruption procedure showed behavioral pathology that could not be accounted for solely on the basis of diminished acoustic and sensory perception. For example, marked visual deficits were present although the visual pathway, including tectum, was rostral to the level of brainstem surgery and appeared histologically normal. The animals showed a loss of affect, an excessive amount of oral activity with a tendency toward hyperphagia, stereotyped behavior characterized by incessant wandering, sniffing, and visual searching. While the animals could learn simple conditioned responses they showed a poor level of retention from one day to the next. Sprague *et al.* (27,28) interpreted these symptoms as a result of forebrain deafferentation. Without patterned input to higher centers via the specific sensory pathways the remaining portion of the nervous system seemed incapable of supporting normal adaptive behavior. The bizarre nature of this behavior led these authors to compare it with autistic performance which they felt shared many of the same aberrant qualities.

On the basis of data obtained from sensory restriction studies, Melzack (20) likewise was led to compare the resultant abnormal behavior which developed with aspects of autism and of childhood hyperactivity. Puppies raised to adulthood under conditions of severe sensory restriction showed high levels of behavioral arousal and hyperactivity, impairment in sensory responsiveness and discrimination, stereotyped behavior, and inability to inhibit irrelevant responses. These abnormalities were irreversible, even after the animals had lived for months in a normal environment. Prolonged disruptive effects of early sensory restriction have also been found in primates (23), which continue to respond inappropriately and apparently fail to discriminate significant stimuli for many months after being restored to a normal environment.

We are presently attempting to extend these studies which relate disturbed sensory inflow to behavioral pathology. In our experiments kittens are being raised in isolation chambers under conditions of severe sensory restriction, or after lateral brainstem transection of the ascending acoustic and somatic systems, or after medial brainstem lesions of reticular formation areas through which these modalities ascend. Intermittent behavioral tests will be carried out as the animals mature and a roster of both behavioral and electrophysiological experiments will be completed on the young adult animals. Although perhaps most relevant to the present conference, this study is not yet sufficiently advanced to provide any data, except for the fact that the kittens survive these brainstem lesioning procedures.

To summarize briefly the thrust of my discussion to this point, emerging clinical and experimental data are beginning to suggest that the brainstem may be an important part of the functional matrix from which normal mental development and behavior evolve. Although the brainstem has not been a focal point in considering etiologies of mental retardation, nor even in analyses of adaptive behavior, information processing within both the brainstem sensory nuclei and the adjacent reticular formation may indeed be one of the most critical and relevant areas for such investigations. Since partial deafness and premature births are represented more prominently among the mentally retarded than in the normal population, we must wonder whether these statistics are importantly correlated with the unique susceptibility of the brainstem auditory nuclei to perinatal anoxia. We must wonder whether some critical amount of cell damage in the initial processing stages of sensory inflow has occurred so as to garble sensory stimuli into redundant noise instead of encoding specific patterns of information. Such garbling of sensory information might, indeed, be more debilitating than complete loss of function within a sensory system. In the latter case, compensatory functions can be assumed by other systems and education can be directed so as to maximize these compensations. Partial damage within one or more sensory nuclei of one of more sensory system, on the other hand, might be difficult to determine clinically and could result in a range of unpredictable behavioral aberrations, depending upon the extent of distortion imposed upon incoming sensory cues.

In my laboratory we are presently exploring the capacity of the brainstem to encode sensory, especially acoustic, stimuli and to modulate the resultant sensory information so as to produce a "learned" response, i.e., a second-order encoding of the sensory stimulus within a greater temporal domain. We have arrived at this present focus on the brainstem only after a considerable amount of wandering through the CNS looking for a model system simple enough to be analyzable, complex enough to support a variety of behaviors, and with some clinical relevance. In earlier studies of normal adult cats behaviorally trained to perform a conditioned leg flexion, we were initially delighted by the many brain loci from which conditioned unit activity could be recorded (5). We became increasingly disenchanted with this situation, however, as we grappled with the analytical problems posed by the web of interacting systems, loops, and circuits which characterize the intact brain. An alternate preparation was that offered by the isolated spinal cord, in which the neural complexity is drastically reduced. Unfortunately behavioral plasticity is likewise reduced and we found that conditioned (as opposed to sensitized) somatic responses were difficult, if not impossible, to establish in spinalized mammals, a conclusion shared by many investigators (4). We then wondered what the minimal "brain" might be from which a convincing behavioral conditioned response could develop.

After reviewing the literature, we found that although considerable attention has been directed toward spinal conditioning, very little work has followed from the intense interest in decorticate conditioning which flourished several decades ago. As reported in this review (4), subsequent to a series of controversial experiments by other investigators, Bromily in 1948 showed that a clear, discriminated conditioned response could be established in the decorticate preparation with confirming brain histology, but only one dog was used for this study; in 1958 Bard and Macht observed anecdotally both habituation and conditioning in the decerebrate cat, but their experiments were not focused on learning capacity and no formal training procedures were utilized.

Because the literature was unclear on the issue of "minimal brain tissue" necessary to support conditioning, and because we were interested in a simplified system in which we could study both sensory information processing and learning, we initiated a behavioral study of adult cats following chronic brain truncations of increasing severity (21). Normative data on the conditioned response of choice, the conditioned eyeblink response, were first collected on a series of intact adult cats. A 75–80 dB, 400-msec tone or

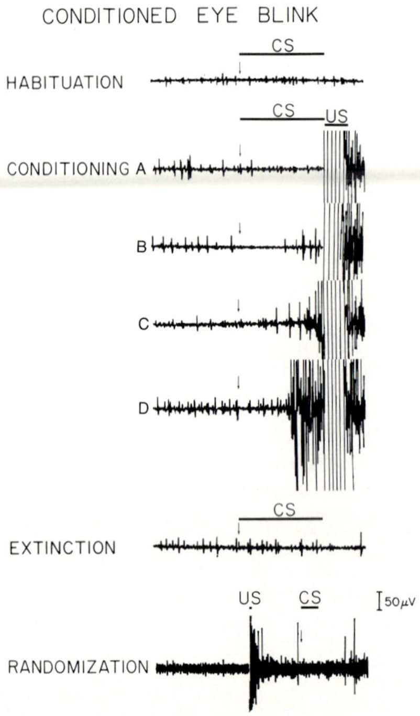

FIGURE 1. Typical development of a conditioned blink response in one cat. CS duration was 400 msec and US duration was 70 msec on all traces. (Note: Bottom trace recorded on a slower time base.) CRs developed only following systematic pairing of CS and US during conditioning trials. They were characterized by a long latency (greater than 100 msec) burst of EMG activity, often superimposed on a suppression of background EMG activity early in training. Traces A through D represent changes in EMG responsiveness to the CS which typically occurred over one to two training sessions. Additional training results in the consistent appearance of sustained, relatively large amplitude CRs. CRs disappeared during extinction and did not reappear during random CS and US presentations. In the bottom trace, the arrow indicates CS onset which induces no response, although a spontaneous EMG potential just precedes the CS. (These records are from a bilaterally hemispherectomized cat but are representative of CR development in both the normal and experimental groups.) From Norman *et al.* (21).

white noise (CS) was paired with a 70-msec shock train to the outer canthus of the eye (US) which produced a cutaneous blink reflex (UR). Trials were separated by 20- to 30-second intertrial intervals and approximately 100 trials were run per session. Electromyogram responses were recorded bipolarly from the orbicularis oculi muscle of the trained eye, as well as from the opposite eye muscle or from muscles elsewhere in the face. A series of procedures was routinely carried out on all animals which included conditioned response acquisition, discrimination between CS+ (reinforced) and CS− (nonreinforced), extinction, and random presentations of CS and US.

In naive animals, no response to the CS was initially present, although with considerably higher stimulus intensities (e.g., 90–110 dB), a 17-msec latency, unconditioned acoustic eyeblink reflex could be elicited. Among the normal nonlesioned cats, CS suppression of ongoing orbicularis oculi EMG activity typically occurred within the first 200 conditioning trials and gradually gave way to a relatively long latency (100 msec) conditioned discharge which became increasingly robust with continued training (Figure 1). During additional training procedures, the conditioned EMG response showed discrimination between CS+ and CS−, discrimination reversal, extinction, and the response did not develop during random presentations of CS and US (Figure 2).

The chronic truncated preparations studied thus far during the various training procedures outlined above are summarized in Table I. Included in this series have been animals with: lesions restricted to the frontal cortex; extensive aspiration of most of the neocortex; bilateral ablation of the caudate

Table I Summary of Conditioning Experiments

Treatment	*Name*	*CR*	*Ext*	*Disc*	*Rand*	*Rev*	*Shift*
Normal	Minuet	×	×	×		×	×
	C-16	×	×	×			
	Chastity	×	×	×	×		
	Daffy	×	×	×	×		
Decortication: frontal cortex	El Rojo	×	×	×		×	
	Freddy	×	×	×	×		
Decortication: neocortex	Zsa Zsa	×	×	×		×	
Caudate ablation	Siete	×	×	×			
	Bobcat	×		×			
Bilateral hemispherectomy	Tiger	×	×	×	×		×
	Cenizas	×	×	×	×	×	
	Puma	×	×		×		×
VPM lesion	Valerie	×	×				
Decerebration	Tigressa	×	×	×	×	×	
	Wrat	×	×	×	×		
	Demian	×	×	×	×		

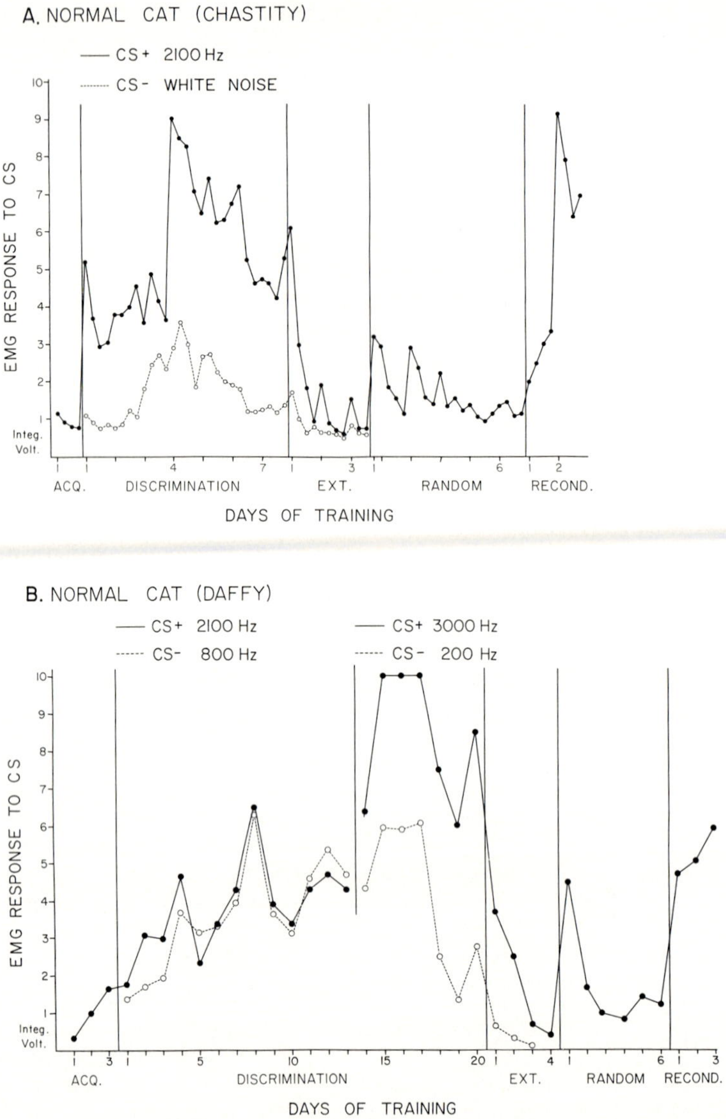

FIGURE 2. Summary of training procedures and typical response levels in normal animals. A. Each point represents the response average of 25 trials. The integrated EMG during the CS period (the CR response measure) is plotted on the ordinate. This animal showed CR acquisition, discrimination between the reinforced CS (CS+), a 2100 Hz tone, and white noise, the discriminative, nonreinforced stimulus (CS−), extinction, a lack of reliable responding during random presentations of CS and US, and finally, reacquisition of the CR during paired CS–US trials. B. Similar data for another normal animal except that averages are for daily sessions. From Norman *et al.* (21).

nuclei; bilateral hemispherectomy, i.e., removal of both cerebral hemispheres, including limbic nuclei, basal ganglia, and internal capsule, leaving the thalamus as the most rostral extension of the CNS; and animals with midcollicular transection of the brainstem, i.e., complete decerebration. All these animals have shown the capacity to acquire a discriminated conditioned

A

B

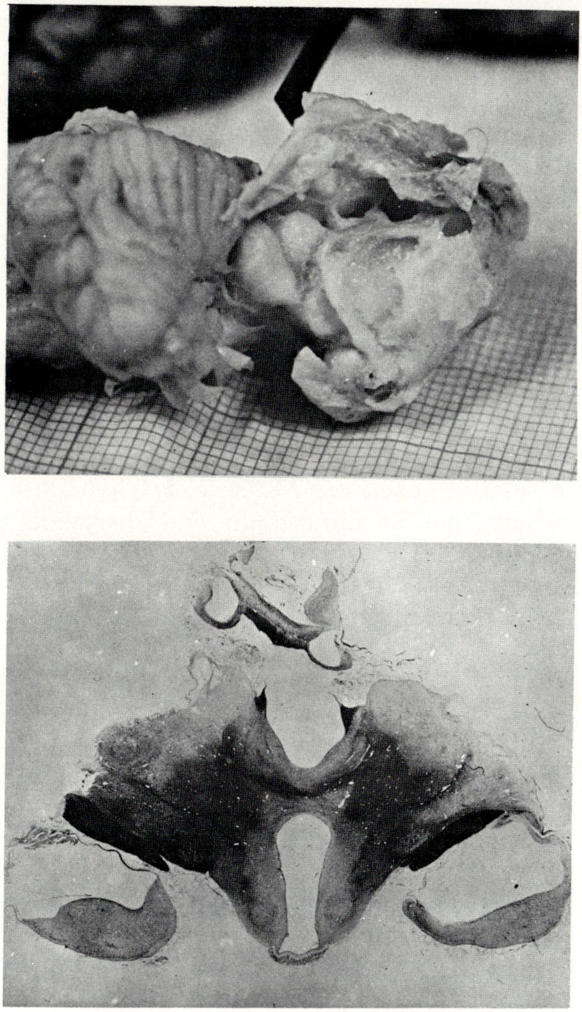

FIGURE 3. The diencephalic brain. A. The brain from one of the chronic diencephalic animals (Tiger) is shown; the hemispheres were removed 4 months prior to termination. The remaining diencephalic stump is devoid of all telencephalic structures. (The probe is lifting a nonfunctional remnant of the fornix.) B. Histology from this animal shows marked degeneration throughout the thalamus. Note the enlarged ventricles and reduced thalamic mass. From Norman *et al.* (21).

response of 100-msec latency, to extinguish this response and not to develop the response during random CS and US presentations (Table I). Although none of the animals showed naive responses to the CS, at higher stimulus intensities (e.g., 90–100 dB), all of the truncated preparations showed the short 17-msec latency, unconditioned acoustic reflex. Data from the most extensively truncated preparations, the hemispherectomized and decerebrate animals, are summarized in Figures 3, 4, and 5. The hemispherectomized cats began to show conditioning within the first 2 weeks postoperatively and once acquisition of the conditioned response was well established, subsequent behavior appropriate to the additional training procedures developed at a normal rate (Figure 4).

In the decerebrate cats a longer postoperative recovery period was necessary before conditioned response acquisition began to appear. During this 4- to 6-week period a fascinating degree of functional recovery occurred; for the sake of brevity I shall dwell only upon those aspects which relate to acoustic responsiveness. For several days following brainstem transection there was a disappearance of acoustic reflex activity. In contrast, reflexes induced by cutaneous stimulation, including the blink reflex, never disappeared although thresholds were transiently elevated immediately after decerebration. Gradually, by the second to third postoperative week, fragmented acoustic startle responses began to reappear but thresholds were high and extremely loud sounds were necessary to elicit any response. By the end of the first month, the orienting response had begun to return with increasingly well-integrated neck, head, and pinna movements. During the second month acoustic reflex thresholds, including that for the 17-msec latency, unconditioned acoustic blink reflex, began to stabilize at levels similar to preoperative values and 100-msec latency conditioned responses began to emerge.

While the conditioned eyeblink responses in the decerebrate animal were less stable than those of the normal cat, they developed with a similar initial suppression of EMG activity during early training followed by the appearance of an EMG discharge 100 msec or more after CS onset. In the three chronic decerebrate animals studied thus far extinction, discrimination between CS+ and CS−, and random CS and US presentation procedures have been carried out. The conditioned response performance during acquisition reached levels of 80 to 90% but did not consistently remain at high levels from one day to the next, although there appeared to be some savings across days. Discrimination between white noise CS+ and 1000 Hz CS− (or 1000 Hz CS+ and white noise CS−) was established, although performance was poorer than normal. During extinction the response diminished; during random CS and US presentations the CS response initially reappeared, but again, it gradually diminished over subsequent trials (Figure 5).

Thus, the chronic decerebrate preparation appears capable of supporting a discriminated conditioned response, although the conditioning is not as clear or robust as in the other less severely lesioned animals that we have studied.

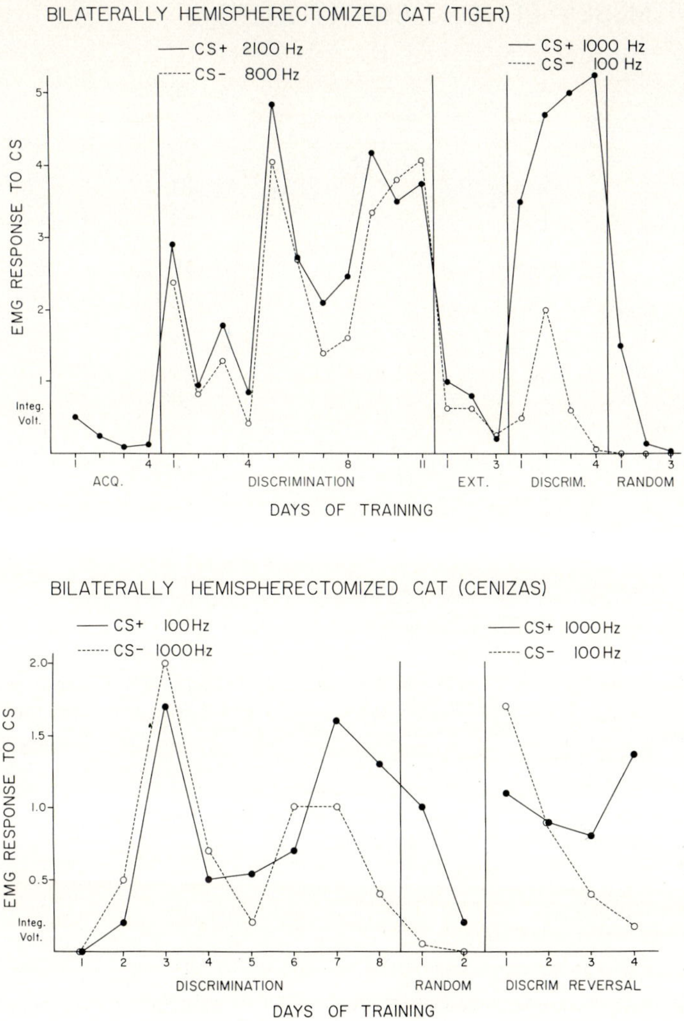

FIGURE 4. Summary of conditioning in two diencephalic cats. Acquisition of conditioned blink response was similar to that of the normal animals. These cats showed the parametric characteristics of conditioning, including discrimination and discrimination reversal, in the absence of all telencephalic structures. From Norman *et al.* (21).

However, the relative simplicity of the isolated brainstem with only one association area (the reticular formation), with access to two sensory modalities (acoustic and trigeminal), and with an easily quantifiable motor output (the eyeblink) make it an intriguing system in which such behavioral phenomena as conditioning, habituation, and functional recovery may be more susceptible to analysis than in the intact brain.

In relevant electrophysiological studies our data thus far are primarily from

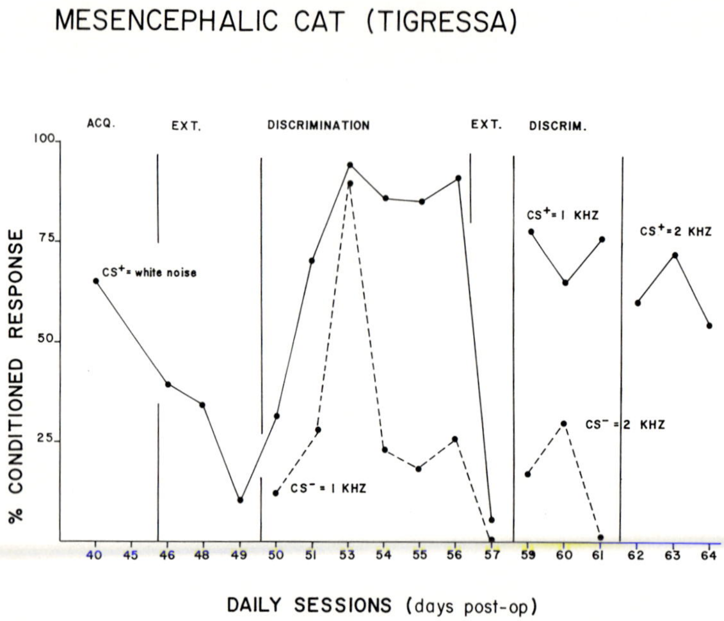

FIGURE 5. This figure expresses percent CR per day during the conditioning training of one decerebrate cat. At the end of the first postoperative month the conditioned response began to look consistent so the response to white noise was extinguished and a discrimination procedure was used. Retraining to the CS+ (1 kHz) was very rapid and was maintained at high levels. The CS− was introduced using a "fading" procedure in which the intensity was initially set below that of the CS+ but was increased gradually over training so that by the end of training the two stimuli were of equal intensity. The stimulus previously used as the CS− was subsequently reinforced and conditioning could be demonstrated. As in other cats, random shock did not provide responses to the CS. From Buchwald *et al.* (8).

the acoustic relay nuclei. We have found that in the acute decerebrate condition unit recordings of ongoing activity and acoustic responsiveness from the cochlear nucleus and inferior colliculus are very similar to the recordings obtained in the implanted, intact cat (6,7,22). Thus, the acute loss of acoustic reflex responsiveness in the decerebrate is not due to a depression of the primary acoustic pathway. On the other hand, the recovery of acoustic reflex function indicates that the necessary circuitry is present in the isolated brainstem. As in other reflex systems, this local circuitry apparently becomes increasingly suppressed as higher thalamic and cortical centers mature and their descending influences become increasingly potent. Release, by decerebration, of the brainstem from these descending influences allows the primitive, or latent, functions of the brainstem to reemerge with a capacity sufficient to support not only acoustic startle and orienting reflexes but an acoustic conditioned response as well. These data poignantly portray the reticular formation as a structure so captivated during maturation by the descending influences of higher centers that its independent associative and reflex functions, perhaps highly significant in shaping neonatal behavior, become largely masked.

While it has long been known that acoustic responses can be recorded from the reticular formation, these have generally been classified as "nonspecific" responses registering novel stimuli through the arousal system rather than subserving any specific acoustic information transfer. On the other hand, in the chronic decerebrate, conditioned discrimination between an acoustic CS+ and acoustic CS− suggests that acoustic information is handled very specifically by the neuropil supporting the production or the withholding of the conditioned response—neuropil which we presently presume to be within the reticular formation. Supportive data for the concept of sensory response specificity in the reticular formation have come from other experiments, the initial purpose of which was to explore acoustic response specificity in the limbic system (2,3). The unit response patterns in hippocampus and amygdala were found to differentiate tones of different frequency or input laterality (2). Subsequently, the source of acoustic input to these sites was investigated by placing lesions either in the brachia of the inferior colliculi to interrupt the primary acoustic pathway, or in the reticular formation of the medial brainstem to interrupt acoustic projections ascending through this system (3). Although an initial, relatively small component of the responses disappeared following the primary acoustic pathway sections, the quality of response specificity was preserved (Figure 6). In contrast, after the reticular lesions, the hippocampal and amygdala acoustic responses largely disappeared (Figure 7). Thus, specific information concerning the nature of the acoustic stimulus was projected to these limbic sites largely through the reticular formation. Taken together, these observations support a conceptualization of the reticular formation as a structure which can receive and transmit acoustic information with retention of specific stimulus coding, rather than simply a degradation of the stimulus into a nonspecific signal of arousal. We are presently pursuing this problem in a mapping study of acoustic response specificity in the chronic decerebrate preparation.

In order to develop a temporal frame of reference for the brainstem structures potentially involved in sensory information processing and learning phenomena, we have also begun to establish what we refer to as "time constants of response plasticity" at different levels of the brainstem system. For example, after an acoustic stimulus has been presented, over what period of time does that stimulus continue to exert an influence; how different is the duration of this influence in the acoustic nerve than in the cochlear nucleus, the inferior colliculus, or the reticular formation? Although a great deal of work has been done in the area of auditory habituation, it has been only within the past decade that the numerous variables leading to artifactual data

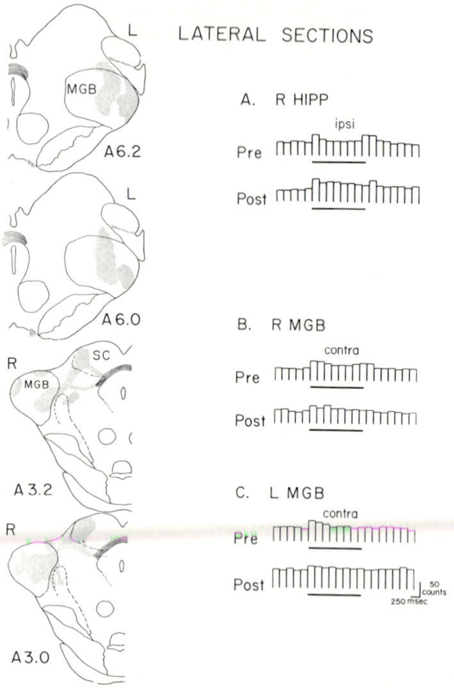

FIGURE 6. Persistence of limbic (hippocampal, HIPP) acoustic response after bilateral damage to primary auditory pathways. Extents of pathway sections are shown in coronal diagrams at slightly different A–P levels on each side (R and L). MGB = medial geniculate body, SC = superior colliculus. A. Multiple-unit discharge frequency histograms from ventral hippocampal site are averaged over five trials. Top trace: Presection excitatory response to ipsilateral 80 dB white noise stimulus (dark bar) is not eliminated after auditory pathway damage (bottom trace). B and C. Five-trial averaged multiple-unit discharge frequency histograms from right and left MGB showing typical presection excitatory responses to contralateral white noise stimulation (top traces) and sharp reduction of postsection (bottom traces) response magnitudes. From Brown and Buchwald (3).

have been recognized and controlled (7). Subsequent experiments have been more carefully carried out but stimulus parameters and response measures have continued to be so varied that for any solid interpretation of the habituation process to emerge a cohesive study of the relevant substrates must be made. In our approach to this problem, a rather wide range of stimulus duty cycles (i.e., stimulus duration/intertrial interval) have been utilized, with a series of 25 successive acoustic stimulation trials at each duty cycle. Single and multiple unit responses were recorded from decerebrated cats maintained under Flaxedil and artificially respired and the percent of response decrement which developed across the 25 trials at each duty cycle was determined. The range of duty cycles extended from very light, i.e., 1-second tones every 10 seconds, to very heavy, e.g., 8.5-second tones every 10 seconds; intensity was held constant at 75 or 80 dB SPL (re 0.0002 dyn/cm^2).

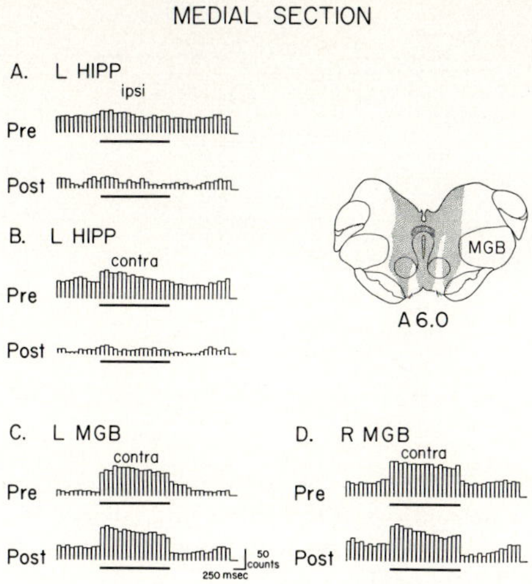

FIGURE 7. Reduction of limbic (hippocampal, HIPP) acoustic responses after medial section of brainstem at geniculate level (A 6.0). Extent of section shown on coronal diagram. MGB = medial geniculate body. A and B. Top traces show five-trial averaged multiple-unit discharge frequency histograms from same ventral hippocampal site before section. Presection excitatory responses (top traces) to ipsilateral (A) and contralateral (B) 80 dB white noise (dark bar) are markedly diminished in postsection (bottom traces). C and D. Five-trial averaged multiple-unit discharge frequency histograms from left and right MGB show typical excitatory responses (top traces) to contralateral 80 dB white noise which are not markedly reduced in postsection (bottom traces). From Brown and Buchwald (3).

The cochlear hair cell microphonic potential recorded from the round window showed no change as a function of any of these duty cycles (7,16). Only during terminal levels of barbiturate did the microphonic potential begin to diminish and with EKG cessation it disappeared. Unit responses recorded from the acoustic nerve also showed marked stability during increasingly heavy duty cycles, with essentially no adaptation as long as 100 msec or more intervened between successive stimuli (Figure 8). During continuous tone stimulation, however, some degree of response decrement appeared but recovery occurred almost immediately after stimulus cessation. At the central level of the cochlear nucleus there was a marked increase in the persistence of the acoustic response trace as indicated by the intertrial interval across which response decrements developed, i.e., at relatively light duty cycles (Figure 9). Thus, in addition to the response pattern encoded by the cochlear nucleus, which functionally distinguishes it from the acoustic nerve, persistence of the acoustic response trace occurs to a qualitatively greater degree in the cochlear nucleus than in the nerve. This difference in response trace persistence can be defined in terms of the duty cycle which produces response changes over successive trials. At the level of the inferior colliculus, greater complexity is encoded into the acoustic responses and a more dramatic degree of response persistence occurs (22). For example, a stimulus duty cycle of 1-second tone/5-

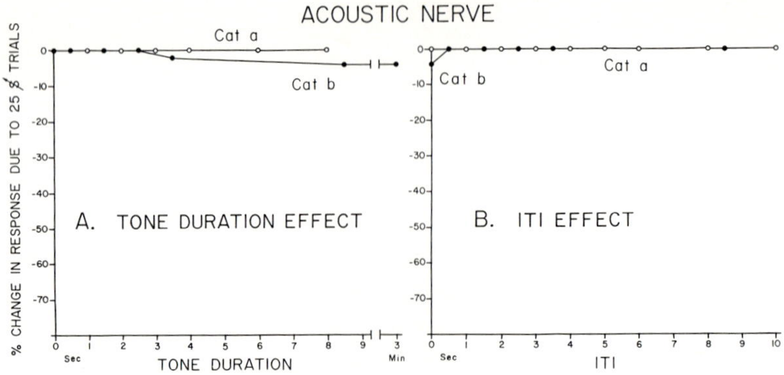

FIGURE 8. For cat a, multiple unit responses at the acoustic nerve did not show any decrement at any tone duration, including continuous tone stimulation. For cat b, small response decrements were observed but were sharply in contrast with the data from the cochlear nucleus shown in Figure 9. From Huang and Buchwald (16).

second intertrial interval produced a response decrement of 80 to 90% in the colliculus, in contrast to the 10 to 20% decrement produced by the same duty cycle in the cochlear nucleus. Both loci are clearly influenced by lighter duty cycles than those necessary to induce changes at the more peripheral auditory stations.

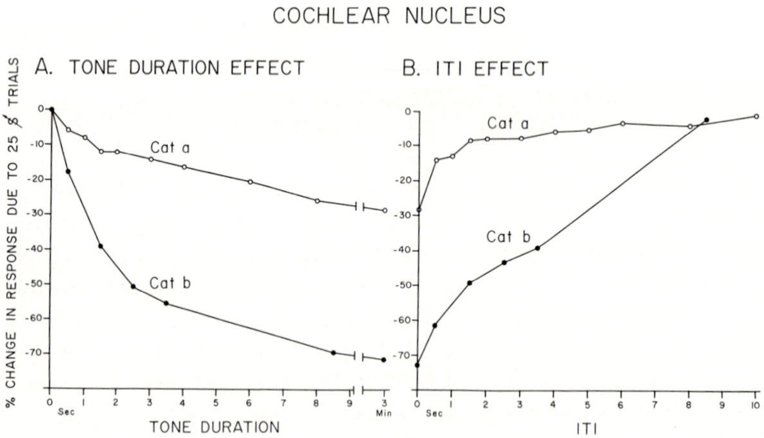

FIGURE 9. A. For a fixed intertrial interval (ITI) of 1.5 seconds, increased tone (80 dB, 3000 Hz) duration enhanced response decrement in cochlear nucleus multiple unit activity during a block of 25 trials. Increasing the tone duration beyond 8–10 seconds had little effect on the percent change. B. Percent change of the cochlear nucleus multiple unit activity became less significant with increasing ITI while tone (90 dB, 3000 Hz) duration is fixed at 1.5 seconds. For ITI beyond 8–10 seconds, the habituation procedure had essentially no effect. From Huang and Buchwald (16).

These data map the temporal domain of excitability and recovery processes, i.e., the persistence of the acoustic response trace, for the acoustic centers tested thus far. By developing similar data for the remaining brainstem acoustic nuclei and for the various areas of the reticular formation which show acoustic responsiveness, we hope to establish a hierarchy of "time constants of response plasticity" within the brainstem. Such a hierarchy would provide a temporal frame of reference for brainstem elements, based on their excitability and recovery processes, and should suggest those regions with lowest modulation thresholds. Those regions particularly sensitive to the repeated stimulation of an habituation paradigm might also be particularly susceptible to the successive convergent sensory inflow of a conditioning paradigm.

In summary, while the various experimental studies I have described are far from completion, we hope that they will expand our present understanding of sensory information processing, the modulation of this processing, and the development of adaptive behavior. As our interests have focused increasingly on the acoustic and reticular brainstem systems, the clinical and experimental data indicating the unique susceptibility of the brainstem sensory systems to perinatal anoxia have seemed increasingly relevant, as has the subpopulation of mentally retarded individuals who are partially deaf with a history of premature birth.

SUMMARY

Emerging clinical and experimental data suggest that the brainstem may be an important part of the functional matrix from which normal mental development and behavior evolve. Although the brainstem has not been a focal point in considering etiologies of mental retardation nor even in analyses of adaptive behavior, information processing within both the brainstem sensory nuclei and adjacent reticular formation may indeed be one of the most critical and relevant areas for such investigations. Data are summarized from several ongoing experiments which are designed to explore the capacity of the brainstem to encode sensory, especially acoustic, stimuli and to modulate the resultant sensory information so as to produce a "learned" response. Such data indicate that in the absence of forebrain or even midbrain structures, a simple conditioned response can be supported by the brainstem. The reticular neuropil is considered particularly important to this response acquisition and is conceptualized as a structure which can receive and transmit acoustic information with retention of specific stimulus coding. It is further suggested that independent associative and reflex functions of the reticular formation may be highly significant in neonatal behavior but, with the development of descending influences from higher centers during maturation, these functions may become largely masked. In order to develop a temporal frame of reference for brainstem structures potentially involved in sensory information processing and learning phenomena "time constants of response plasticity" are being established for different levels of the brainstem system.

ACKNOWLEDGMENTS

This work has been supported by USPHS Grant Nos. NS-05437, HD-04612, HD-05958, and NIH Special Resources Grant No. RR-3.

REFERENCES

1. Berman, D., Karalitzky, A. R., and Berman, A. J. Auditory thresholds in monkeys asphyxiated at birth. *Exp. Neurol.*, 1971, **31:** 140–149.
2. Brown, K. A., and Buchwald, J. S. Acoustic responses and plasticity of limbic units in cats. *Exp. Neurol.*, 1973, **40:** 608–631.
3. Brown, K. A., and Buchwald, J. S. Acoustic projection pathways to limbic sites in the cat. *Anat. Rec.*, 1975, **181:** 319.
4. Buchwald, J. S., and Brown, K. A. Subcortical mechanisms of behavioral plasticity. In: *Mechanisms of Motor Integration.* (J. Maser, Ed). Academic Press, New York, 1972: 99–136.
5. Buchwald, J. S., Halas, E. S., and Schramm, S. Changes in cortical and subcortical unit activity during behavioral conditioning. *Physiol. Behav.*, 1965, **1:** 11–22.
6. Buchwald, J. S., and Humphrey, G. L. Response plasticity in the cochlear nucleus of decerebrate cats during acoustic habituation procedures. *J. Neurophysiol.*, 1972, **35:** 864–878.
7. Buchwald, J. S., and Humphrey, G. L. An analysis of habituation in the specific sensory systems. In: *Progress in Physiological Psychology.* (E. Stellar and J. Sprague, Eds). Academic Press, New York, 1973: 1–75.
8. Buchwald, J. S., Norman, R. J., Villablanca, J. R., Brown, K. A., and Schwafel, J. A. Classical conditioning of the eyeblink response in chronic decerebrate cats. *Proc. 26th Int. Physiol. Cong.*, 1974, **11:** 216.
9. Craigie, E. H. The comparative anatomy and embryology of the capillary bed of the central nervous system. *Res. Publ. Assoc. Res. Nerv. Ment. Dis.*, 1938, **18:** 3–28.
10. Ernhart, C., Graham, F., and Thurston, D. Relationship of neonatal apnea to development at three years. *Arch. Neurol.*, 1960, **2:** 504–510.
11. Faro, M. D., and Windle, W. F. Transneuronal degeneration in brains of monkeys asphyxiated at birth. *Exp. Neurol.*, 1969, **24:** 38–53.
12. Fisch, L. The aetiology of congenital deafness and audiometric patterns. *J. Laryngol. Otol.*, 1955, **69:** 479–493.
13. Gottfried, A. W. Intellectual consequences of perinatal anoxia. *Psychol. Bull.*, 1973, **80:** 231–242.
14. Hall, J. G. On the neuropathological changes in the central nervous system following neonatal asphyxia. With special reference to the auditory system. *Acta Otolaryngol., Suppl.*, 1963, **188:** 331–338.
15. Hall, J. G. The cochlea and cochlear nuclei in neonatal asphyxia. A histological study. *Acta Otolaryngol., Suppl.*, 1964, **194:** 6–93.
16. Huang, C.-M., and Buchwald, J. S. Multiple unit responses in cochlear nucleus and acoustic nerve during acoustic habituation procedures. *Anat. Rec.*, 1974, **178:** 379–380.
17. Hyman, A., Parker, B., Berman, D., and Berman, J. Delayed response deficits in neonatally asphyxiated rhesus monkeys. *Exp. Neurol.*, 1970, **28:** 420–425.

18. Kodman, F. The incidence of hearing loss in mentally retarded children. *Am. J. Ment. Defic.*, 1957, **62:** 675–678.
19. Lloyd, L. L., and Reid, M. J. The incidence of hearing impairment in an institutionalized mentally retarded population. *Am. J. Ment. Defic.*, 1967, **71:** 746–763.
20. Melzack, R. Effects of early experience on behavior: Experimental and conceptual considerations. In: *Psychopathology of Perception.* (P. H. Hoche and J. Zubin, Eds.). Grune & Stratton, New York, 1965: pp.271–299.
21. Norman, R. J., Villablanca, J. R., Brown, K. A., Schwafel, J. A., and Buchwald, J. S. Classical eyeblink conditioning in the bilaterally hemispherectomized cat. *Exp. Neurol.*, 1974, **44:** 363–380.
22. Regan, D., and Buchwald, J. S. Single unit response decrements in the inferior colliculus of decerebrate cats during repeated acoustic stimulation. *Proc. Soc. Neurosci.*, 1974, **4:** 389.
23. Riesen, A. H. Plasticity of behavior: Psychological aspects. In: *Biological and Biochemical Bases of Behavior.* (H. F. Harlow and C. N. Woolsey, Eds). Univ. of Wisconsin Press, Madison, 1958: pp. 425–450.
24. Saxon, S. V. Effects of asphyxia neonatorum on behavior in the rhesus monkey. *J. Genet. Psychol.*, 1961, **99:** 277–282.
25. Saxon, S. V. Differences in reactivity between asphyxial and normal rhesus monkeys. *J. Genet. Psychol.*, 1961, **99:** 283–287.
26. Sechzer, J. A. Memory deficits in monkeys brain damaged by asphyxia neonatorum. *Exp. Neurol.*, 1969, **24:** 497–507.
27. Sprague, J. M., Chambers, W. W., and Stellar, E. Attentive, affective and adaptive behavior in the cat. *Science*, 1961, **133:** 165–173.
28. Sprague, J. M., Levitt, M., Robson, K., Liu, C. N., Stellar, E., and Chambers, W. W. A neuroanatomical and behavioral analysis of syndromes resulting from midbrain lemniscal and reticular lesions in the cat. *Arch. Ital. Biol.*, 1965, **101:** 225–295.
29. Towbin, A. Mental retardation due to germinal matrix infarction. *Science*, 1969, **164:** 156–161.
30. Windle, W. F. Neuropathology of certain forms of mental retardation. Experiments on monkeys illustrate probable mechanisms of brain damage in human infants. *Science*, 1963, **140:** 1186–1189.
31. Windle, W. F. Brain damage at birth. *JAMA*, 1968, **206:** 1967–1972.
32. Windle, W. F., Jacobsen, H. N., de Arellano, R., and Combs, C. M. Structural and functional sequelae of asphyxia neonatorum in monkeys (*Macaca mulatta*). *Res. Publ. Assoc. Res. Nerv. Ment. Dis.*, 1962, **39:** 169–182.

11A

Discussion: Neurophysiological Substrates of Behavioral Habituation and Conditioning

CHARLES D. WOODY
Mental Retardation Research Center,
University of California Los Angeles,
Los Angeles, California

The observations reported by Dr. Buchwald are of considerable significance. The ability to produce auditory cued conditioned responses in a mesencephalic preparation sheds light on problems that have been previously raised by Bard and Macht (2) and by Mering of the Soviet Union (18). Before proceeding to further specific comments, however, I should like to address a few remarks to various dubiously related, but relevant aspects of the more general question of neurophysiological substrates of conditioning.

CONDITIONING IS DEFINITIONALLY OVERSIMPLIFIED, THE UNDERLYING PROCESSES ARE COMPLEX

Our task as neurobiologists is to simplify. But our nature, it seems, is to oversimplify. Also, science tends initially to be descriptive, and descriptive science, itself, can be oversimplistic. We may be just approaching the point where our understanding concerning conditioned behavior permits an awareness of some oversimplifications in this field.

Let us examine details of two particularly meritorious attempts to define aspects of classical conditioning. One states, reasonably enough, that an essential feature of classical conditioning involves the reliable evocation of a measurable unconditioned response by an unconditioned stimulus (13). This descriptive characterization must now be qualified in light of studies in which conditioning has been attempted in preparations in which the peripheral efferent nerves have been crushed. In such preparations, the unconditioned peripheral motor response does not occur during training, yet the animals learn a conditioned response which is indistinguishable from the usual type of conditioned behavior (3,7).

Another definitional attempt is appropriately concerned with the presence or absence of a response to the conditioned stimulus (CS) prior to training (16). The problem here is that the physiological level of the response in question may itself require stricter definition. That is, one may need to distinguish between responses at the level of postsynaptic potentials, nerve action potentials, muscle action potentials, and finally gross movement. Postsynaptic potentials are very likely generated in motor neurons by many types of CSs delivered in *naive* animals (35). Unitary action potentials generated by or in a single neuron in the motor cortex can lead to a measurable peripheral myographic response (34). Since neither of the above need be associated with any observed gross movement, one wonders if the generally accepted usage of "observable behavioral response" in the context of conditioning theory requires some modification. In addition, specific attempts to distinguish between alpha conditioning and classical conditioning on the basis of the presence or absence of observed responses prior to training should also note Pavlov's observations of salivary responses to metronome CSs in some of his animals prior to training (20).

Probably the complex nature of processes underlying conditioning also contributes to definitional confusion. An analogous problem has long been obvious in research on "schizophrenia" and the same may undoubtedly be said for "mental retardation." Even the application of some ostensibly simple, electrophysiological investigative techniques may be more complex (11,29) than some might recognize.

PARTITIONING COMPLEX PROCESSES ACCORDING TO SUBSETS OF UNDERLYING, CONSEQUENTIAL OPERATIONS MAY HELP THEIR ANALYSIS

What possible solutions may be sought to these problems? Most useful approaches (cf. 16,20) require recognition of consequential relationships between the underlying process-substrates and the observed behaviors. Thus, perhaps, the present session might have been entitled "Neurophysiological Substrates *Are* Behavioral Habituation and Conditioning."

It would appear useful to partition "learning" or "conditioning" into subsets of measurable "behavioral" operations deriving consequentially from corresponding sets of underlying processes or substrates mediated through selected populations of neurons. To take a specific example, the following partitioning may help to characterize conditioned blink reflexes resulting from pairing click-CS with glabella tap US.*

a. Certain specific stimuli such as the CS evoke the conditioned response after training while other stimuli do not (9).

b. The motor response evoked after conditioning is a specific one involving measurably specific patterns of muscle activity (37, cf. Figure 5).

c. Some changes must occur within the CNS such that the same physical stimulus which fails to produce a specific response prior to training does so afterward (33,36).†

DESCRIPTIONS OF SOME POTENTIALLY RELEVANT PROCESSES AND OPERATIONS

What processes and substrates might relate significantly to the above operations? A partial listing of some which might profitably be considered at present follows:

Temporal Contiguity

Processes that promote and underlie the development of persistent changes in affected neurons are poorly understood at present. However, "temporal contiguity," i.e., the specific temporal association between paired stimuli, appears to influence them significantly (see also 8). Temporal contiguities of 200–400 msec between associated stimuli appear to be near the optimum delays for efficient development of some key changes subserving conditioning (23). Note, however, that longer temporal contiguities are optimal for the development of other types of conditioning, such as those studied by Dr. Garcia (12). Differences in still other aspects of temporal contiguity, for example, the difference between trace and delayed conditioning, may produce other striking differences in the operational consequences of stimulus association (14).

Anatomical Representation

Another aspect of processes underlying conditioned behavior concerns their anatomical representation. Ostensibly and superficially similar conditioned behaviors can depend, anatomically, on quite different parts of the brain.

*Specific, related physiological operations are described in detail elsewhere (9,32–40).

†Some responses may occur initially, but they are of questionable motor specificity and do not persist with repeated stimulus presentation in contrast with the persistent, specific responses observed after training.

Small differences in stimulus character and temporal contiguity can, for example, lead to strikingly different operational consequences for the development of conditioned blinking, including differences in response latency and anatomical representation (cf. 4–6,40). Some types of conditioned blinking clearly depend upon processes subserved by neurons of rostal cortex (32,36). In contrast, blink conditioning of the type reported by Dr. Buchwald appears to depend upon processes subserved by neurons at brainstem levels. Those interested in cortical function may find the former type of conditioning of particular relevance, while those interested in performance subserved by isolated brainstem will prefer to investigate the latter. It is, parenthetically, paradoxical that the conditioned response in the "simpler" brainstem preparation, which might be expected to employ simpler circuitry, is of five to ten times longer reflex latency than is that in the intact preparation. The question of the minimal reflex circuitry (6) useful for physiological investigation is problematic. Response latencies as short as 12–20 msec (35,39) are much longer (even after subtracting known conduction delays) than the 0.3–0.6 msec required for each *synaptic* delay along the response pathway and hence still too long for some useful approaches to circuit analysis (21).

"Physiological Locus": Presynaptic Changes, Postsynaptic Changes, and Growth of New Connections

A third point of relevance to biological processes subserving conditioning is the "physiological locus" of the processes. We might wish to distinguish between various types of process-loci. One would involve pre- or intrasynaptic changes which could affect synaptic potency. With possible exceptions (e.g., "long-lasting" habituation phenomena in *Aplysia*) such processes appear to be concerned primarily with short-lasting changes. These include posttetanic potentiation, presynaptic inhibition, and common heterosynaptic facilitation (30). Rather analogous mechanisms may subserve habituation (10,26–28).

Another process-locus involves postsynaptic mechanisms which could affect cellular excitability. Although the work is still in its preliminary stages (34,36), there is some indication that such mechanisms may be involved in establishment of the motor specificity of some types of conditioned blinking.

Still another class of processes concerns those to do with new growth and differentiation of cells and their connections as described in earlier chapters in this volume. The role of such processes in adult learning remains to be demontrated. In complex computer automata, something must be held constant once adaptive, complex, learning-like processes are begun (1,19,22,24). My present bias as to what is held relatively constant in the adult human favors neuroanatomical connections which would, as set forth genetically and developmentally, provide appropriate bases for later interactions. The problem of how then would "switching functions" be accomplished in informational transactions within the adult brain is, as will be seen, easily resolved.

Functional Ensembles of Neurons

A fourth point characterizing processes subserving conditioning concerns the stochastic interaction of functionally related populations of neurons. It appears increasingly likely that coding and transmission of information relevant to the performance of very simple conditioned reflexes are subserved via changes in synaptic potency or cellular excitability over functionally related ensembles or sets of units (32). Unfortunately, it may be difficult to measure precisely changes in the processes of a single unit relevant to complex consequential behavioral operations because the magnitude of such changes appears to be quite small (34). Identification and sampling of many such elements within functionally related neuronal populations may be necessary if one is to demonstrate such changes. Identification and sampling of such functional ensembles appear to be afforded in cat motor cortex by establishing the motor projection of the neurons and in sensory cortex by establishing their sensory receptivity (9,33,37,38).

Temporal-spatial summation or ensemble averaging over functionally related neuronal populations is one medium through which the operational consequences of altered neuronal process-substrates is manifest. Notions that learning and memory might be subserved by diffuse processes have been around for some time (15,17,20). Ideas concerning coding (and "switching") of information via the *stochastic interactions* of neural ensembles are also not new (25,31). One wonders if comparable processes exist to be identified by those working in the area of cell growth and differentiation or in other areas within the field of research on mental retardation.

Substances and Mechanisms

A final consideration concerning processes underlying behavior concerns substrates underlying the processes themselves. Although in the last decade and a half progress has been made toward understanding some electrophysiological processes potentially involved with learning and plasticity, none of these processes is as yet explained biochemically. For process there is mechanism, and understanding of mechanism surely must depend upon knowledge of involved biochemical substrates and their interactions. It is just as easy for this to be overlooked in the content of psychophysiological investigation as it is for those who would define the substrates to overlook the proper psychophysiological context.

In conclusion, recognition of the complexity of processes and substrates that underlie conditioning is necessary if we are to formulate and pose the questions that must be asked, investigatively, to advance our understanding of conditioned behavior. There is also need to secure adequacy of measurement in attempting investigative solutions to any posed questions. Model or simplified systems and partitioning of complex processes according to their consequential operations may be useful in this regard, but one must nonetheless beware of oversimplification.

REFERENCES

1. Arbib, M. A. *Brains, Machines, and Mathematics.* McGraw-Hill, New York, 1964: 41–49.
2. Bard, P., and Macht, M. B. The behavior of chronically decerebrate cats. In *Ciba Foundation Symposium on the Neurological Basis of Behavior.* (G. E. W. Wolstenholme and C. M. O'Connor, Eds.). Little, Brown, Boston, Massachusetts, 1958: 55–75.
3. Beck, E. C., and Doty, R. W. Conditioned flexion reflexes acquired during combined catalepsy and de-efferentation. *J. Comp. Physiol. Psychol.,* 1957, **50:** 211–216.
4. Black-Cleworth, P. Conditioned blink acquired by pairing click and electrical stimulation of facial nerve. In: *Cellular Mechanisms Subserving Changes in Neuronal Activity.* (C. D. Woody *et al.,* Eds.). Brain Information Service/Brain Research Inst., UCLA, Los Angeles, 1974: 111–118.
5. Buchwald, J. S. Classical conditioning of the eyeblink response in the simplified mammalian central nervous system. In: *Cellular Mechanisms Subserving Changes in Neuronal Activity.* (C. D. Woody *et al.,* Eds.). Brain Information Service/Brain Research Inst., UCLA, Los Angeles 1974: 143–151.
6. Buchwald, J. S. Neurophysiological substrates of behavioral habituation and conditioning. Chapter 11, this volume.
7. Crow, T. J., and Woody, C. D. Acquisition of a conditioned eyeblink response during reversible denervation of orbicularis oculi muscles in the cat. *Brain Res.,* 1973, **64:** 414–418.
8. Doty, R. W. Discussion. In: *Brain Mechanisms and Learning.* (A. Fessard *et al.,* Eds.). Blackwell, Oxford, 1961: 659.
9. Engel, J., Jr., and Woody, C. D. Effects of character and significance of stimulus on unit activity at coronal-pericruciate cortex of cat during performance of conditioned motor response. *J. Neurophysiol.,* 1972, **35:** 220–229.
10. Farel, P. Habituation and persistent PTP of a monosynaptic response. In: *Cellular Mechanisms Subserving Changes in Neuronal Activity.* (C. D. Woody *et al.,* Eds.). Brain Information Service/Brain Research Inst., UCLA, Los Angeles 1974: 45–56.
11. Freeman, J. A., and Stone, J. A technique for current density analysis of field potentials and its application to the frog cerebellum. In: *Neurobiology of Cerebellar Evolution and Development.* R. Llinas, Ed.). Amer. Med. Ass. Educ. & Res. Found., Chicago, Illinois, 1969: 421–430.
12. Garcia, J., and Ervin, F. Gustatory-visceral and telereceptor-cutaneous conditioning: Adaptation in internal and external milieus. *Commun. Behav. Biol.,* 1968, **1:** 389–415.
13. Gormezano, I. Classical conditioning. In: *Experimental Methods and Instrumentation in Psychology.* (J. B. Sidowski, Ed.). McGraw-Hill, New York, 1966: 385–420.
14. Gormezano, I. The interstimulus interval and mechanisms for CS-CR functions in classical conditioning. In: *Cellular Mechanisms Subserving Changes in Neuronal Activity.* (C. D. Woody *et al.,* Eds.). Brain Information Service/Brain Research Inst., UCLA, Los Angeles 1974: 97–110.
15. Hebb, D. O. *The Organization of Behavior.* Wiley (Interscience), New York, 1949.
16. Kandel, E. R., and Spencer, W. A. Cellular neurophysiological approaches in the study of learning: *Physiol. Rev.,* 1968, **48:** 65–134.
17. Lashley, K. S. See: *The Neuropsychology of Lashley.* (F. A. Beach *et al.,* Eds.). McGraw-Hill, New York, 1960.

18. Mering, T. A. *Aspects of Conditioned Reflex Closure Involving Auditory Analyzers.* Med. Publ. House, Moscow, 1967: 1–155.
19. Minsky, M., and Papert, S. *Perceptrons. An Introduction to Computational Geometry.* MIT Press, Cambridge, Massachusetts, 1969.
20. Pavlov, I. P. *Conditioned Reflexes.* (G. V. Anrep, Transl. and Ed.). Oxford Univ. Press, London and New York, 1927.
21. Renshaw, B. Activity in the simplest spinal reflex pathways. *J. Neurophysiol.*, 1940, **3:** 373–387.
22. Rosenblatt, F. *The Perceptron.* Cornell Aeronaut. Lab., Cornell University, Ithaca, New York, 1958: Rep. UG-1196-G-1.
23. Schneiderman, N., and Gormezano, I. Conditioning of the nictitating membrane of the rabbit as a function of CS-US interval. *J. Comp. Physiol. Psychol.*, 1964, **57:** 188–195.
24. Selfridge, O. G. *Pandemonium: A Paradigm for Learning.* Armed Services Technical Information Agency (ASTIA) 1960: AD 236251; also JA-1140 (1958).
25. Siebert, W. M., and Communications Biophysics Group. *Processing Neuroelectric Data.* MIT Press, Cambridge, Massachusetts, 1959.
26. Spencer, W. A., Thompson, R. F., and Neilson, D. R., Jr. Response decrement of the flexion reflex in the acute spinal cat and transient restoration by strong stimuli. *J. Neurophysiol.*, 1966, **29:** 221–239.
27. Spencer, W. A., and Thompson, R. F., and Neilson, D. R., Jr. Alterations in responsiveness of ascending and reflex pathways activated by iterated cutaneous afferent volleys. *J. Neurophysiol.*, 1966, **29:** 240–252.
28. Spencer, W. A., Thompson, R. F., and Neilson, D. R., Jr. Decrement of ventral root electrotonus and intracellularly recorded PSPs produced by iterated cutaneous afferent volleys. *J. Neurophysiol.*, 1966, **29:** 253–274.
29. Stevens, C. F. *Neurophysiology: A Primer.* Wiley, New York, 1966: 161–173.
30. Tauc, L. Transmission in invertebrate and vertebrate ganglia. *Physiol. Rev.*, 1967, **47:** 521–593.
31. Woody, C. D. *Some Aspects of Information Processing in the CNS.* Honor's Thesis, Harvard Medical School, Cambridge, Massachusetts, 1962.
32. Woody, C. D. Aspects of the electrophysiology of cortical processes related to the development and performance of learned motor responses. *Physiologist*, 1974, **17:** 49–69.
33. Woody, C. D. Mechanisms underlying blink conditioning in the cat. In: *Cellular Mechanisms Subserving Changes in Neuronal Activity.* (C. D. Woody *et al.*, Eds.). Brain Information Service/Brain Research Inst., UCLA, Los Angeles 1974: 5–12.
34. Woody, C. D., and Black-Cleworth, P. Differences in excitability of cortical neurons as a function of motor projection in conditioned cats. *J. Neurophysiol.*, 1973, **36:** 1104–1116.
35. Woody, C. D., and Brozek, G. Changes in evoked responses from facial nucleus of cat with conditioning and extinction of an eye blink. *J. Neurophysiol.*, 1969, **32:** 717–726.
36. Woody, C. D., Carpenter, D., Knispel, J. D., Crow, T., and Black-Cleworth, P. Prolonged increases in resistance of neurons in cats motor cortex following extracellular iontophoretic application of acetylcholine (ACh) and intracellular current injection. *Fed. Proc.*, 1974, **33:** 399.
37. Woody, C. D., and Engel, J., Jr. Changes in unit activity and thresholds to electrical microstimulation at coronal-pericruciate cortex of cat with classical conditioning of different facial movements. *J. Neurophysiol.*, 1972, **35:** 230–241.
38. Woody C. D., Vassilevsky, N. N., and Engel, J., Jr. Conditioned eye blink: Unit activity at coronal-precruciate cortex of the cat. *J. Neurophysiol.*, 1970, **33:** 851–864.
39. Woody, C. D., and Yarowsky, P. J. Conditioned eye blink using electrical stimulation of coronal-pericruciate cortex as conditional stimulus. *J. Neurophysiol.*, 1972, **35:** 242–252.
40. Woody, C., Yarowsky, P., Owens, J., Black-Cleworth, P., and Crow, T. Effect of lesions of cortical motor areas on acquisition of conditioned eye blink in the cat. *J. Neurophysiol.*, 1974, **37:** 385–394.

Table II Parts of the Brain That Evidenced Learning at Stage II[a]

Brain Part	N[b]
1. Nonspecific thalamus	28
2. Posterior diencephalon	11
3. Central midbrain	17
4. Ventral nucleus	22
5. Dentate gyrus	35
6. Internal capsule	40
Questionable Evidence at this Stage	
1. Middle cortex	28
2. Posterior nucleus	11

[a] At the same time as behavioral signs of learning appeared. Stage II = learning at 20–30 trials.
[b] N = number of cases tested.

Table III Parts of the Brain That Evidenced Learning at Stage III of Behavior Learning[a]

Brain Part	N[b]
1. Posterior nucleus (or stage II)	11
2. Preoptic (excitatory)	11
3. Anterior midbrain	4
4. Caudate	8
5. Globus pallidus	16
Questionable Evidence at this Stage	
1. Lateral nucleus	13
2. Posterior cortex	13

[a] Stage III = learning at 30–40 trials.
[b] N = number of cases tested.

Table IV Parts of the Brain That Did Not Evidence Learning until Stage IV of Behavior Learning[a]

Brain Part	N[b]
1. Posterior cortex (or stage III)	12
2. Medial geniculate	9
3. Lateral nucleus (or stage III)	13
4. Middle cortex (or stage II)	28
5. Anterior pons (to cerebellum)	14
6. CA 3 (hippocampus)	38

[a] Stage IV = learning at 40–50 trials.
[b] N = number of cases tested.

Table V Parts of the Brain That Did Not Evidence Learning until Stage V of Behavior Learning[a]

Brain Part	N[b]
1. Frontal cortex	22
2. Dorsomedial nucleus	17
3. CA 1 (hippocampus)	34
4. Subiculum (hippocampus)	40

[a] Stage V = learning at 50–70 trials.
[b] N = number of cases tested.

learned responses in the association centers of the thalamus lost their dubiousness and became pronounced.

At phase four, when the behavior became smooth and fast, new responses appeared for the first time in the auditory cortex (see Table IV). There were also important upsurges in responses recorded from the medial geniculate, from the association cortex, from the pontine region which forms a link between cortex and cerebellum, and also from the main field of the hippocampus, that is, the CA 3 field.

During the fifth phase as behavioral changes became complete, there were still three parts of the brain which seemed to go on learning (see Table V). The first of these was the frontal cortex. The second was the dorsomedial nucleus of the thalamus which is correlated with the frontal cortex. The third was the main output field of the hippocampal cortex, that is, the CA 1 field. Because motor cortex and frontal association cortex are overlapped in the rat, it is not clear whether this late learning (after behavior learning was complete) was correlated with these motor output functions or with association functions. However, it is tempting to suppose that it was association centers that were involved and that this was some kind of consolidation process.

While these data validated some older ideas about the different functions of different areas, their main importance was to show that a main requirement of the method would work. The method needed different brain areas to "learn" at different rates. They did so and the differences seemed to be large ones.

AUDITORY TUNING

Training caused the signal to branch off into new pathways at almost every auditory station. It also caused preexisting responses in the auditory stations to be modified, usually to be amplified or enhanced. Besides both of these, there was also a substantial change in the background firing rate, the so-called spontaneous discharge rate of neurons in some of the auditory stations.

The Lower Auditory Centers

Responses recorded from the eighth nerve, the cochlear nucleus, and the superior olive all began within 3 msec of the arrival of the auditory signal at the ear (see Figures 5 and 6). The average data taken from 19 highly responsive probes in the cochlear nucleus and the eighth nerve did not show any important effects of training. The same was true for ten responsive probes implanted in the superior olive. However, there were individual cases where improvement, even in the first 1–3-msec part of the cochlear nucleus response, did occur (see Figure 7). The probes were responsive in the first place, highly responsive. The improvement amounted to about 30%. Because these were small proportionately, and because they did not show up in the overall average, I would have some inclination to doubt whether the real effects of conditioning reached down this far. However, because of data from Weinberger's laboratory (Norman M. Weinberger, University of California, Irvine, private communication) that evoked potential changes occurred in the cochlear nucleus in the curarized cat, I take them seriously and will explore these centers further.

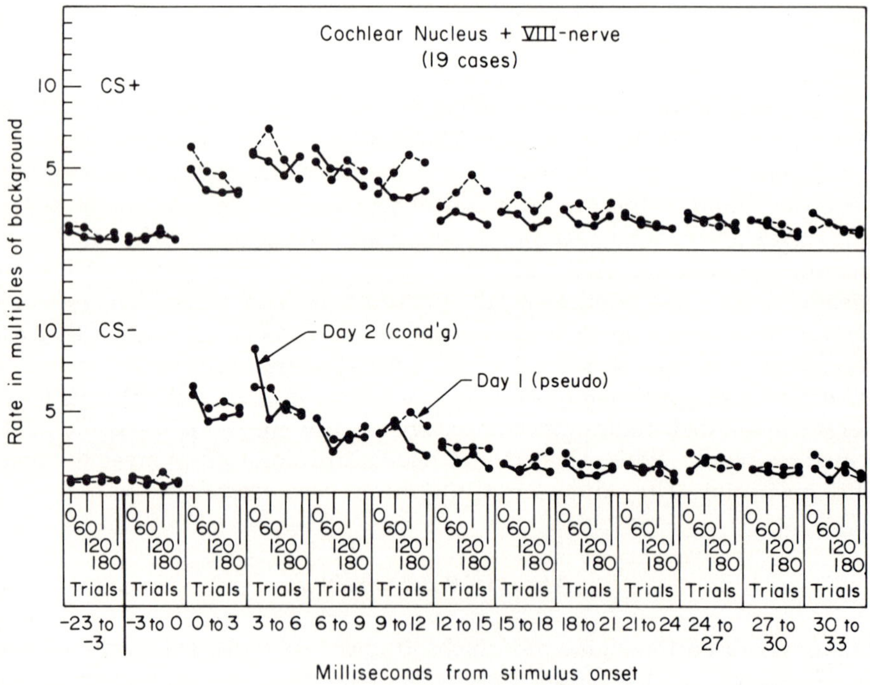

FIGURE 5. Average cochlear nucleus and eigth nerve response during pseudoconditioning (– – – –) and conditioning (———). Each group of four points stands for the neuron firing rate in a particular latency interval. Each of the points is the score for a particular 60-trial block. For the solid curves, the first point is the 60 trials before conditioning, and the other three are the successive blocks of conditioning.

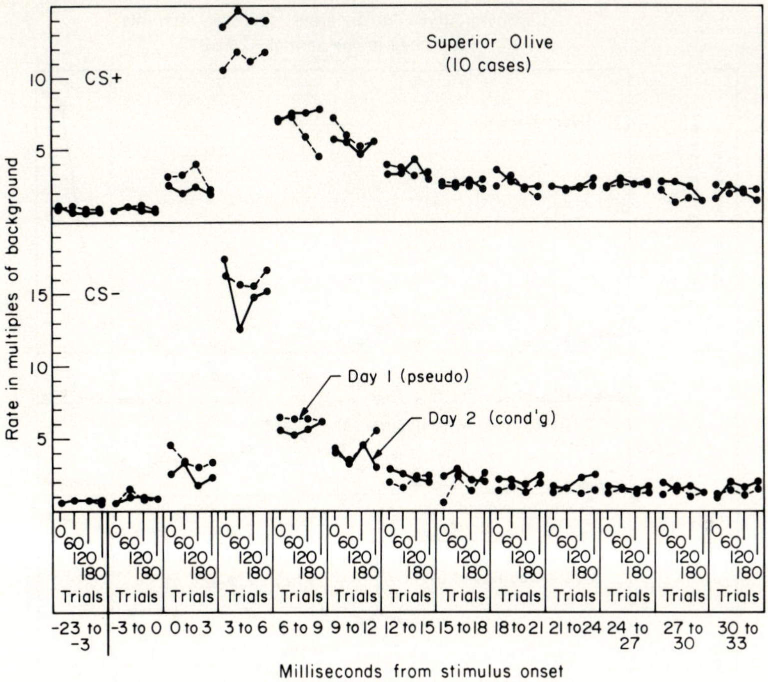

FIGURE 6. Average superior olive response during pseudoconditioning (– – – –) and conditioning (———). The details are the same as in Figure 5.

The Inferior Colliculus

At the level of the inferior colliculus, the response to the auditory signal began during the second 3-msec interval after arrival of the signal at the ear, but it reached its peak 3 to 6 msec after that. The average taken from 47 responsive probes implanted in the inferior colliculus showed an augmentation by conditioning of the average peak response (see Figure 8). This occurred in spite of the fact that in a full third of the cases, there was a substantial trend in the opposite direction. When averages were taken from a specially selected 21-member subgroup from which all cases without the main effect were eliminated, several main trends were obvious (see Figure 9). First, the average response of these neurons was about doubled during the second 60 responses of conditioning. Second, increased responsiveness appeared even in the 3–6-msec latency time period; thus the improvement could not have been fed back after the message had advanced to higher centers. Third, there was a tendency at the end of the day, at a time when motivation was lower, for the responses in the inferior colliculus to fall off. Fourth, there was no appreciable trend of any kind on day 1 during pseudoconditioning. Fifth, although there was no trend of change in the course of pseudoconditioning, there was a sub-

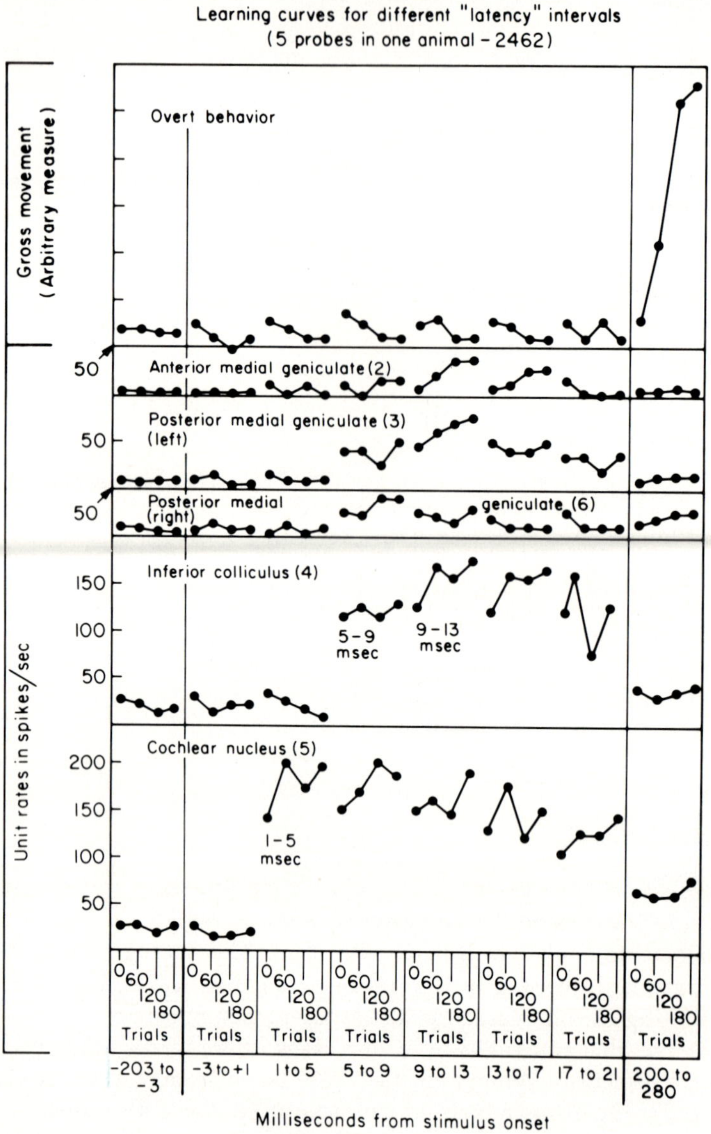

FIGURE 7. Behavioral response and five individual brain probe responses for the same rat during conditioning. The details are as in Figure 5.

stantial improvement between pseudoconditioning on the first day and pseudoconditioning on the second day. This was not a chance occurrence. It was not restricted to just these 21 cases, as you will see later. What caused this substantial change?

Something which occurred on the first day must have had an effect even

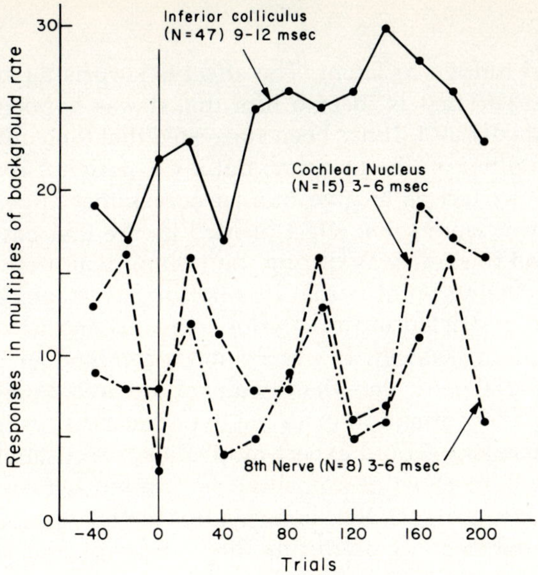

FIGURE 8. Average responses for the inferior colliculus, cochlear nucleus, and eighth nerve during conditioning. Each curve is for just one latency interval (as marked); this was the one that showed the greatest improvement during conditioning. The trials before and after the start of conditioning are marked on the baseline.

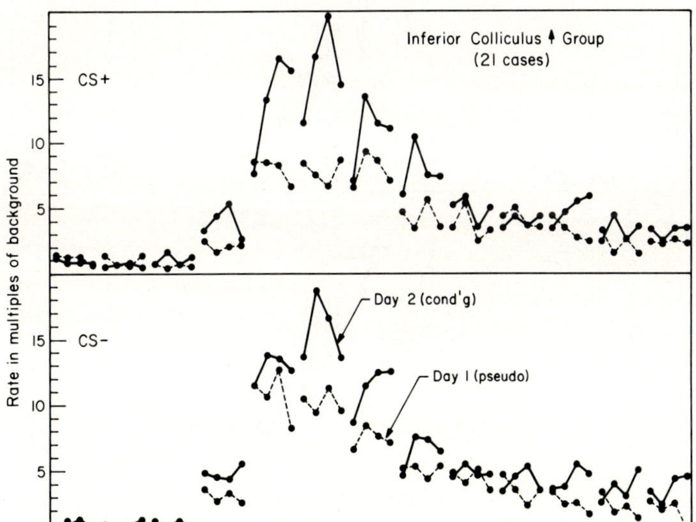

FIGURE 9. Average response of 21 "augmented" inferior colliculus probes during pseudoconditioning (– – – –) and conditioning (———). The details are the same as in Figure 5.

though it stayed hidden or latent. The effect is surprising and interesting for several reasons. The first is that no hint that it was happening could be observed in the data of day 1. It has been suggested that there might be two effects canceling one another on the first day; but my experience is that the canceling could not be so perfect as to give the flat curves that appeared. Therefore it looks to me as if it were some effect planted by the first day's training which then consolidated in some way during the 11-hour wait between experiments. The second interesting point is that it is not by any means a general effect in the brain. It was restricted to the inferior colliculus and to very closely linked parts of the auditory system. It was far more common in the colliculus and maybe in the medial geniculate than in any of the linked neighbors. It did not occur in the reticular formation or in the hypothalamus, or in any of the parts of the brain where one would expect motivational arousal effects. It seems to me that if it were an effect of a positive association between this signal and food, or of a negative association between this signal and food (both of which could be conceived as going on during the first day of pseudoconditioning), it

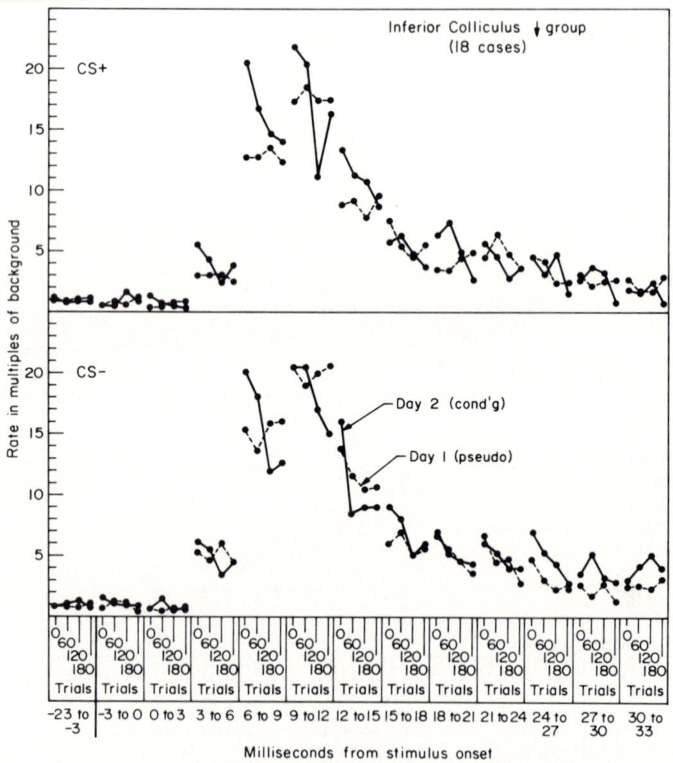

FIGURE 10. Average response of 18 "diminished" inferior colliculus probes during pseudoconditioning (– – – –) and conditioning (———). The details are the same as in Figure 5.

should have been reflected one way or another in arousal or motivational regions. Our other data give good evidence that motivational and arousal emanating from a signal do get reflected in hypothalamus and in the reticular formation. Therefore I am inclined to reject these and to believe that this effect in the auditory system has something to do with familiarization; the animal becomes familiar with this stimulus and possibly "learns" to perceive it. The seeds are planted on the first day. But the effect has a delayed onset. This is a speculation that will need to be tested by eliminating the other possible motivational influences.

The averages from 18 colliculus cases whose responses were diminished by conditioning gave a picture that was inverse in several respects (see Figure 10). There was a 30–50% diminution in the peak response. That the diminution was caused by conditioning was attested by its absence on day 1. Like the augmentation it occurred even in the 3–6-msec latency interval, and it was attenuated during the last 60 trials of the day. In one respect, however, these opposed cases were not the inverse. There was the same substantial rise in amplitude between the day-1 pseudoconditioning tests and day-2 pseudoconditioning tests. The day 1 − day 2 difference was thus the most dependable finding we have come upon so far (whatever it may mean).

The Nucleus of the Trapezoid Body

Whatever else it may mean, it suggests that something happened on day 1 which was not exhibited in the responses of neurons in the inferior colliculus. Were there any neurons that showed substantial response changes on day 1? Yes. The most marked of these occurred in an auditory station below the colliculus in the anatomical chain but coming after the colliculus in the latency chain (see Figure 11). It could be a station that receives messages after they have circuited through the upper brain and then returned, although it looks to be in a place to receive collaterals from neurons of the cochlear nucleus (and maybe even from the eighth nerve). This is the nucleus of the trapezoid body. It is on the boundary of the decussating nerve fibers on their way from the cochlear nucleus to the superior olive. It is adjacent to the nucleus gigantocellularis of the medullary reticular formation, and the latency of its auditory responses (6–12 msec) and their plasticity seem to label it as a part of the reticular formation. It is tempting to suppose it receives collaterals from the trapezoid auditory fibers but that its plastic synapses somehow slow down the message. That's really a romantic notion with little likelihood, but it is attractive all the same. A group of 13 cases chosen more or less anatomically were averaged. There was a shade of a response here at 3–6 msec. A better but still minimal response at 6–9 msec, and then a definite response at 9–12 msec. Even the 9–12 msec response was pretty much absent at the beginning of pseudoconditioning. It grew over the course of the day. The overall response

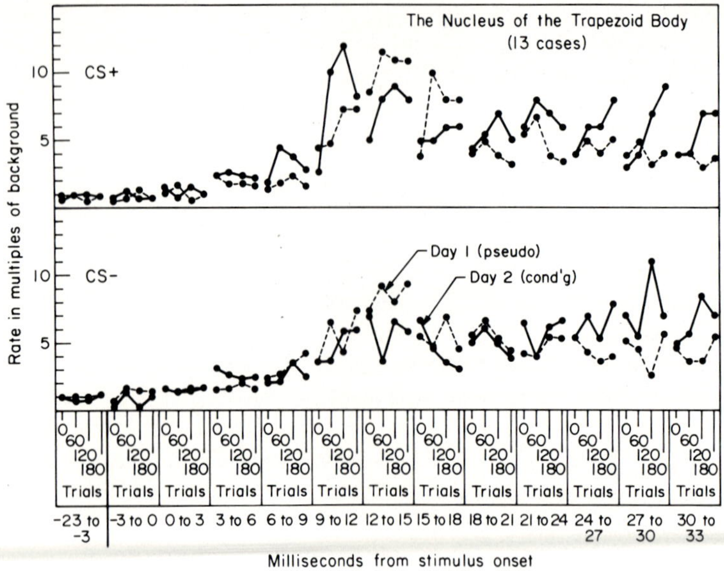

FIGURE 11. Average trapezoid nucleus response during pseudoconditioning (----) and conditioning (———). The details are the same as in Figure 5.

gained so much in size as to suggest an order of magnitude change during the pseudoconditioning procedure. The improvement that accrued during the course of the pseudoconditioning trials then disappeared completely during the day 1–day 2 interval but reasserted itself on the second day. The improvement during pseudotraining and the loss during the time between sessions made this the inverse of the inferior colliculus. But both areas pointed to a happening on the first day.

The Thalamus

The neurons of the posterior thalamic nucleus were far less responsive to these mild tones (20 dB) with "stabilized auditory images" than they were to the intense tones (70–80 dB) from a wall loudspeaker which had been used in previous experiments (2). The average response at the height of conditioning was barely double the background rate (see Figure 12). In this case, however, there was no sign of the response in the averages from day 1. The latency of these responses, however, fell between 15 and 18 msec. This put them substantially behind new responses in other parts of the brain and permitted the interpretation that conditioned responses here have a secondary status.

In individual cases with probes on the boundary between the medial geniculate and the posterior nucleus there were much earlier learned responses (with 9–13-msec latency) which also arose *de novo* from previously unre-

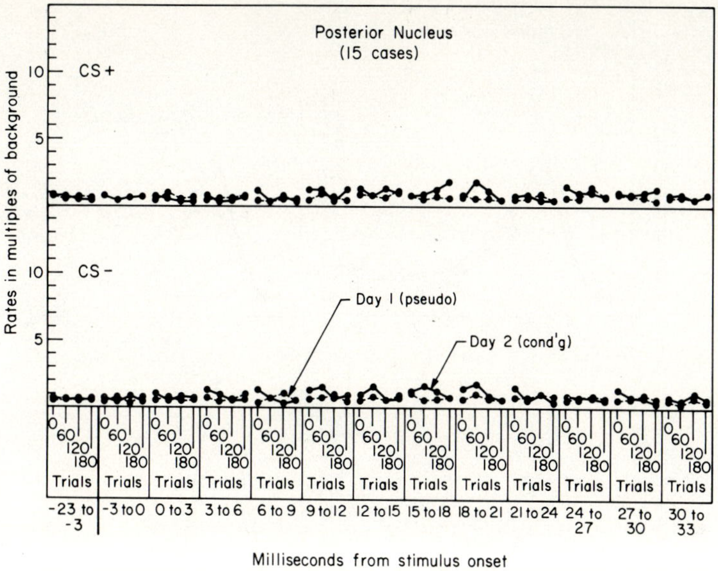

FIGURE 12. Average posterior nucleus response during pseudoconditioning (– – – –) and conditioning (———).

sponsive probes during the course of conditioning (see Figure 7). I am not yet in a position to give a general picture of the data for the medial geniculate and the auditory cortex. The data are collected but the probes still need to be located, categorized by response, and averaged.

The Reticular System

Data from a similar, but not identical, experiment of Montplaisir (9) showed that neurons of the pontine reticular formation had learned responses whose latencies also fell in the 9–10-msec range. In this case, pseudoconditioning and conditioning tests were made successively on the same day (120 trials of pseudoconditioning followed by 120 trials of conditioning) and there were intense auditory signals from loudspeakers mounted about 1 foot from the head. The peak response of these neurons came 6–9 msec after the onset of the signal (5–8 msec after its arrival at the ear). This response was already substantial even before conditioning (amounting to about 7 times the background firing level). It was not changed appreciably by habituation. But it was doubled by conditioning (see Figure 13). The effect was large and the data were convincing because they were all gathered on one day. Did these account for the changes in the auditory centers? It is unlikely that they could account for the changes in the inferior colliculus. The latter appeared in the 3–6-msec interval even

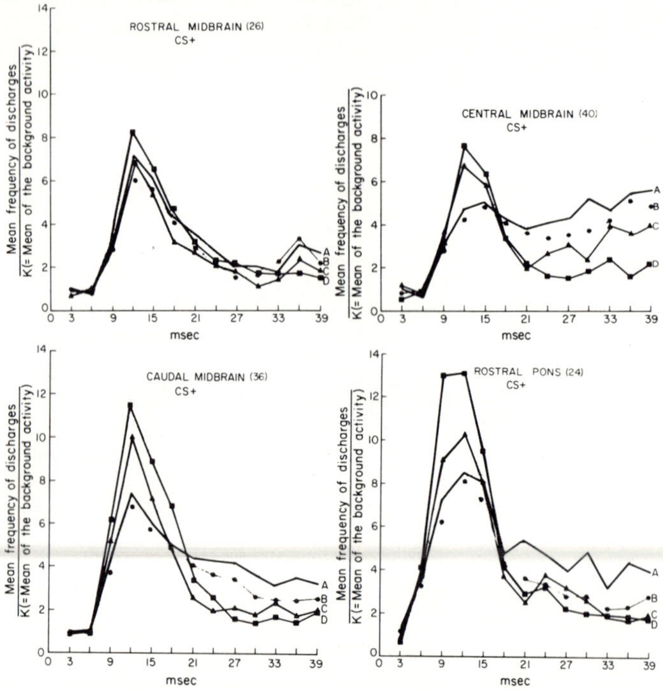

FIGURE 13. Averaged responses for different groups of reticular formation probes during pseudoconditioning and conditioning. On the baseline are marked the end times of the latency intervals. There were 120 trials before conditioning and 120 trials during conditioning. A = first 60 trials before. B (●) = second 60 before. C (▲) = first 60 of conditioning. D (■) = final 60.

with a very mild tone; and these appeared in a 5–8-msec interval with a very intense tone. Thus they did not likely stand behind the colliculus changes.

DYNAMIC TRACES

What do you suppose did stand behind the changes in the inferior colliculus, and those in other lower auditory centers? My first guess would be that there was some special bombardment emanating from the cortex and that the kind of switches involved were dynamic ones that would flop back after the cessation of the cortical process.

The message from the cortex might be either an excitatory or an inhibitory one. And it might be applied either like presynaptic inhibition, or postsynaptically as either a facilitatory or inhibitory input. If training changed the background firing level of cortical units and if these innervated the auditory input channels, this would suffice to explain some of the changes observed.

My first guess would be that each channel from the ear to the cortex (whether it be a frequency channel or a channel based on some other auditory feature) might have, not only its private line to the cortex, but the specialized cortical cells at the end of the line might be in a position both to respond to and to gate the signals in the channel. This is guessed mainly on the basis of anatomical evidence that seems to show this kind of organization. If a small set of cortical cells were involved, they might be hard to find.

To answer the question of whether anything like this happens, I have to refer back to the older data which, as I said previously, were flawed. These are the learning curves for the different brain areas which sum all neuronal activity during the CS–US interval and thus are susceptible to contamination by movements. As previously, I justify use of these data by the fact that data from all brain areas should be equally contaminated by movements, and yet the different brain areas gave quite different changes during learning.

Did the cortex show any changes in background activity during learning? Was it different in this regard from other parts of the brain? The answer on both scores is "yes." Let us look at changes in background rates during conditioning. The background level of movement (see Figure 2) is seen to decline during the period of conditioning (this is sad, because it puts a pall over the cortex data). Although movement scores exhibited this change in background level, it was not reflected in many of the brain centers. In the motivation centers, arousal centers, and extrapyramidal motor centers, training caused only brief changes in background firing rate and left them well within control ranges (see Figure 3). The main effect of training in these cases was to cause a widening gap between the firing rate caused directly by stimulation and the background firing rate. Only in the cortex was there a stable and sustained change in the background firing rate itself (see Figure 4). During the first two stages of training, this was the only change observed in the cortex. There was about a 25% decline in the average background spiking rate of these auditory cortex neurons. At first, the activity rate during the CS–US interval fell along with the background. They stayed parallel for the first, second, and third stages (during the period when interest, attention, and then purpose were already beginning to characterize the learned behavior). This leaves the impression that if cortex participated at all during this period, it did so by its changes in background firing, not by its changed responses. Then, during the fourth and later stages, the responses to the auditory signal began to rise, even though the background rates remained depressed. It was appealing to suppose therefore that these neurons in auditory cortex first reduced their background rate (or perhaps their connection to other irrelevant noises) and then increased their connection to the special auditory signal that had just acquired a new meaning. While it is of course possible that slowing of these cortex neurons was just a reflection of the behavioral change, another possibility must also be taken seriously. The decreased spontaneous discharge rate might be part of an

siveness to the CS− and a gain to the CS+, the events could not be ascribed entirely to the motive change.

What part of the brain mediated this behavioral improvement? The answer is that no part of the brain tracked the behavioral changes very well. Tests were made with probes in the cortex, in the hippocampus, and in the nonspecific centers of the thalamus. Only in the cortex were there day 1 to day 2 improvements in responsiveness to the CS+; but in this case there were also lesser improvements in the response to the CS− (see Figure 15). The latter would be looked on as "spontaneous recovery" of an extinguished response if it appeared in behavior. However, it did *not* appear in the behavior, and taken together with the improvement in the cortex response to the CS+ it looked like a special property of cortical connections might be to grow (or to grow back—like weeds). In any event, the cortex yielded correlates of the behavior to the CS+ but not of that to the CS−. Were there any correlates of behavior loss to the CS−? Yes. These occurred in both hippocampus and in the thalamic recordings (see Figure 16). In hippocampus, the response to the CS+ stayed in place during the time-out period. But the response to the CS− disappeared. In thalamus there was a special change on day 1 that deserves comment. The responsiveness to both the CS+ and the CS− improved when

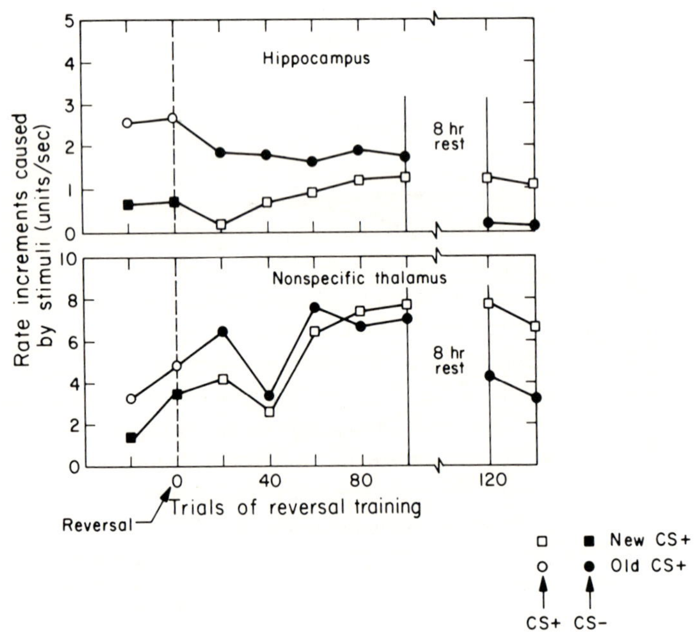

FIGURE 16. Hippocampus and thalamus unit responses before and after reversal of CS+ and CS−. The details are the same as in Figure 15. The data are from as yet unpublished work by J. Disterhoft and M. Segal.

the reversal experiment began. This suggested that things became especially interesting to this part of the brain when there was associative switching going on. In any event, thalamus, like hippocampus, yielded some loss of responsiveness to the CS− during the time-out, but no gain to the CS+.

These three observations of changes during time-out were not aimed at this problem. They need repetition, therefore, with careful controls. Just observing such changes does not point directly to a growth or consolidation of connections. But the fact that they take such different shapes and directions in different parts of the brain (even in very closely connected parts of the brain as in the parts of the hippocampal circuit) makes them very promising. If there are some connections that are planted by learning and which then grow as a function of time, it should be easy to discover them. And if there are entirely temporary changes that disappear as a function of time it may even be possible to identify them.

SUMMARY

The aim is to find some switches in the brain and to characterize them if possible as either temporary and requiring some reverberatory process or as more stable and structural.

There were five assumptions involved: (a) that the very large population of neurons in the brain could be effectively sampled in a limited set of experiments; (b) that a middle kind of electrodes could direct themselves to a sufficiently stable single unit population to permit extended conditioning experiments; (c) that averaging could be used to eliminate the effects of all unwanted variables that were not correlated with the main auditory signals; (d) that latency mapping would permit the tracing of a signal even through the multiple-channeled pathways of the brain (and would help us to identify switching points); (e) that a middle kind of conditioning (not Pavlovian entirely nor Skinnerian entirely) could be used to get us the rapid learning of a Skinner experiment with the clear CS of a Pavlovian one.

To permit the separation of the links of a message chain to help us find a larger number of the plastic coupling points it was hoped that different parts of the brain would "learn" at different rates. This did happen to some degree, different functional systems in the brain showing their changes at times when their functions were most relevant; hypothalamus changed when the signal was reacquiring interest. The arousal system changed when the signal caused orienting responses. The extrapyramidal system changed when the signal caused purposive behavior.

After this, the search for the shortest latency new responses led surprisingly, or not (depending on your point of view), to the very early stations of the auditory system. Clear learned responses were not proved for the shortest latency components of the responses in the first and second stations (the cochlear nucleus and the superior olive), but they were not excluded either. Learning did characterize the first (3–6 msec) part of some responses in the inferior colliculus. In this case it was mainly an amplification of a preexisting response already of substantial magnitude before training. In the medial geniculate, learned brain responses with a latency of 9–12 msec arose *de novo*. In the nucleus of the trapezoid body and the reticular formation there were learned responses of similar latencies.

Interesting response changes occurred during pseudoconditioning in the inferior colliculus and the trapezoid nucleus. The colliculus had stable responses on the first day, but then a marked improvement demonstrated after an 11-hour rest period. This suggested some latent change created or planted on the first day which then was developed or consolidated during the intertest interval. The trapezoid body responses showed learning scores that were almost as good on the first day during pseudoconditioning as on the second day during conditioning. But in this case the improvement was lost during the long intertest interval.

A search for dynamic processes, i.e., changes in background firing rates, that could account for the changes in lower auditory centers pointed in preliminary tests to the auditory cortex where conditioning was accompanied by a drop in the general background firing rate.

Finally, changes that occurred during an 11-hour intertest interval suggested that the time-out method may distinguish dynamic from structural traces: the dynamic ones might disappear with time; the structural ones may well grow or become consolidated. The experiments demonstrating such effects so far are contaminated to some degree because there was a major change in the motive state during the time-out periods. But planned experiments aimed explicitly at this should pay good dividends.

REFERENCES

1. Disterhoft, J. F. Unit response in the auditory system and posterior thalamus of rat during classical conditioning and extinction. *Proc. 2nd Annu. Meet. Soc. Neurosci.*, 1972: 84.
2. Disterhoft, J. F., and Olds, J. Differential development of conditioned unit changes in thalamus and cortex of rat. *J. Neurophysiol.*, 1973, **35:** 665–679.
3. Disterhoft, J. F., Stuart, D. K., and Olds, J. Emergence of changed unit responses in the auditory system of the alert rat during classical conditioning. *Fed. Proc.*, 1973, **32:** 383.
4. Frank, K., and Fuortes, M. G. F. Presynaptic and postsynaptic inhibition of monosynaptic reflexes. *Fed. Proc.*, 1957, **16:** 39–40.
5. Globus, A., and Scheibel, A. B. The effect of visual deprivation on cortical neurons: A Golgi study. *Exp. Neurol.*, 1967, **19:** 331–345.
6. Kornblith, C., and Olds, J. Unit activity in brain stem reticular formation of the rat during learning. *J. Neurophysiol.*, 1973, **36:** 489–501.
7. Linesman, M. A., and Olds, J. Activity changes in rat hypothalamus, preoptic area, and striatum associated with Pavlovian conditioning. *J. Neurophysiol.*, 1973, **36:** 1038–1050.

8. Llinas, R., and Nicholson, C. Electrophysiological properties of dendrites and somata in alligator Purkinje cells. *J. Neurophysiol.*, 1971, **34:** 532–551.
9. Montplaisir, J., and Olds, J. Conditioned responses in the reticular formation. *Proc. 3rd Annu. Meet. Soc. Neurosci.*, 1973: 115.
10. Olds, J. Brain mechanisms of reinforcement learning. In: *Pleasure, Reward and Preference.* (D. E. Berlyne and K. B. Madsen, Eds.). Academic Press, New York, 1973: 35–63.
11. Olds, J., Disterhoft, J. F., Segal, M., Kornblith, C., and Hirsh, R. Learning centers of the rat brain mapped by measuring the latencies of conditioned unit responses. *J. Neurophysiol.*, 1972, **35:** 209–219.
12. Olds, M. E. Short-term changes in the firing pattern of hypothalamic neurons during Pavlovian conditioning. *Brain Res.*, 1973, **58:** 95–116.
13. Rescorla, A. Pavlovian conditioned inhibition. *Psychol. Bull.*, 1969, **72:** 77–94.
14. Segal, M. Flow of conditioned responses in the limbic telencephalic system of the rat. *J. Neurophysiol.*, 1973, **36:** 840–854.
15. Segal, M., Disterhoft, J. F., and Olds, J. Hippocampal unit activity during classical aversive and appetitive conditioning. *Science*, 1972, **175:** 792–794.
16. Segal, M., and Olds, J. Behavior of units in hippocampal circuit of the rat during learning. *J. Neurophysiol.*, 1972, **35:** 680–690.
17. Wiesel, T. N., and Hubel, D. H. Comparison of the effects of unilateral and bilateral eye closure on cortical unit responses in kittens. *J. Neurophysiol.*, 1965, **28:** 1029–1040.

12A

Discussion: "Operant Sensitization" and Some Remarks on Unit Recording in Conscious Animals

S. STEFAN SOLTYSIK

Mental Retardation Research Center,
University of California Los Angeles,
Los Angeles, California

I admire Dr. Olds' work and am especially fond of his "organizing ideas." They may not represent the only logical outcome of his observations, but they do, indeed, emerge as a very elegant and highly inspiring product of both his data and his personal taste and biases. And I share them wholeheartedly, the more so that many of them fit so neatly with my own prejudices which I acquired while experimenting in the field of classical and instrumental conditioning. For lack of time, I shall mention only one idea that was generated by behavioral experiments carried out in Warsaw and for which I have found in Dr. Olds' data a converging of evidence coming from the electrophysiological experiments. The idea of changing threshold for a stimulus rewarded with food has been developed during the instrumental conditioning of "involuntary" responses, and in this discussion, I intend to couple it with Dr. Olds' demonstration of what he calls "receptor tuning."* Following early experiments of Fedorov (1), Yakovleva (9), and Kupalov (5), Jankowska, and I (4) observed that when a tactile stimulus (eliciting a scratch reflex) is rewarded with food, a hyperesthesia develops in the location of the stimulation. It may occasionally develop to such an extent that the animals ignore food for a while and continue

* Earlier studies by Hernandez-Péon *et al.* (3), Galambos (2), and others who used evoked potential techniques were clouded by the controversy over uncontrolled variations of the auditory input due to the animal's changing position of the head in relation to the source of sound (6). Dr. Olds copes with this problem by delivering the sound through a divided tube attached to the head of the animal.

striving to remove an imaginary object from the skin. This lowering of threshold for reflexes from a receptive field, the stimulation of which was paired with a reward, is restricted to the experimental situation and is not carried over to the home cage. It is, however, under the control of a drive, and the animal must be hungry for this phenomenon to occur reliably. These features prompt me to suggest a name for the phenomenon, namely, "operant sensitization."

Dr. Old's data showing an enhancement of unit response to an auditory stimulus in the cochlear nucleus, if not in the cochlear nerve itself, after this stimulus was consistently paired with food, gives strong support to one of three possible mechanisms. Fedorov and Yakovleva faithfully recalled Pavlov's theory of instrumental conditioning and located the learning change in the connection between cortical taste and kinesthetic (for a scratch response in this case) analyzers. Kupalov (5) also considered the involvement of sensory cortex representing tactile receptive field for a scratch reflex. Jankowska and Soltysik (4) on the basis of the observation that the training resulted in an increased frequency of not only the rewarded scratch reflex, but also other reflexes from the same receptive field (such as shaking the head and pricking the ears) hypothesized that the facilitation must occur at the very low relay stations in the afferent pathway. It is worthwhile to point out in this connection that such "operant sensitization" occurring due to, as I now like to believe, "receptor tuning" may offer some clues to both positive and negative findings in the elusive field of visceral operant conditioning. The findings of Russian authors and ourselves* show that it is possible to bring under operant control an involuntary reflexlike response if the experimental design favors the development of "operant sensitization," namely, if a reward follows a stimulus that elicits this response. Dr. Old's concept of "receptor tuning" extended also, of course, to low afferent relays, although not yet explaining how it occurs, gives the evidence of why and where in the CNS the sensitization is brought about. On the other hand, failures in visceral conditioning of this kind might be related to the experimental design which ignores the stimuli controlling a given "involuntary" response.

To conclude my afterthoughts, I would like to express my sincere admiration for the ingenious way Dr. Olds executes single neuron recording during a 2-day long learning procedure. It is not the sharpness of his electrodes, but the acuity at the other end of the recording equipment that enables him to scan the brain in search for plastic changes on the level of single or almost single units. But admitting that collecting data with his method offers tremendous assets, I would like to express my belief that the traditional way of extracellular single unit recording may also have its virtues. One sees less with a

* The credit for the first attempts of operant conditioning of a scratch reflex should be given to Thorndike (7), who described behavior of cats which were allowed to escape from the cage by scratching themselves.

sharp microelectrode, but may spot more details in behavior of the same cell throughout the recording epoch. To illustrate this and to contribute to this meeting by presenting new data, let me show you just two units, one from the caudate nucleus and one from a globus pallidus of a monkey which performs a task involving a delay of an instrumental response (Figure 1). The trial lasts long enough to observe changes in the firing rate of a unit during several consecutive epochs of the entire behavioral sequence: (a) during the control period "C" prior to the onset of a light stimulus, (b) immediately after the stimulus onset "S," (c) during the delay "D," (d) during the last 2 seconds before a response when the anticipatory or preresponse behavior occurs "Pre-R," (e) during the first second after the response "Post-R," and finally, (f) during the feeding behavior "F." By averaging the records of several trials, the exact course and statistical reliability of impulse rate modulations was assessed. Figure 2 shows a caudate unit [the dorsolateral part of the caudate at the A 21 according to the "Stereotaxic Atlas" of Winters, Kado, and Adey (8)] averaged over 25 behavioral trials. Typically, it exhibited a very low firing rate, but showed an unusual correlation with several phases of behavior: probably an on-response to light, increased and levelled firing rate during the delay, rise of firing before the response and a high peak immediately after a response. Only 20% of our caudate units have shown such an interest in more than two epochs. Half of the caudate neurons in our monkeys do not modulate firing rate during the trial, and of the remaining half, a great majority show modulations associated only with one or two of the enumerated epochs of the behavioral sequence. The pallidal units (Figure 3) are different in several ways. They have much higher firing rates and almost all of them show modulation of firing frequency associated with at least 2 or 3 phases of

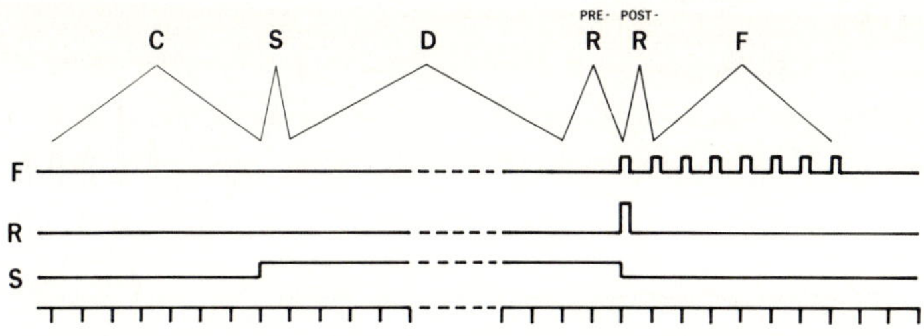

FIGURE 1. The schematic representations of a trial shows how the entire sequence of events was divided into epochs, or behavioral responses. The trial starts with presenting a light stimulus which continues until the animal pulls the bar; only the response performed after 8 seconds from the onset of light is rewarded. Typically, the monkey, after an orienting response to the light, waits 8 to 12 seconds and then responds. Somewhat arbitrarily, we enumerated 5 behavioral epochs: C, the control period prior to the light stimulus; S, 1 second after the onset of light; D, the delay; Pre-R, two seconds before the responses; Post-R, 1 second after the response; and F, drinking the juice. The deviation of firing rate (measured in 500 msec bins) exceeding three standard deviations was considered as a significant response.

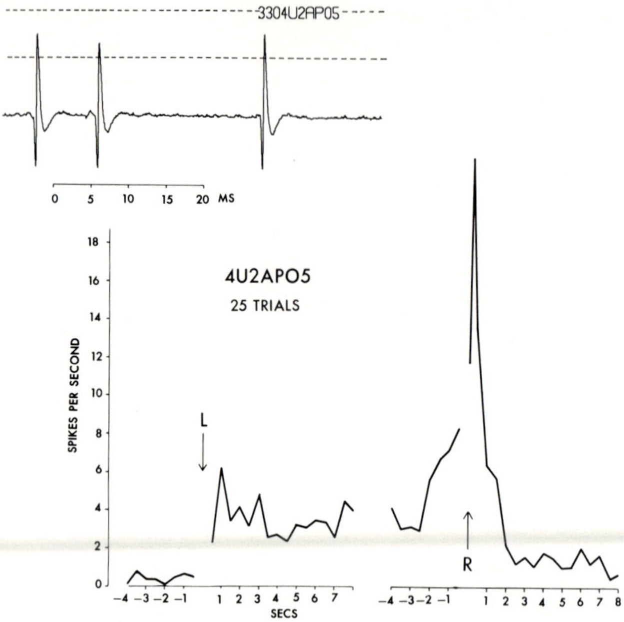

FIGURE 2. The firing rate changes during the trial in a caudate neuron. This is an atypical caudate unit showing significant deviations from the slow intertrial firing level during several epochs.

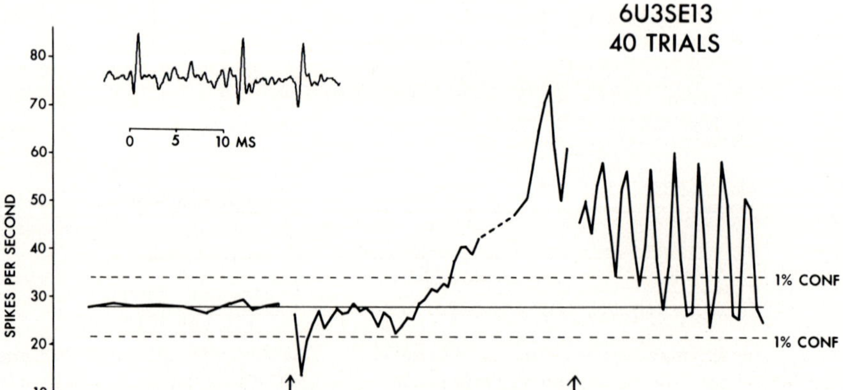

FIGURE 3. Pallidal unit from the border of internal and external segment. Typically, this unit shows changes of firing frequency during many epochs and particularly, a rhythmic oscillation during drinking grape juice, delivered in 1/second jets into the mouth.

the same behavioral sequence. Perhaps the most striking is the tendency of our pallidal units to follow faithfully the rhythm at which we deliver the jets of juice into the monkey's mouth as a reward. Note that the unit firing is averaged over 40 trials and the oscillations during drinking exceed 20 spikes per second.

The point I want to make is that caudate neurons reflect in their firing rates only one or at most two aspects of a complex behavioral sequence, whereas pallidal units show modulations in the firing rate correlated with several phases of the same behavioral sequence. Since both caudate and pallidum show considerable heterogeneity in neuronal firing, these details of unit behavior might easily get lost with recording technique not strictly limited to one unit at a time.

ACKNOWLEDGMENT

The data presented above are from work conducted jointly with N. A. Buchwald, C. D. Hull, T. Fekete, and A. Uyeda.

REFERENCES

1. Fedorov, V. K. Basic principles of mutual influences between various motor reactions. (In Russian.) *Fiziol. Zh. SSSR,* 1952, **38:** 559–565.
2. Galambos, R. Electric correlates of conditioned learning. In: *The Central Nervous System and Behavior.* First Conference. (M. A. B. Brazier, Ed.). Josiah Macy, Jr. Found., Madison Printing Co., Madison, New Jersey, 1959: 375–415.
3. Hernandez-Péon, R., Scherrer, H., and Jouvet, M. Modifications of electrical activity in cochlear nucleus during "attention" in unanesthetized cats. *Science,* 1956, **123:** 331.
4. Jankowska, E., and Soltysik, S. Motor conditioned reflexes established from unconditioned motor reflexes reinforced by food. (In Russian.) In: *Tsentral'nye i Perifericheskie Mekhanizmy Dvigatel'noi Deyatel'nosti Zhivotnykh.* Izd. Akad. Nauk SSSR, Moscow, 1960: 61–69.
5. Kupalov, P. S. Involuntary reactions to conditioned food stimuli. (In Russian.) In: *Trudy Ob'edinennoi Sessii, Posv. 10-letiu so dnia Smerti I.P. Pavlova.* Izd. AMN SSSR, Moscow, 1948: 67–78.
6. Marsh, J. T., Worden, F. G., and Hicks, L. Some effects of room acoustics on evoked auditory potentials. *Science,* 1962, **137:** 280–282.
7. Thorndike, E. L. *Animal Intelligence.* Macmillan, New York, 1911.
8. Winters, W. D., Kado, R. T., and Adey, W. R. *A Stereotaxic Brain Atlas for Macaca nemestrina.* Univ. of California Press, Berkeley, 1969.
9. Yakovleva, V. V. Establishment of conditioned reflexes to a complex kinesthetic stimulus (to the so-called involuntary movements). (In Russian.) *Zh. Vssh. Nerv. Deiat.,* 1952, **2:** 305–316.

AGE

Stages of Cognitive Development

The concept of stages in human cognitive development is most closely identified with the work of Jean Piaget (28,39). Although the observation that human beings demonstrate increasing competence for intellectual abilities with age is perhaps as much a statement of universal experience as of scientific fact, there exists an extensive experimental literature on the subject. A particularly interesting example of age-dependent changes in intellectual functioning is that of conservation—in Piagetan terms, the ability to maintain a concept of equality in the face of sensory appearances. For instance, if a quantity of water is poured from a container of one size and shape into another of different dimensions, adults and children above the age of 6 or 7 will understand that the quantity of water in the second container is exactly the same as in the first container. Quite reliably, however, children under the age of 6 or 7 will believe that there has been a change in quantity (4,5,52).

One need not adhere to the conceptual framework of Piaget to find evidence of chronological steps in cognitive development. Satz and Van Norstrand (46) have recently reviewed some of the evidence indicating sequential and hierarchical development of perceptual, spatial, and verbal skills with age. Lenneberg (34) has also presented evidence for ontogenetic milestones in the emergence of language. Although developmental psychologists differ greatly on a number of issues related to the child's acquisition of conceptual skills (6,8,28,40), the evidence from a variety of sources forces recognition of an orderly and successive attainment of intellectual achievements with age.

In contrast to the plentiful bounty of studies on cognitive development in children, very few studies have been concerned with this subject in laboratory animals. For facts about cognitive development in infrahuman primates, we must turn to the pioneering investigations of Harlow (25,26). From such studies we know that infant monkeys can be conditioned to avoid shock as early as the fourth day of life and can learn to perform simple spatial and visual discriminations within the first few weeks of life. However, monkeys do not demonstrate full maturation of object discrimination capacity until they are 5 months of age. At about this same time, monkeys begin to perform delayed-response problems but adult levels of proficiency apparently are not reached until the end of the first year of life and beyond. Maturation of the skills involved in learning-set performance may not be complete until the end of the second year of life and even by 3 years of age, monkeys have not yet shown adult-level efficiency in learning still more complex oddity problems. According to Harlow (25), 4 or 5 years may not be an unreasonable estimate for the length of time required for monkeys to achieve full intellectual maturity. These findings may be regarded as evidence for stages of cognitive development in monkeys paralleling those in man.

Structural Considerations

It seems reasonable to assume, and indeed, has been so assumed widely, that the maturation of the nervous system underlies the emergence of ever increasingly complex mental activities. Yet, it is difficult to say precisely which parameters of the central nervous system mature when, and in what structures, to permit a child to conserve quantity or to allow a monkey to locate a reward that has been concealed from view. Many studies of central nervous system maturation quite reasonably pertain to events either of the embryonic or early postnatal periods [e.g., studies of the thalamus (11,44,56); of the cortex (9,31,41) of connections (10)]. Although modern techniques are replacing classic methods in unraveling the intricacies of neurogenesis, cell migration, and cell differentiation (1–3,12,43,47), these anatomical events still antedate functional maturity, at least in the primate, by months and years. Events, like myelination, that do extend into the postnatal years are known only in broad outline. Thus, Flechsig (15) described the basic plan by which myelination of the sensory and motor regions of the primate brain precede myelination of the association areas—a plan which Geschwind (16) has related to the phylogenetic origins of language. Yakovlev and Lecours (55) elaborated on cycles of myelinogenesis. Fiber systems of brain regions may myelinate early or late in fetal life and whether originating early or late, myelination may proceed rapidly or slowly. The cycle of myelinogenesis, they suggest, is an important parameter of regional maturation and may extend, in the case of intracortical neuropil of association cortex, into and past the third decade of life.

With respect to long-term development, it is difficult to say that we have gone far beyond the broad outlines layed down by Flechsig (15) and Yakovlev and Lecours (55). Many gaps remain in the knowledge of the structural features that are elaborated in the interval between birth and functional maturity to confer upon the association cortices, for example, their ultimate functional capacities and evidence of a neurological basis for stages of cognitive development is, as yet, unspecific and indirect.

Neural Basis of Cognitive Development

Since children and monkeys demonstrate increasingly complex cognitive capacity at different stages of development, it should at least be possible to demonstrate correlative maturation of particular neural structures with advancing age. Behavioral observations of monkeys raised from infancy without certain parts of their frontal lobes have provided some evidence that cortical areas of the primate brain do develop at different times after birth and in relation to the development of cognitive skills (7,19,20,36). It would appear from these studies that the orbital prefrontal cortex, for example, becomes functionally significant at or before 1 year of age, while the dorsolateral prefrontal cortex shows a slower and more protracted course of development.

Evidence for the late development of the dorsolateral cortex is shown in Figure 1. The curves present the mean scores (with ranges) for independent groups of operated and unoperated monkeys tested on delayed response for the first time when they were 12, 24, or an average of 31 months of age. In all experimental subjects, the dorsolateral prefrontal cortex as described in Goldman (19) had been removed bilaterally at least 10 months prior to testing. The lesions were completely comparable in the two groups of monkeys tested at the earliest and latest ages (19). The monkeys tested at 24 months are still alive and their lesions have therefore not been analyzed. Comparing the performance of the operated and unoperated groups at 31 months of age confirms the well-known finding that dorsolateral prefrontal lesions result in severe impairments on delayed response. However, the degree of impairment produced by such lesions declines with decreasing age—at 24 months of age, some monkeys with dorsolateral prefrontal areas removed in infancy perform as well as unoperated controls while others are severely impaired. Still earlier, at 12 months of age, the effect of the lesion virtually disappears as operated monkeys perform as well as unoperated controls. Figure 2 presents findings for another related measure, delayed alternation, given to the same animals approximately three months later at 15, 27, and 34 months of age. Again, the significance of the dorsolateral cortex for behavior changes with age. While the scores of operated and unoperated monkeys overlap considerably at 15 months of age, by 27 months, there is complete separation between the scores of the two groups. At 34 months of age, the divergence is more pronounced.

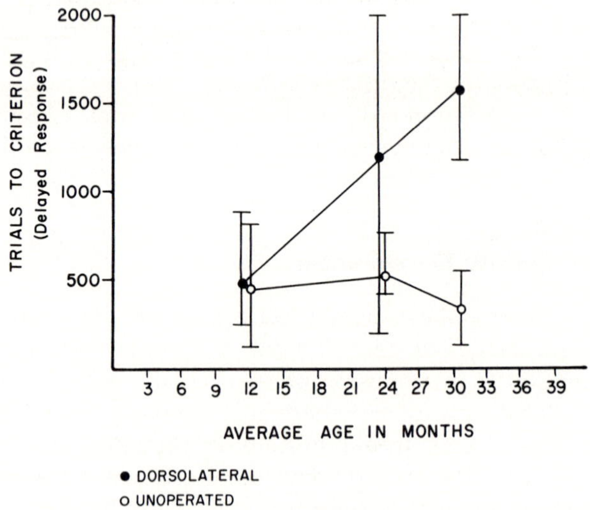

FIGURE 1. Curves showing mean delayed response performance of operated and unoperated groups at 12, 24, and an average of 31 months of age. Each point is based on four monkeys except in the case of the 12-month unoperated control group where $n = 9$. Brackets indicate ranges.

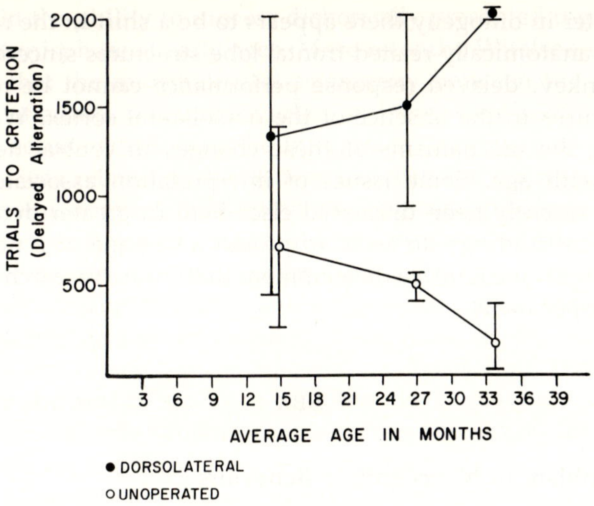

FIGURE 2. Curves showing mean delayed alternation performance of the same groups as in Figure 1 approximately 3 months later at 15, 27, and an average of 34 months of age. Brackets again indicate ranges.

At this last age, operated monkeys, without exception, fail to learn the task within the limits of training while the unoperated monkeys achieve criterion performance in an average of 170 trials. The finding that the differences between the two groups continues to increase beyond 2 years of age indicates that the dorsolateral cortex does not become fully functional until after 2 years of age. The additional fact that operated monkeys show increasing rather than static deficits with age further indicates that normally structures other than the dorsolateral cortex may mediate delayed-response behavior before the dorsolateral cortex matures.

Some suggestions as to which structures may be important at earlier stages of development is given by considering the status of brain structures other than the dorsolateral cortex at selected points along the age continuum described in Figures 1 and 2. Monkeys given orbital prefrontal lesions in infancy have been tested on delayed response and delayed alternation at 12 and 15 months of age, respectively (19,36). Monkeys raised from infancy with lesions in the anterodorsal sector of the head of the caudate nucleus (22) and in the dorsomedial nucleus of the thalamus (21) have similarly been studied under identical conditions at the same ages. All such groups were impaired on delayed alternation and all but the group with thalamic lesions were impaired on delayed response at 12 and 15 months of age, when monkeys with dorsolateral lesions were not. These findings provide evidence that the orbital prefrontal cortex, the head of the caudate nucleus and the dorsal thalamus are functionally mature at the 1-year stage of development and could mediate delayed response functions

41. Rabinowicz, T. Quantitative appraisal of the cerebral cortex of the premature infant of 8 months. In: *Regional Development of the Brain in Early Life.* (A. Minkowski, Ed.). Davis, Philadelphia, Pennsylvania, 1964: 91–124.
42. Raisman, G., and Field, P. M. Sexual dimorphism in the neuropil of the preoptic area of the rat and its dependence on neonatal androgen. *Brain Res.,* 1973, **54:** 1–29.
43. Rakic, P. Neurons in rhesus monkey visual cortex: Systematic relation between time of origin and eventual disposition. *Science,* 1974, **183:** 425–427.
44. Rose, J. E. The ontogenetic development of the rabbit's diencephalon. *J. Comp. Neurol.,* 1942, **77:** 61–129.
45. Rosenzweig, M. R. Effects of environment on development of brain and behavior. In: *Biopsychology of Development.* (E. Tobach, Ed.). Academic Press, New York, 1971: 303–342.
46. Satz, P., and Van Norstrand, G. K. Developmental dyslexia: An evaluation of a theory. In: *The Disabled Learner: Early Detection and Intervention.* (P. Satz and J. Ross, Eds.). Univ. of Rotterdam Press, Rotterdam, 1973: 212–248.
47. Sidman, R. L. Autoradiographic methods and principles for study of the nervous system with thymidine-H^3. In: *Contemporary Research Methods in Neuroanatomy.* (W. J. H. Nauta and S. O. E. Ebbesson, Eds.). Springer-Verlag, Berlin and New York, 1970: 252–274.
48. Sluckin, W. *Imprinting and Early Learning.* Aldine, Chicago, Illinois, 1965.
49. Towbin, A. *The Pathology of Cerebral Palsy.* Thomas, Springfield, Illinois, 1960.
50. Valenstein, E. S., Cox, V. C., and Kakolewski, J. W. Sex differences in hyperphagia and body weight following hypothalamic damage. *Ann. N. Y. Acad. Sci.,* 1969, **157:** 1030–1046.
51. Valenstein, E. S., Kakolewski, J. W., and Cox, V. C. Sex differences in taste preference for glucose and saccharin solutions. *Science,* 1967, **156:** 942–943.
52. Wallach, L. On the bases of conservation. In: *Studies in Cognitive Development, Essays in Honor of Jean Piaget.* (D. Elkind and J. H. Flavell, Eds.). Oxford Univ. Press, London and New York, 1969: 191–219.
53. Wender, P. *Minimal Brain Dysfunction in Children.* Wiley, New York, 1971.
54. Witelson, S. F., and Pallie, W. Left hemisphere specialization for language in the newborn: Neuroanatomical evidence of asymmetry. *Brain,* 1973, **96:** 641–646.
55. Yakovlev, P. I., and Lecours, A. R. The myelogenetic cycles of regional maturation of the brain. In: *Regional Development of the Brain in Early Life.* (A. Minkowski, Ed.). Davis, Philadelphia, Pennsylvania, 1964: 3–70.
56. Yamadori, T. The developmental study of the thalamic nuclei in the Japanese fetus. *Kobe J. Med. Sci.,* 1961, **7:** 1–25.

13A

Discussion: Effects of Caudate Nuclei Removal versus Frontal Cortex Lesions in Kittens

JAIME R. VILLABLANCA

*Mental Retardation Research Center,
University of California Los Angeles,
Los Angeles, California*

I will briefly report on our results in kittens with large brain lesions, either cortical or subcortical. It did not take us very long to become aware of the many technical difficulties and potential shortcomings of the lesion method as applied to the study of the developing brain; the many difficulties and unavoidable hardships pertaining to the research in this area render Dr. Goldman's studies even more meritorious.

Our interest has focused on studying the effects of cortical versus subcortical brain lesions in newborn animals, as well as in comparing the magnitude and characteristics of recovery of the resulting defects with those of similar lesions inflicted in the adult animal. In the long range, our aim is the better understanding of the mechanisms involved in recovery processes following early injury to the brain.

A review of the literature reporting the effects of cortical lesions in newborn animals indicates, in general, that such injuries cause much less severe functional deficit and allow much more recovery than similar lesions inflicted in adulthood (1,3,4,7,11,12,18,20,22,24–26).

The knowledge regarding the effects of subcortical experimental brain lesions in the newborn is more limited since far fewer reports dealing with this problem have been published (10,13,15,17,23). An influential piece of work in this area has been the report by Kling and Tucker (17) that lesions destroying 10–50% of the caudate nuclei in newborn monkeys produced devastating neurobehavioral effects. Furthermore, the deterioration of the monkeys was progressive, since four of the animals died within 6 weeks and the remaining three, with the smallest lesions, were maintained with great difficulties for up to 3 months. Since lesions of comparable extension have been performed in adult monkeys (2,6,21) without the deleterious consequences observed in the newborn, the conclusion resulting from this experiment was that subcortical brain lesions inflicted early in life have a much worse outcome than similar lesions inflicted in adulthood and are also relatively more detrimental than early cortical lesions.

Dr. Goldman (9), as well as other authors (14,16,18), has presented evidence indicating that the time course of the effect of early brain injury may not be as simple as that suggested above, i.e., steady progressive recovery or steady progressive deterioration of function. Instead, according to their data, a reversal of the trend prevalent up to a given point in time may occur along with further development. This important observation strongly emphasizes the need for a long follow-up of the experimental animals, into adulthood if possible, in order to be able to make meaningful statements. Unfortunately, not complying with this requirement may be an important drawback in many of the developmental brain lesion studies up to now.

We have attempted to test in newborn kittens the possibility raised by the Kling and Tucker experiments quoted above that the early lesion of a subcortical structure, like the caudate nucleus, may have a more marked impact upon neurobehavioral development than pure cortical damage. The cortical area selected for comparison was the frontal region. The results of similar lesions to these structures in adult cats, reported elsewhere in this volume (27), have provided us with a baseline for evaluating the kittens lesion effects as well as of the age variable in the final outcome of the injuries. Our strategy has been to ablate as much of the caudate or frontal cortical areas as possible in order to avoid masking compensatory effects by remaining portions of these structures and with the intention of initially disclosing gross functional defects. Hopefully, the eventually larger, unequivocal defects resulting from extensive ablations will guide us in the future in a finer grain analysis of the consequences of localized lesions.

The surgical techniques used to ablate the caudate nuclei, as well as the frontal cortical areas in kittens, were similar to those used in adult cats (27).

A battery of neurological tests was applied periodically to all operated kittens and to their littermate controls to assess their neurobehavioral status. In addition to the items in the description of our similar studies in adult cats (27), the following aspects were also assessed: tail position, opening of eyelids, blink reflexes, auditory startling and orienting, rooting reflex, play activity, thermoregulatory shivering, and pendular head movements. The kittens' gross behavior has been assessed during frequent observations in their home cages, with their littermates and mother, and in an open field in the laboratory. In addition, the development of the kittens' motor activity has been quantified (19) by recording their movements in an open field (by means of a sensitive force transducer, from birth to 21 days, or by using multiple photocell beams, from days 21 to 62) and their basic learning abilities have been evaluated in a T-maze where the animals were trained to make a black-white discrimination and to perform a position reversal task. Some of the kittens are now being tested in a passive-avoidance paradigm and the older ones are beginning the bar pressing training, previously used to study adult BAc or BFr cats (28).

Very briefly, the results are as follows:

1. Bilateral removal of the caudate nuclei has been successfully accomplished in 14 kittens (BAc), and bilateral removal of the frontal cortical areas has been performed in five kittens (BFr). The average age of all lesioned animals at the time of surgery was 18.3 days, with a minimum of 7 and a maximum of 35 days. Four of the BAc kittens died at 68, 88, 105, and 115 days after surgery, respectively, because of intercurrent diseases similarly affecting their littermates. The remaining ten BAc kittens, as well as all the BFr kittens, are still alive and in good health. To date, the average survival time of all animals is 98 days, with three of the BAc kittens having reached puberty (over 7–10 months of age).

2. The only histological material available to date belongs to the four deceased kittens mentioned above. Two of these brains showed almost complete removal of the caudate nuclei (95 and 100% of caudate tissue removed, respectively), with little damage to other brain areas (Figure 1), whereas the other two brains had a partial, asymmetric ablation.

3. All kittens were up, walking, and nursing, either the same day of surgery or the following day; only five of them required supplemental tube feeding for 1–3 days.

4. Ten of the BAc kittens exhibited a behavior similar to the "compulsory approaching syndrome" (CAs) seen in adult BAc cats (27). This was an impressive change, particularly in the smallest kittens, since prior to surgery they stood and walked hesitantly and weakly, and yet the day following surgery they would eagerly and strongly approach and follow the investigator or an object in a stereotyped manner for many minutes; they would also come back to the investigator when repeatedly pushed away, as did the adult BAc cats. The main difference between the CAs in the kitten when compared with similar phenomenon in the adult cat was its shorter duration; indeed, in the kitten the CAs was usually clearly present from 1 to 4 days and thereafter progressively decreased such that by the tenth postoperative day it was no longer present. A fainter, shorter lasting, auditory approach could be elicited, whereas no manifestations of tactile approaching could be induced in the BAc kittens.

In the four kittens for whom the brains were available for histology, there was a clear, positive correlation between the amount of caudate removal and the magnitude of the CAs; one of them, with only about 30% of caudate nuclei removed, did not exhibit any CAs at all, whereas the syndrome was very pro-

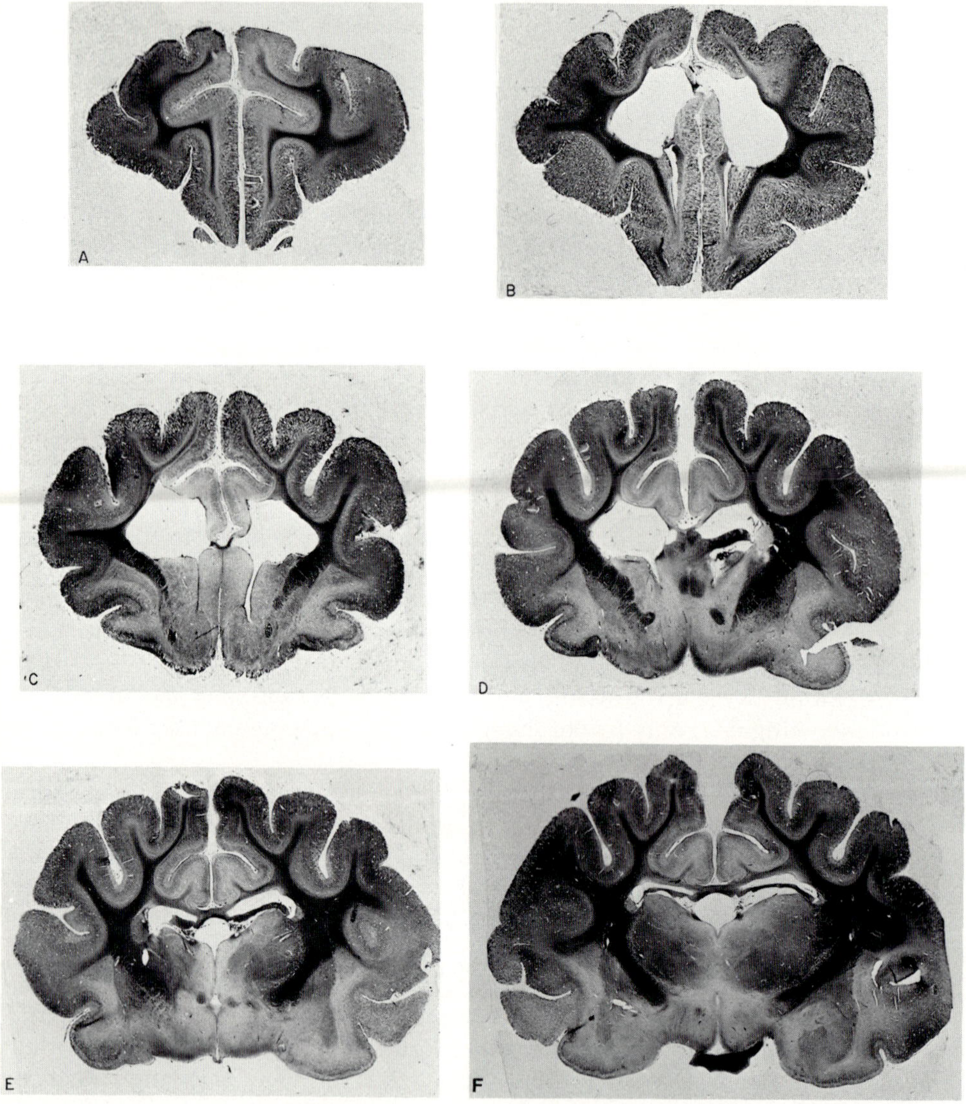

FIGURE 1. Histological sections of the brain of a kitten at 133 days of age with bilateral removal of the caudate nuclei performed at 18 days of age. Weil-stained frontal sections at frontal (A–B), septal-fornix (C–D), and anterior thalamic (E–F)levels.

nounced in the two kittens with almost total removal. The BFr kittens did not exhibit any stereotyped approaching; however, most kittens in both groups displayed stereotyped visual tracking of pendular motion, similar to BAc and BFr adult cats (27), which also persisted for a short period (1–4 days).

5. Neither the BAc nor the BFr kittens have shown any gross neurobehavioral abnormalities after the early postoperative period had elapsed. However, there is some indication that the maturation of several neurological parameters under observation may be delayed; these findings are being verified in ongoing studies.

The comparison with their littermates at each testing session has been the most reliable criterion to evaluate the performance of the brain-lesioned kittens, since part of our normative data on intact kittens was in discrepancy with similar data from other investigators (1,8). The development of the limb placing reactions, particularly the contact placing reaction, deserves special mention in this respect. Our experience has been that this is a function which develops progressively in normal kittens and does not become fully mature until the third or fourth month of age. A similar, although delayed time course, occurred in the operated kittens. This finding, which is consistent with the marked inability of young kittens to walk on planks or approach edges without falling, is in contrast with reports from other authors (1,5,8) that the contact placing reaction is developed during the first days of life.

6. The BAc kittens readily learned the basic T-maze discrimination task. However, they behave differently from their littermates in that they had difficulties in learning the reversal aspects of the task, as demonstrated by their strong tendency to persist in the response producing the last reinforcement, a perseverative defect also exhibited by the adult BAc cats (28). The preliminary data on motor activity measurements have not revealed gross differences in the development of the motor activity patterns of BAc and BFr kittens in relation to their littermates (19).

In summary, the above data suggest that in the cat: (a) subcortical brain lesions in infancy do not produce any more severe defects than early cortical injuries do; (b) although both cortical and subcortical brain lesions are followed by a striking recovery, our ongoing observations indicate that there may be a retardation in neurological maturation; and (c) finally, these experiments demonstrate that, unlike the findings in monkeys (17), bilateral, almost total ablation of the caudate nuclei can be done in kittens and these animals can be maintained in good health for indefinite periods of time.

ACKNOWLEDGMENT

Supported by USPHS Grant Nos. MH-07097, HD-05958, and HD-04612. This research was carried on in collaboration with Drs. R. J. Marcus, C. E. Olmstead, and M. S. Levine, Department of Psychiatry, UCLA.

REFERENCES

1. Amassian, V. E., Ross, R., and Donat, J. Development of contact placing and thalamocortical organization in kittens. *Fed. Proc.*, 1971, **30:** 434.
2. Battig, K., Rosvold, H. E., and Mishkin, M. Comparison of the effects of frontal and caudate lesions on delayed response and alternation in monkeys. *J. Comp. Physiol. Psychol.*, 1960, **53:** 400–404.
3. Beach, F. A. The neural basis of innate behavior: Relative effects of partial decortication in adulthood and infancy upon the maternal behavior of the primiparous rat. *J. Genet. Psychol.*, 1938, **53:** 109–148.
4. Benjamin, R. M., and Thompson, R. F. Differential effects of cortical lesions in infant and adult cats on roughness discrimination. *Exp. Neurol.*, 1959, **1:** 305–321.
5. Bignall, K. E., and Schramm, L. Behavior of chronically decerebrated kittens, *Exp. Neurol.*, 1974, **42:** 519–531.
6. Davis, G. D. Caudate lesions and spontaneous locomotion in the monkey. *Neurology*, 1958, **8:** 135–139.
7. Doty, R. W. Functional significance of the topographical aspects of the retino-cortical projection. In: *The Visual System: Neurophysiology and Psychophysics.* (R. Jung and H. Kornhuber, Eds.). Springer-Verlag, Berlin and New York, 1961: 228–245.
8. Fox, M. W. Reflex development and behavioral organization. In: *Developmental Neurobiology.* (W. A. Himwich, Ed.). Thomas, Springfield, Illinois, 1970: 553–580.
9. Goldman, P. S. Functional development of the prefrontal cortex in early life and the problem of neuronal plasticity. *Exp. Neurol.*, 1971, **32:** 366–387.
10. Goldman, P. S., and Rosvold, H. E. The effects of selective caudate lesions in infant and juvenile rhesus monkeys. *Brain Res.*, 1972, **43:** 53–66.
11. Goldman, P. S., Rosvold, H. E., and Mishkin, M. Selective sparing of function following prefrontal lobectomy in infant monkeys. *Exp. Neurol.*, 1970, **29:** 221–226.
12. Harlow, H. F., Akert, K., and Schlitz, K. A. The effects of bilateral prefrontal lesions on learned behavior of neonatal, infant and preadolescent monkeys. In: *The Frontal Granular Cortex and Behavior.* (J. M. Warren and K. Akert, Eds.). McGraw-Hill, New York, 1964: 126–148.
13. Isaacson, R. L., Nonneman, A. J., and Schmaltz, L. W. Behavioral and anatomical sequelae of damage to the infant limbic system. In: *The Neuropsychology of Development.* (R. L. Isaacson, Ed.). Wiley, New York, 1968: 41–78.
14. Kennard, M. A. Reorganization of motor function in the cerebral cortex of monkeys deprived of motor and premotor areas in infancy. *J. Neurophysiol.*, 1938, **1:** 477–496.
15. Kling, A. Behavioral and somatic development following lesions of the amygdala in the cat. *J. Psychiatr. Res.*, 1965, **3:** 263–273.
16. Kling, A. The effect of cerebral ablation in infant monkeys on motor and cognitive function. In: *Physical Trauma in Mental Retardation.* (C. R. Angls and E. A. Baring, Eds.). U.S. Dept. of Health, Education, and Welfare, Washington, D. C., 1970: 197–205.
17. Kling, A., and Tucker, T. J. Effects of combined lesions of frontal granular cortex and caudate nucleus in the neonatal monkey. *Brain Res.*, 1967, **6:** 428–439.
18. Kling, A., and Tucker, T. J. Sparing of function following localized brain lesions in neonatal monkeys. In: *The Neuropsychology of Development.* (R. L. Isaacson, Ed.). Wiley, New York, 1968: 121–145.
19. Levine, M. S., Hull, C. D., and Buchwald, N. A. Development of motoric activity in kittens. *Proc. Soc. Neurosci.*, 1974, **4:** 305.
20. Raisler, R. L., and Harlow, H. F. Learned behavior following lesions of posterior association cortex in infant, immature and preadolescent monkeys. *J. Comp. Physiol. Psychol.*, 1965, **60:** 167–174.
21. Rosvold, H. E., and Delgado, J. M. R. The effect of delayed-alternation test performance of

stimulating or destroying electrically structures within the frontal lobes of the monkey's brain. *J. Comp. Physiol. Psychol.*, 1956, **49:** 365–372.

22. Scharlock, D. P., Tucker, T. J., and Strominger, N. L. Auditory discrimination by the cat after neonatal ablation of temporal cortex. *Science*, 1963, **141:** 1197–1198.
23. Schneider, G. E. Mechanisms of functional recovery following lesions of visual cortex or superior colliculus in neonate and adult hamsters. *Brain, Behav. Evol.*, 1970, **3:** 295 –323.
24. Tsang, Y.-C. Maze learning in rats hemidecorticated in infancy. *J. Comp. Psychol.*, 1937, **24:** 221–253.
25. Tucker, T., and Kling, A. Differential effects of early vs. late brain damage on visual duration discrimination in cat. *Fed. Proc.*, 1966, **25:** 207.
26. Tucker, T. J., and Kling, A. Differential effects of early and late lesions of frontal granular cortex in the monkey. *Brain Res.*, 1967, **5:** 377–389.
27. Villablanca, J., and Marcus, R. J. Effects of caudate nuclei removal in cats. Comparison with effects of frontal cortex ablation. Chapter 10, this volume.
28. Villablanca, J. R., Olmstead, C. E., and Marcus, R. J. Perseverative instrumental behavior in caudatectomized cats. *Proc. Soc. Neurosci.*, 1974, **4:** 461.

14
Prenatal Nutrition and Neurological Development

JOHN DOBBING
Department of Child Health,
University of Manchester,
Manchester, England

INTRODUCTION

The decision to investigate the effects of infant malnutrition on the developing brain imposes on the researcher an unusually high standard of social and scientific responsibility when it comes to interpreting his results; for the subject involves him in the interrelation between man's most important human faculty, that of higher mental function, and our greatest manmade scourge: the malnutrition of most of the world's children. The following remarks are put forward in an attempt to counteract some of the more extravagant claims of animal experimenters in this uniquely human field.

Experimental projects will inevitably be conducted on animal species, usually the rat, and experience shows that it is not difficult to produce results which can easily be grossly misleading when uncritically interpreted for politicians, planners, and grant-giving bodies. Thus animals underfed during fetal and neonatal life whose brains are permanently small and with too few cells have found their human counterparts in the fertile imagination of many who have not ever considered the real significance (or otherwise) of the finding. The extrapolation has often been made without even wondering whether a modest reduction of total brain cells or of brain weight may be of any real significance, especially if that brain resides in a smaller body. Add to this the very great uncertainties of studies of animal behavior from which rats are happily pronounced to be "emotional," of "short memory" or with "learning birth whether the latter occurs at the immature stage (rat), the mature (guinea pig), or at an intermediate (human) stage of brain growth (Figure 1). Thus expressions such as "the fetal brain" or "the neonatal brain" are valueless unless the species be specified and the brain growth characteristics of that species known.

A particularly heinous travesty is frequently perpetrated when the effects of malnutrition on neuronal cell division are being considered. Experimentally it is extremely convenient that birth in the rat marks the close of the main phase of cerebral neuronal multiplication, before glial mitosis has seriously begun. This means, in general terms, that any effect of maternal malnutrition in this species on the mitotic rate of brain cells will selectively affect neurons rather than glia; and the level of DNA in a newborn rat brain will be quite directly related to number of neurons.

The temptation has therefore been great, and for some irresistible, to use rats for experiments to accentuate the importance of maternal malnutrition on brain development. Various nutritional regimens have led to smaller newborn rat brains with smaller numbers of neurons, and the general extrapolation has been made that human maternal malnutrition will be similarly important for the human neuronal multiplication.

This conclusion is likely to be completely false and probably constitutes a serious and very misleading misapplication, to humans, of the experimental findings in animals, even supposing that small reductions in neuronal number matter.

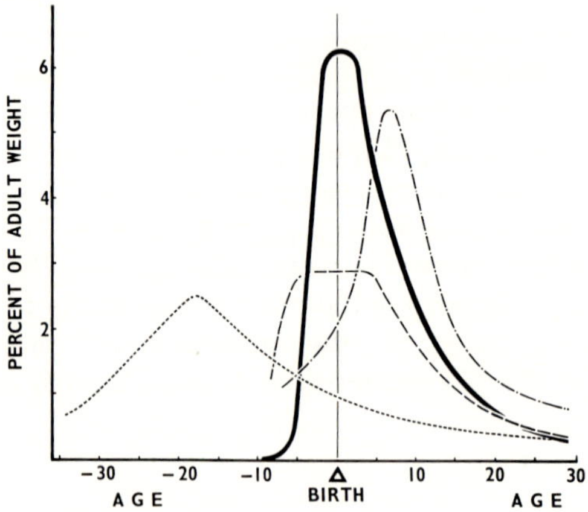

FIGURE 1. Velocity of human brain growth (wet weight) compared with that in other species. Prenatal and postnatal age is expressed as follows: human (————) in months (12); guinea pig (----------------) in days (9); pig (————————) in weeks (5); rat (—·—·—·—·—·—·—) in days (11).

RAT COMPARED WITH HUMAN FETAL LIFE

The error arises quite simply from the following considerations. It is well known that fetal growth susceptibility to maternal malnutrition in both rat and man is virtually confined to the last third of pregnancy. Whether because the fetus is too small relative to the mother in the middle third of pregnancy or for other less obvious reasons the "malnourished" human fetus, whether in multiple pregnancy or otherwise, seems to grow quite well until about 28 gestational weeks. At this time it begins to lose ground rapidly as it attempts to increase its size relative to both the mother and to the placenta. It is during the third trimester only that growth restriction is detectable in the otherwise normal malnourished fetus. From this it is clear that although neuronal multiplication in the rat occurs in the highly vulnerable last one-third of fetal life, in the human it occurs in the highly protected second trimester when growth processes are extremely unlikely to be inconvenienced by placental insufficiency. If this be true, we are therefore absolutely prevented from comparing human fetal malnutrition with rat fetal malnutrition in terms of neuronal multiplication.

The falseness of the comparison can be pushed still further. It must be remembered that the equivalent human brain age of the rat brain at birth cannot be much later than 18 weeks of human gestation (see later), and that the equivalent rat brain age to that at birth, at human full term, is about 5–7 rat postnatal days. It must follow that newborn rats showing the 20 or 30% body weight deficits so common in the experimental literature would be equivalent to human fetuses at 18 weeks gestation showing similar body weight deficits. Such severe deficits of human fetal growth in the second trimester have never been reported, even in very unusual highly pathological circumstances; and this makes these rat "models" valueless except to the specific investigation of rats. The very lowest full-term birth weight of a human nutritionally "small-for-dates" baby is about half the normal average weight, and any growth retardation due to a failure of supplies in these cases has occurred during the third trimester, after the end of the main stage of neuronal multiplication. A more correct model to study the human malnourished fetus would therefore be to take newborn rats of normal weight and reduce their growth rate during their first 5–7 postnatal days, to a degree no greater than is necessary to achieve half the normal weight at that time. This would clearly not disturb the major period of multiplication of neurons in their brains, any more than would be likely in humans, but it may well affect the more important subsequent steps of dendritic and synaptic growth outlined above.

A strong plea must therefore be made that unless one is erecting models for those severe nonnutritional conditions which slow fetal growth in the second human trimester, one should probably not malnourish the rat fetus in order to study the effects of maternal malnutrition on human fetal brain growth. It

hexose-containing lipids, cerebroside and su
is a much easier lipid to estimate reliably in
and although it is much less specific, its ac
relation to that of cerebroside, arriving befo
tioned earlier, the spurt in cholesterol synth
tiplication, since it is synthesized by them, a
phases of the brain growth spurt.

Figure 8 shows its increase in human fo
although its end point is not very well defin
almost to 4 years of age, followed by a very
growth spurt proper, which includes myelin
be considered to continue well into the fourt

NEURONS AND

It has already been mentioned in describi
of mammalian brain growth that the major
occurs before the numerically larger phase
adult number of neurons is achieved very ea
tain regions. Theoretically, therefore, any gr
in numbers of cells of all types should exhib
division. Such a phenomenon has not been
laboratory species studied, although it was i
non was first described by histologists. It no
the two phases in "DNA counts" may be d
consequent rapidity of developmental pro
whom such events take only a few hours
require almost hourly monitoring of con
frequent observations on aspects of later dev
of cell multiplication. However, in humans a
such as the cow, the time scale is much more
humans are the first slowly growing speci
quantitatively described using "DNA count
cell division have been quantitatively reveal

Figure 9 shows a "high power view" of th
shown in Figure 6. Cell multiplication cle
phases with a remarkably sharp cut-off poin
almost certain that the period from 10 to
human neuroblast multiplication, differenti
curring toward the end of this time. Glial
cupies the remainder of the multiplicative
postnatal year.

2. Barlow, P. The influence of inactive chromosomes on human development. *Humangenetik*, 1973, **17:** 105–136.
3. Davison, A. N., and Dobbing, J. The developing brain. In: *Applied Neurochemistry*. (A. N. Davison and J. Dobbing, Eds.). Blackwell, Oxford, 1968: 253–286.
4. Davison, A. N., and Peters, A. *Myelination*. Thomas, Springfield, Illinois, 1970.
5. Dickerson, J. W. T., and Dobbing, J. Prenatal and postnatal growth and development of the central nervous system of the pig. *Proc. R. Soc. Lond.* [*Biol.*], 1967, **166:** 384–395.
6. Dobbing, J. Undernutrition and the developing brain. In: *Developmental Neurobiology*. (W. A. Himwich, Ed.), Thomas, Springfield, Illinois, 1970: 260–261.
7. Dobbing, J. Undernutrition and the developing brain: The relevance of animal models to the human problem. *Am. J. Dis. Child.*, 1970, **120:** 411–415.
8. Dobbing, J., Hopewell, J. W., and Lynch, A. Vulnerability of developing brain. VII. Permanent deficit of neurons in cerebral and cerebellar cortex following early mild undernutrition. *Exp. Neurol.*, 1971, **32:** 439–447.
9. Dobbing, J., and Sands, J. Growth and development of the brain and spinal cord of the guinea pig. *Brain Res.*, 1970, **17:** 115–123.
10. Dobbing, J., and Sands, J. Timing of neuroblast multiplication in developing human brain. *Nature* (*Lond.*), 1970, **226:** 639–640.
11. Dobbing, J., and Sands, J. Vulnerability of developing brain. IX. The effect of nutritional growth retardation on the timing of the brain growth-spurt. *Biol. Neonate*, 1971, **19:** 363–378.
12. Dobbing, J., and Sands, J. Quantitative growth and development of human brain. *Arch. Dis. Childhood*, 1973, **48:** 757–767.
13. Dobbing, J., and Smart, J. L. Early undernutrition, brain development and behaviour. In: *Clinics in Developmental Medicine*. No. 47. (S. A. Barnett, Ed.). Heinemann, London, 1973: 16–36.
14. Hertzig, M. E., Birch, H. G., Richardson, S. A., and Tizard, J. Intellectual levels of school children severely malnourished during the first two years of life. *Pediatrics*, 1972, **49:** 814–824.
15. Miller, R. W., and Blot, W. J. Small head size after *in utero* exposure to atomic radiation. *Lancet*, 1972, **2:** 784–787.
16. Richardson, S. A. Ecology of malnutrition: Non-nutritional factors influencing intellectual and behavioural development. *Pan American Health Organization, Scientific Publication, 1972, No. 251:* 101–110.
17. Winick, M. Changes in nucleic acid and protein content of the human brain during growth. *Pediat. Res.*, 1968, **2:** 352–355.
18. Winick, M., and Noble, A. Cellular response in rats during malnutrition at various ages. *J. Nutr.*, 1966, **89:** 300–306.

15

The Futility of Comparative IQ Research

JOHN GARCIA
Department of Psychology,
University of California Los Angeles,
Los Angeles, California

This conference is entitled "Brain Mechanisms in Mental Retardation," but paradoxically there has been little discussion of one central issue. Presumably the term "mental retardation" refers to a reduced "mental age" or MA, the troublesome numerator in that well-known equation MA/CA = IQ where CA is the chronological age and IQ is the intelligence quotient of the subject under consideration. This equation has the elegant simplicity of the Einsteinian $E = MC^2$ and its sociopolitical implications are about as explosive as a nuclear reaction. Nevertheless, we must deal with the concepts of mental age and IQ and the operations by which they are measured, if we are to understand the meaning of the term "mental retardation" and its significance or lack of significance in our research programs.

To avoid another endless controversy we must eschew the broad issues such as the one raised by Jensen at the very onset of his 1969 paper in the *Harvard Review* (15), i.e., "Compensatory education has been tried and it has apparently failed." The provocative form of the statement leads to disputes which cannot be decided by scientific inquiry. Substitution of any catch phrase, such as National Defense, Police Protection, Automotive Transportation, Environmental Conservation, for Compensatory Education would start an endless debate on any topic. To reach a decision, we need to raise more mundane questions, such as: Specifically how is intelligence measured? How is an IQ test made up? What sort of responses increase (or decrease) the IQ test scores?

tion of information and complex skills is what most people considered intelligence to be. In the final analysis, however, intelligence as defined by items selected from the anthropometric laboratory by the hereditarians were deemed a failure, because they were not predictive of success in the academy or the market place, however well they may have fared in the playing field or the ballroom.

CORE CURRICULUM AND STANDARD PUPILS AS *sine qua non* FOR IQ

Environmentalists, i.e., the established school authorities, were in effect allowed to define "intelligence" in the "successful" approach to mental testing as initiated by Alfred Binet in France and carried on in this country by Lewis Terman and Maud Merrill at Stanford University (25). The Stanford-Binet test, by virtue of the monumental amount of applied research, became the definitive measure of IQ against which most other IQ tests are evaluated. It is imperative that we examine what kind of intelligence this test measures.

The first practical stratagem devised by Binet and employed by Terman was to select items predictive of progress in school. Furthermore, the items reflected only that segment of the curriculum which the school authorities deemed to be important, namely the reading, writing, and arithmetic of the "core" curriculum. The effect of this arbitrary decision was to exclude items drawn from the "special" classes such as the art studio, musical conservatory, and the machine shop from the IQ test thus relegating these abilities forever into the sphere of "special" abilities, and in effect reducing the measured intelligence of people whose skills and vocations lay in these spheres. Artists, musicians, and machinists, like Black Americans, need not be intelligent; they only need "specialized" talents to be successful. Yet in judging the intellectual level of prehistoric man, cave paintings, musical instruments, and handicrafts were accepted without question as marks of advanced intelligence. As illustrated in Figure 1, this process has given us the popular conception of the human mind.

The second practical stratagem devised by the mental testers was the "standardization group." They recognized that American school children at the turn of the century formed a motley group with parents of different social, ethnic, and language groupings. Since one could only be sure that children of white English-speaking parents had the full opportunity to become conversant in the language and problems used in the core curriculum, these children were selected as the sample on which the test items were validated or standardized. Children from other biosocial groups were excluded, making the original Stanford-Binet a middle class "Anglo" IQ, to use that loose biosocial category without prejudice. It should not be surprising that vocabulary items based on

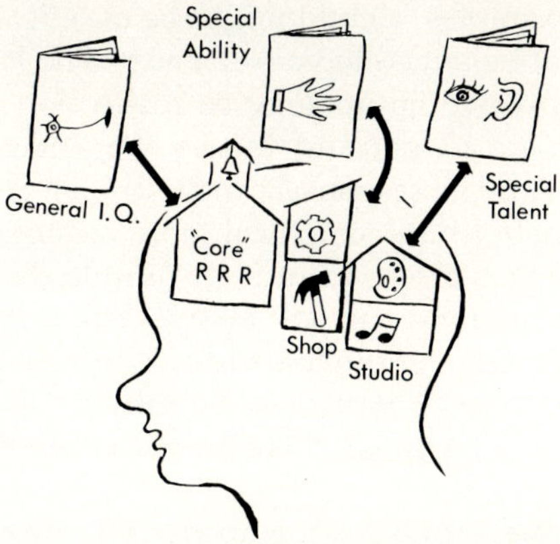

FIGURE 1. The structure of the turn-of-the-century school curriculum, the construction and labeling of tests, and the popular conception of the child's mind reflect one and the same cultural phenomenon. This myth assumes a central role for general intelligence and peripheral roles for special (motor) abilities and special (sensory) talents without independent neurophysiological verification. The same prejudice tracks the minority child into special courses deemed appropriate for his inherited characteristics without regard for the evidence necessary for genetic inference.

common English usage proved to be the most efficient subtest in this IQ test. To use this test and other group tests based primarily on Anglo vocabulary on other minority groups for comparative purposes, one must make the assumption that all groups have had equal opportunity and motivation to learn the same words. Needless to say, these assumptions invariably lead to controversy.

ITEM SELECTION AND THE CRITERION GROUP

The third practical stratagem employed by the mental testers was to write items designed to yield a direct monotonic relationship to increasing age, which is to say, that an item must be passed by progressively larger numbers of older children. Now many items have an inverse or U-shaped function. For example, "Black is a color; true or false?" is apt to be a difficult and confusing item for very young children who have not mastered reading or for college students who have mastered the distinction between hue and brightness. Grade school children, familiar with the crayon box, would have no difficulty in marking the item "true." Such an item would have to be rejected or scored in several ways in order to force a direct monotonic function with age necessary for the measurement of intelligence.

It is most instructive to examine items and the scoring guidelines in the manual for the Stanford-Binet. There one can see how IQ scores are generated.

To paraphrase a few examples, a child might be asked, "What would you do if you lost something that belonged to your friend?" The key instructs us that the correct answer must involve an apology or restitution or both. This is what middle class children are taught and this is the answer which increases in frequency with age. All other responses, including an attempt to deal with the friend's feelings, no matter how insightful, only reduce the subject's IQ score. Not all the correct answers are so intuitively simple. For example, the subject might be asked "How are loud and soft alike?" The response, "Both affect the ear," is scored correct. On the other hand, "You can hear both of them" is incorrect. At another point, a knife can be either "sharp" or "very sharp," however, a mile can only be "long." The answer "too long" reduces the subject's measured IQ.

The correct answer may appear to be arbitrary to anyone who believes that an IQ test should directly measure reasoning capacity or intellectual power, but the IQ test merely determines whether the child's answer resembles the answer of the average urban Anglo child of his age. If it resembles that of an older child, he is superior in IQ. This general technique of comparing the subject's answer to the most frequent answer given by a criterion group is employed in many tests. Multiphasic psychiatric tests do not measure thought disturbance to achieve their diagnostic ends, they merely compare the subject's answers with that of groups diagnosed as schizophrenic, manic, paranoid, etc. Vocational tests do not measure the subject's capacity or even interest in a vocation or profession, they merely match his answer to those given by the established members of the vocation or profession. Any item, whether it deals with values, hobbies, appetites, or whatever, is acceptable just as long as it distinguishes one insanity from another, or one profession from the others. Of course, if the members of a given profession happen to be of another sex or ethnic group, the subject's chances to be counselled into that profession are greatly reduced, not necessarily because he has no interest or potential in the profession, but because he does not respond to irrelevant items in the same way that the professional does (1).

WHY NOT MEASURE LEARNING DIRECTLY?

Since previous exposure to the IQ content and the testing situation is such a crucial variable in IQ performance, one is inclined to ask "What happens when these practice effects are controlled?" Jensen provides some evidence in his rather remarkable review. He points out that in conventional IQ tests, the child's performance depends upon what he has learned at home or elsewhere before he comes in to take the test, and that it is possible to devise items that show "how fast a child can learn something new and unfamiliar right in the test situation." Commenting on such performance upon various tasks (e.g., memory for digits presented aloud, learning lists of familiar objects, associating pairs of objects, recalling names or objects presented randomly), Jensen writes, citing a half dozen of his own publications, ". . . lower class children, whether white, negro or Mexican-American, perform as well on these direct learning tests as do middle-class children. Lower class children in the IQ range of about 60 to 80 do markedly better than middle class children who are in this range of IQ."

However, Jensen does not go on to exploit a new line of reasoning. Instead he depreciates his own learning studies for the incredible reason that the data have a low correlation with IQ which, of course, is precisely what you would expect if IQ performance favors prior learning to which the children were differentially exposed. He then cites data from his own laboratory to show that if testing conditions are changed, the lower class children are again disadvantaged. In essence, children are now presented with objects which were selected so that they could be classified into one of four categories: animals, furniture, clothing, or foods. Now the middle class children utilizing this categorical clustering selected by middle class testers were superior in recall performance. Jensen goes on to note that the recall of categorized lists correlates with IQ, i.e., with what they knew before they came into the test situation. Lower class children show "some idiosyncratic clustering" but do not "spontaneously" use the appropriate categories in recall, despite the fact that post-test interviews indicated that they knew the names of the categories.

Obviously, categorical clustering is a memorizing strategy that can be learned by association, but in this review there was no report of attempts to teach new and unfamiliar categorical clusters to both classes of children. Instead Jensen relegates the learning of new and unfamiliar tasks to Level I (associative learning ability) and the spontaneous use of "Anglo" categories in recall to Level II (problem solving ability) solely on the basis of correlation with IQ data. Thus the syllogistic operational trap is sprung. Intelligence is what IQ tests measure. IQ tests measure what is learned before one comes to the test situation. Learning in the test situation is not a measure of true intelligence.

In summary, IQ items are not validated on an abstract notion of "truth" or because they measure "intellectual" capacity. They are validated by a correlational technique designed to reflect progress of Anglo children through a core curriculum designed by Anglo educators. This correlation depends not only on the test items but also upon the subjects who were tested. There is no reason to assume that such a test would be suitable to measure the same function in another biosocial group. For example, if the progress of Black children is to be measured, then the items must be selected for them in the same empirical way that they were selected for the White group. The failure to select and search diligently for items which empirically reflect progressive change with age in Black Americans makes any test, even those which now include Black Americans in standardization groups, of dubious validity.

Naturally the Anglo educators and mental testers selected their own subculture and the progress of the children of their own biosocial group as the *sine qua non* for the definition of intelligence. All biosocial groups, civilized as well as primitive, tend to view themselves as human and others as somewhat less than human. At the turn of the century, most segments of European and American society tended to view the non-Europeans as the "White man's burden" and even the most progressive American educators were confident that the school, an essential part of the American "melting pot," would in time convert the outsiders into core Americans. Apparently this optimism is waning as it becomes apparent that biosocial groups tend to maintain cultural continuity and integrity over centuries. It is surprising that with today's methodological and technical sophistication, data gathered with tests designed to place individuals within their own social group are used to draw comparisons between groups.

WHY MEN AND WOMEN ARE EQUAL IN INTELLIGENCE

The dilemma which faces anyone who attempts to compare intelligence of two biosocial groups can best be illustrated by comparing the test performance of males and females. On the average, males excel on items involving speed and coordination of gross motor activities, spatial tasks, mechanical problems, and arithmetic reasoning; females fare better on tasks involving fine motor skills, perceptual skill, memory, numerical computation, and verbal fluency (2).

Both the biological and the social argument are called forth to account for these differences. The biologically inclined point to differences in body structure, musculature, and hormonal factors. The natural child-bearing and rearing functions dictated that women were biologically bound to the protected center of the primitive village while the stronger and faster males were more effective in dealing with dangers of hunting and fighting at the perimeter of the tribal territory. Thus evolution can be viewed as favoring sexual differences. The socially inclined point to the obvious differences in social training. Women are rewarded for accepting the feminine role and ridiculed for attempting to acquire mechanical and quantitative skills. They are denied educational and professional opportunities in the man's world by law as well as custom. Since no one can define intelligence as an entity independently of test results, this piquant controversy goes on and on.

The mental testers dealt with this problem in their characteristic practical fashion. Figure 2 makes it clear that if too many "male items" were included in a test battery, males would have a higher intelligence score on the average and if too many "female items" were included, females would have the higher intelligence. In keeping with the social trends toward equality of the sexes, Lewis Terman and Maud Merrill (25) assumed that the intelligence of males and females was on the average equal, and balanced the number and weight of

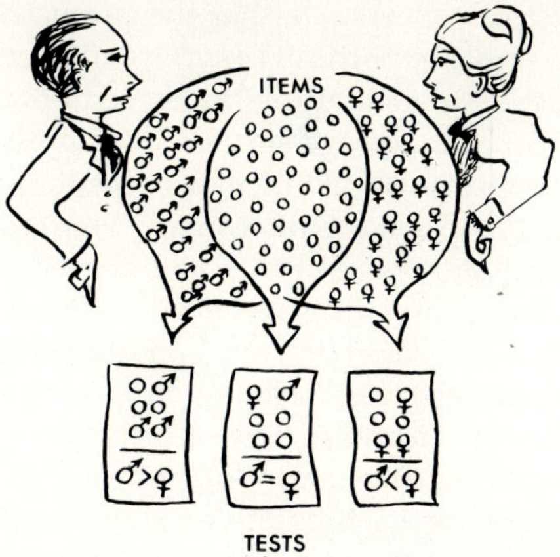

FIGURE 2. A virtually infinite number of items can be written which presumably measure intelligence. Some favor men, some favor women, and some favor neither sex as the overlap in the two spheres indicates. Lewis Terman and Maud Merrill balanced their tests to equate the sexes by arbitrary selection of items. The same rationale holds for Black versus White differences in responding to test items. Since the gene pools underlying races overlap and contain enormous numbers of genes affecting intellectual performance, a similar value judgment would be necessary if a small finite sample of genetic factors were to be selected as a eugenic criterion for intellectual improvement.

the male and female items. For instance, in the 1937 Stanford-Binet, items that showed a large sex difference were excluded while items which only slightly favored one sex were balanced by items favoring the opposite sex to an equal degree. The deviation intelligence procedure maintains this equality through the use of separate norms for males and females.

These sex differences consistently appear in the Graduate Record Examination (GRE) where men do better in "quantitative subtests" and women do better in "verbal subtests." Here again comparative group judgments are avoided by assuming equal weights for quantitative and verbal subtests and by measuring each individual's performance in relation to the performance of a group of the same sex (17). Thus the IQ of women is equal to that of men on the average because intelligence testers design their tests that way.

One could treat other biosocial differences in the same way. What if for example, Chicano children score lower than Anglo children on a test composed of "Anglo items." We need not agonize about heredity and environment. We merely need to write some "Chicano items" which reflect the progress of Chicano children. We can then balance the Chicano items with the Anglo items in a single test, or we can make up a Chicano test and standardize it for Chicano progress, then presto, Chicanos would be equal to Anglos in intelligence.

Now some proponents of mental testing piously express a concern that such inclusion of Chicano items and Black items will attenuate the predictive value of the IQ test. It is just as conceivable that the predictive value may be ultimately enhanced when equal opportunity is afforded to minority people. In any case, it is again instructive to look at this in terms of males versus females. In the grade schools girls on the average surpass boys of the same age by a wide margin in academic performance, yet men are accepted into graduate university training almost to the exclusion of women. The biologically inclined say that girls mature faster than boys, but that young men are less emotional and more adaptive thus a better risk in graduate work than women. The socially inclined say that the grade school culture is more compatible with the little girls' social role while the graduate school admissions are biased in favor of the adult male social role. However, the mental testers assigned the same average IQ and the same distribution of IQs to boys, girls, men, and women without apparent concern for its predictive value in grade school or university. Unfortunately, they were not in the position to assign equal pay for equal work, or equal opportunity to place equally intelligent women into professional schools. As a result IQ scores are more predictive of male success than female success (26).

THE ASSUMED "GROWTH" AND "DECLINE" OF INTELLIGENCE WITH AGE

When an individual intelligence test is presented to groups of subjects of differing ages it is found that the number of items passed increases with age, leveling off between the ages of 16 to 26 years, and then there is a steady decline with advancing years. This is not a direct observation of the growth and decline of intellectual function. Intelligence tests were designed to yield this picture of intellectual growth because it fitted the *a priori* notions of intellectual growth held by the mental testers and school authorities.

Obviously, an intelligence test composed of items selected to reflect school progress should yield a peak in intellectual development at the precise age when people are leaving school. The longer the subjects are out of school the worse they should do on school tests because people forget some skills and acquire others as they enter new fields. This decline in the slope of intelligence can be as logically attributed to the discontinuity of their environment, as to some loss in intellectual function. By other standards, ability to deal with the extraschool environment seems to continue to grow. For example, most auto insurance companies have decided on an empirical actuarial basis that ability to deal with the problems of survival on the highways is not fully developed until age 25. If one searched for items which reflected increasing ability to deal with the extraschool environment and "blended" these items in with the school items, intelligence would seem to continue to grow monotonically beyond age 16 (see Figure 3) (29).

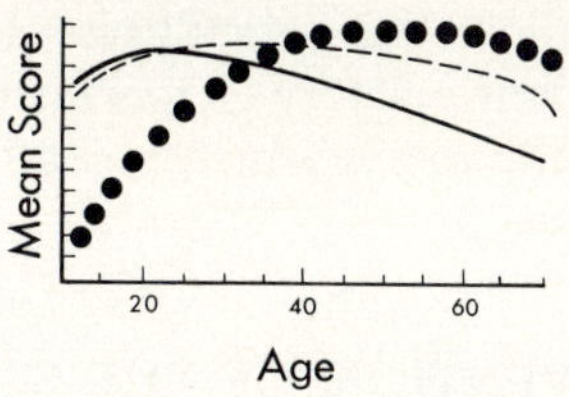

FIGURE 3. The solid line is the "curve of average decline of mental ability with age" presented by Wechsler (29). Significantly it closely approximates the curves obtained with tests of school activities: block design, price arrangement, digit span, and digit symbol. The dashed line indicates the same function obtained with tests more meaningful to adults: information, vocabulary comprehension, and arithmetic. The dotted line is our speculation on the probable results of a test assessing the adaptive responses to the highway patrol and internal revenue service, to credit and property demands, and to irksome social responsibilities at work and home.

An examination of the original Stanford-Binet testing kit reveals that this blending tactic was employed to deal with the discontinuity of environment when the child leaves home and enters school. Items involving sensory-motor tasks reflecting the home environment, such as naming toys and following instructions, are qualitatively different from the scholastic items. These items were selected and standardized on preschool children so as to yield a smooth monotonic function with age during the transition from preschool years to school years when mean mental age is plotted. However, the discontinuity of environment makes the prediction of future intelligence from these preschool tests to the scholastic tests less reliable than prediction within the scholastic test series.

The simple fact is that adults do less well with increasing age on tests designed for children and that adults with relatively low IQ scores are often successful even in academic professions, because long-term adaptive persistence to obtain hard-won skills and goals in the adult world cannot be predicted from a test made up from "paper and pencil" items to be solved within minutes. For "practical" reasons, test items have to conform with the segmented educational recitation activities in a classroom setting. Items have to be brief so that many items can be given and the IQ obtained in one sitting. Quite naturally it has been found that IQs obtained in this way are more closely related to activities of an accountant than the activities of a lumberjack,* more closely related to the skill of a bridge player than that of a quarter-

* Herrnstein (12) presents a list ranking civilian occupations according to IQ. At the top of the list are accountants and auditors (IQ = 127) who work in a situation on tasks which resemble the IQ situation. At the bottom of the list are lumberjacks and teamsters (IQ = 91) whose skills, abilities, and technical language are considered too "specialized" for IQ test items. Obviously, both groups are highly specialized, i.e., adapted to their particular niche. The question of which group is more likely to survive successfully depends whether the survival test is conducted in the urban counting house or the north woods. Such considerations forced the mental testers to abandon the conceptionalization "intelligence is adaptive" in favor of "intelligence is whatever our test measures."

back. Since these items reflect the subculture of the student, teachers and professors are apt to view their mastery as meritorious, but except for TV quiz programs, there are few occupations which resemble the peculiar niche of the student taking an intelligence test.

THE INVENTION OF THE STABLE IQ

It was immediately obvious to the mental testers that infants, children, youths and adults belonged to separate biosocial groups which differed in biological maturation and level of socialization. Appropriate tests were designed for each group and a scale was sought which would make all groups equivalent in intelligence despite age differences. The mental testers wanted a numerical score which would remain constant for each individual as he grew older and accumulated more years and education.

First the intelligence quotient (IQ) was devised by the simple assumption that the mean mental age (MA) of each group was equal to its actual chronological age (CA). When the MA is divided by the CA and multiplied by 100 the result is the IQ. For any age group the mean IQ is equal to 100. The child who performs at a higher MA than the average for his group receives an IQ proportionally higher than 100, and the child who performs lower than his age group receives an IQ lower than 100. Obviously this lower score could either be due to "biological immaturity" or "inferior training."

The IQ device appears rational until the measured MA reaches a leveling off after age 16. After this point if CA continues to increase then IQ becomes progressively lower. This was solved in a bold fashion by the mental testers who set a ceiling on actual age (CA) to conform to the ceiling on measured MA. Nevertheless people continue to grow older and do worse on IQ tests. This depressing state of affairs was handled in a more sophisticated way when the MA/CA ratio was dropped in favor of the deviation IQ where the IQ of any age group is assumed to be 100 and the variation of individuals of any group is assumed to be symmetrically distributed with a standard deviation of 16. However, when people are tested and retested IQ scores tend to fluctuate widely despite these efforts to stabilize them over age. One study found that between the ages of 6 to 18 years approximately 60% of the individuals retested had changed 15 IQ points or more. Approximately 10% had changed 30 IQ points or more (13). A more recent study indicates that the average IQ change from infancy to adolescence is nearly 30 points or enough to change the classification of a child from "normal" either up to "genius" or down to "moron" (19).

THE DILEMMA OF THE CULTURE-FREE TEST

Let us now consider the dilemma which faces any researcher who attempts to compare the intelligence of different cultural and social groups. The notion of a "culture-free" test is illusory, because each item in such a test would have to be tested on members of at least two different cultural groups. If, on the average, the performance of one group on a given item is superior to that of the other group, one may conclude that the item is culturally biased in favor of that group and, therefore, should be eliminated from the "culture-free" test. If this criterion is accepted then no item which differentiates between the two groups is acceptable and, in effect, the two groups are declared to be equal in intelligence as measured by the test. Widespread testing of the item in a variety of cultures does not assist us, since whenever differences are found, "cultural bias" is always a possible explanation. The alternative conclusion that a given item reflects a true difference in intelligence between groups requires an independent criteria of mental capacity. Such criteria are precluded by the circular operational definition "intelligence is what the intelligence test measures." Each item in an intelligence test reflects the environmental development of a skill completely confounded with hereditary capacity to acquire that skill. No amount of social research and no level of statistical analysis can ever unravel that biosocial confounding.

THE DILEMMA OF HEREDITY VERSUS ENVIRONMENT STUDIES WITH HUMAN SAMPLES

A similar dilemma faces the researcher who attempts to determine the relative influence of heredity or environment within a single biosocial group. Ideally the researcher would like to attribute 100% of the difference in IQ scores of his sample of children proportionally either to the influence of "family" and or to the influence of "home."* In most cases, family and home are confounded, that is children are raised in the family home, so the researcher usually deals with foster children where children of one family are raised in the home of another. The first problem that arises is that the foster child has been nurtured within the environment of the mother's body and environmental influences of disease, nutrition, and trauma during this period have already left their mark on him forever. Subtle deprivations of protein, hormones, oxygen, or minerals during this period could reduce a potential genius to an imbecile. These are environmental influences which the foster child brings to his new home. This confounding of heredity and environment can never be completely unraveled by studies of the foster child.

The second problem arises from the placement practices of adoption agencies. They select appropriate homes for their foster children. For experi-

* While this notion may be defended by appeals to the statistical procedures of analysis of variance, it does not make any sense genetically speaking, to say as Herrnstein does . . . "that the genetic factor is worth 80 percent and that only 20 percent is left to everything else." Estimates of the heritability of a trait do not yield estimates of how much that trait will be influenced by environmental changes.

tion to defend against illness (9). The evolutionary significance of this behavior has already been discussed and need only be summarized here. Taste information is vital if the rat is to select nutrients effectively and avoid toxins, thus maintaining the integrity of his internal homeostatic environment. However, in its natural history the species has never had to cope with auditory sounds that led to illness. On the other hand, in the natural external environment, rats make good use of auditory cues to avoid the painful attacks of predators upon their cutaneous surface. But taste cues are not particularly informative when it comes to avoiding predators (see Figure 4).

Lesions made in the ventral hippocampus or the lateral septum disrupt the noise-shock learning making the animal less intelligent in coping with the external world, which is not surprising. It is surprising that the same lesions facilitate flavor-illness learning making the animals more intelligent in coping with internal problems (20). If we were to summate the effects across both tasks we would conclude that the lesions had no effect upon general intelligence. It is the concept of general intelligence that makes this type of analysis ludicrous. Whenever we damage animals by whatever method, protein starvation, vitamin deficiency, or drugs, we are apt to be confronted by incongruous results if we view adaptive behavior as a general function. Our treatments will have specific effects upon specific motive systems, on specific integrative systems, and on specific perceptual systems which cannot be

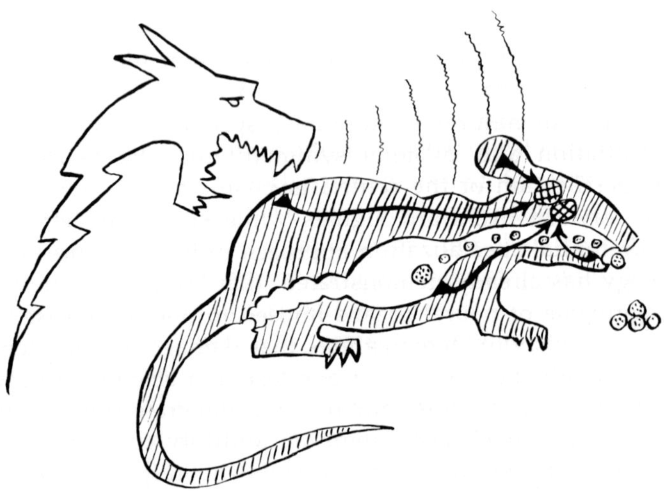

FIGURE 4. Rats quickly and appropriately adapt to noises followed by peripheral pain or to flavors followed by illness. Conversely these animals are relatively insensitive to noise-illness and flavor-pain contingencies. Moreover, specific brain lesions may disrupt one form of adaptation while enhancing another making a notion of general adaptation untenable. Survival appears to depend upon a variety of specialized input–output systems selected by differential evolutionary pressures and controlled by differential neurological and genetic mechanisms.

accounted for by a single factor. Behavior, like other body functions, must be differentiated into its component elements and related to specific neural structures. General intelligence is about as useful for this purpose as *élan vital* is to diagnostic medicine.

REFERENCES

1. Anastasi, A. *Psychological Testing.* Macmillan, New York, 1954.
2. Anastasi, A. *Differential Psychology.* (3rd ed.) Macmillan, New York, 1958.
3. Bolles, R., and Seelbach, S. Punishing and reinforcing effects of noise onset and termination for different responses. *J. Comp. Physiol. Psychol.*, 1964, **58:** 127–131.
4. Bridgman, P. W. *The Logic of Modern Physics.* Macmillan, New York, 1927.
5. Burt, C. The inheritance of intelligence *Am. Psychol.*, 1958, **13:** 1–15.
6. Cattell, J. M. Mental tests and measurements. *Mind,* 1890, **15:** 373–381.
7. Dobrzecka, C., Szwejkowska, G., and Konorski, J. Qualitative versus directional cues in two forms of differentiation. *Science,* 1966, **153:** 87–89.
8. Galton, F. *Hereditary Genius.* Macmillan, New York, 1869.
9. Garcia, J., and Koelling, R. A. Relation of cue to consequence in avoidance learning. *Psychon. Sci.*, 1966, **4:** 123–124.
10. Garcia, J., McGowan, B., and Green, K. Biological constraints on conditioning. In: *Classical Conditioning: Current Research and Theory.* (A. H. Black and W. F. Prokasy, Eds.). Appleton, New York, 1972: 3–27.
11. Heber, R., Garber, H., Harrington, S., and Hoffman, C. Rehabilitation of families at risk for mental retardation. Unpublished research report, University of Wisconsin, Milwaukee.
12. Herrnstein, R. IQ. *The Atlantic,* 1971, **228:** 43–58.
13. Honzik, M. P., Macfarlane, J. W., and Allen, L. The stability of mental test performance between two and eighteen years. *J. Exp. Educ.*, 1948, **17:** 309–324.
14. Huxley, A. *Brave New World.* Harper, New York, 1932.
15. Jensen, A. R. How much can we boost IQ and scholastic achievement? In: *Environment, Heredity, and Intelligence.* Harvard Review Reprint Ser. No. 2. Harvard Univ. Press, Cambridge, Massachusetts, 1969: 1–123.
16. Kamin, L. J. *The Science and Politics of IQ.* Earlbaum Associates, Potomac, Maryland, 1974; *Heredity, Intelligence, Politics and Psychology.* Invited address to the Eastern Psychological Association, Washington, D.C., May, 1973.
17. Lannholm, G. V., and Schrader, W. B. *Predicting Graduate School Success: An Evaluation of the Effectiveness of the Graduate Record Examination.* Educational Testing Service, Princeton, New Jersey, 1951.
18. Lashley, K. S. *Brain Mechanisms and Intelligence.* Univ. of Chicago Press, Chicago, Illinois, 1929.
19. McCall, R. B., Appelbaum, M. I., and Hogarty, P. S. Developmental changes in mental performance. *Monogr. Soc. Res. Child Dev.*, 1973, **38:** 1–83.
20. McGowan, B. K., Hankins, W. G., and Garcia, J. Limbic lesions and control of the internal and external environment. *Behav. Biol.*, 1972, **7:** 841–852.
21. Page, E. B. Miracle in Milwaukee: Raising the IQ. *Educ. Res.*, 1972, **1:** 8–16..
22. Pavlov, I. P. *Lectures on Conditioned Reflexes.* International Publishers, New York, 1928.
23. Rosenthal, D. *Genetic Theory and Abnormal Behavior.* McGraw-Hill, New York, 1970.
24. Seligman, M. E. P., and Hager, J. L. *Biological Boundaries of Learning.* Appleton, New York, 1972.
25. Terman, L. M., and Merrill, M. A. *Stanford-Binet Intelligence Scale.* (3rd ed.) Houghton, Boston, Massachusetts, 1960.

26. Terman, L. M., and Oden, M. H. *The Gifted Child Grows Up*. Stanford Univ. Press, Stanford, California, 1947.
27. Tryon, R. C. A theory of psychological components—an alternative to "mathematical" factors. *Psychol. Rev.*, 1935, **42:** 425–454.
28. Tryon, R. C. Genetic differences in maze-learning ability in rats. *39th Yearb. Natl. Soc. Stud. Educ.*, 1940, Part I: 111–119.
29. Wechsler, D. *The Measurement and Appraisal of Adult Intelligence*. Williams & Wilkins, Baltimore, Maryland, 1958.
30. Wilcoxon, H., Dragoin, W., and Kral, P. Illness-induced aversions in the rat and quail: Relative salience of visual and gustatory cues. *Science*, 1971, **171:** 826–828.

Metabolic Defects in Development

zyme. Finally, if the kidney contains a different isozyme from the liver, then the kidney enzyme may remain unaffected in phenylketonuria.

In an attempt to determine if mammalian kidney enzyme is the same or different from that of the liver, the physical, catalytic, and immunological properties of the kidney enzyme were compared with the properties of the enzyme from liver (4).

The physical properties of kidney and liver phenylalanine hydroxylase from rat were compared by (a) gel filtration and (b) sucrose gradient centrifugation. (a) When rat liver phenylalanine hydroxylase is passed through a Bio-Gel A-5 column, two bands of activity are eluted. If either band is run again through the column the same elution profile results. This indicates that the enzyme exists in two different molecular weight forms which are interconvertible. Rat kidney enzyme, when passed over the same column produces a very similar elution pattern. This shows that the kidney also has two different molecular weight forms, the molecular weight of each being similar to those of the liver enzyme. (b) Sucrose gradients (5–20%) were run in the absence or presence of 5 m*M* phenylalanine. Enzyme was preincubated for 20 minutes, either with buffer alone or with buffer containing phenylalanine, before being applied to the appropriate gradient. It has been reported that phenylalanine increases the sedimentation velocity of rat liver phenylalanine hydroxylase (16). In the gradients without phenylalanine the rates of sedimentation of the kidney and liver enzymes were the same. In the presence of phenylalanine the peak of activity sedimented more rapidly, leaving a trailing shoulder. This effect is also observed with the kidney enzyme to the same extent as with the liver enzyme.

The catalytic and immunological properties were determined for kidney and liver phenylalanine hydroxylase from both man and rat. The comparison of species served as a measure of the sensitivity of the methods for distinguishing between enzymes from different organs of the same species.

The apparent Michaelis constants (K_M) (6) were measured for phenylalanine, the pseudocofactor, 6,7-dimethyltetrahydropterin, and the natural cofactor, tetrahydrobiopterin. All of the Michaelis constants were determined at least in triplicate (Table IV). In each case the liver and kidney values agree within experimental error. However, the K_M's for phenylalanine and 6,7-dimethyltetrahydropterin also show no species dependence. On the other hand, the K_M for tetrahydrobiopterin shows a 2–3-fold difference between species, but has identical values for the K_M with liver and kidney enzyme of the same species. This is of special interest since the dihydroxypropyl group of tetrahydrobiopterin, which the pseudocofactor lacks, is responsible not only for the tight binding of the natural cofactor, but is also involved in allosteric regulation of the enzyme (1,2). It is not surprising therefore that species differences are more readily detected with the natural cofactor. There is also a species difference in the ratios of maximum velocity with natural cofactor to the max-

Table IV Kinetic and Immunological Properties of Phenylalanine Hydroxylase from Liver and Kidney of Man and Rat

Property	Rat		Human	
	Liver	Kidney	Liver	Kidney
K_M Phenylalanine (mM)[a]	0.83 ± 0.05	0.95 ± 0.16	0.62 ± 0.06	0.84 ± 0.16
K_M Me_2H_4-pterin (mM)[b]	0.101 ± 0.014	0.107 ± 0.005	0.154 ± 0.018	0.144 ± 0.043
K_M H_4-biopterin (mM)[b]	0.023 ± 0.002	0.021 ± 0.003	0.057 ± 0.014	0.057 ± 0.014
V_M H_4-biopterin[c] / V_M Me_2H_4-pterin	4.5	4.5	2.0	2.0
Milliliter antiserum/mU enzyme for 50% inhibition[d]	0.008	0.008	0.2	0.2

[a] Apparent Michaelis constants were determined at pH 7.4 and 27°C. The K_M for phenylalanine was measured at 0.2 mM Me_2H_4-pterin, with phenylalanine concentration varied from 0.2 to 4.0 mM.

[b] The K_M's for Me_2H_4-pterin and H_4-biopterin (tetrahydrobiopterin) were measured at 1 mM phenylalanine, with Me_2H_4-pterin varied from 0.02 to 0.5 mM, and H_4-biopterin varied from 0.01 to 0.2 mM.

[c] Ratio of the apparent maximum velocity with H_4-biopterin as cofactor to the apparent maximum velocity with Me_2H_4-pterin as cofactor.

[d] See legend to Figure 1 for experimental details.

imum velocity with pseudocofactor, but for the different tissues of the same species the values are the same.

The immunological properties of the kidney and liver enzymes were compared on the basis of their reactivity with antibodies to rat liver phenylalanine hydroxylase. Enzyme was incubated with increasing amounts of antiserum. The precipitate formed was removed by centrifugation, and the supernatant was assayed for remaining activity. The amount of antiserum required to give 50% inhibition of the rat kidney enzyme was identical to that required for the rat liver. The enzyme from the two human tissues was then titrated with rat liver enzyme antiserum. Both human liver and human kidney required 25 times more antiserum than did the rat enzymes, to give 50% inhibition (Figure 1, Table IV). Thus, although distinguishing between species, these immunological studies were unable to distinguish between enzymes from kidney and liver of the same species.

By all of the above criteria we have not been able to differentiate the kidney from the liver enzyme, either from man or from rat. We are at present developing methods to allow a comparison of the electrophoretic properties of the kidney and liver enzymes. The ultimate method of comparison will be the amino acid sequence of the enzymes from the two tissues.

Some of the milder forms of phenylketonuria might be explained by retention of phenylalanine hydroxylase activity in the kidney. Although in normal individuals it appears that only 2% of the total body phenylalanine hydroxyl-

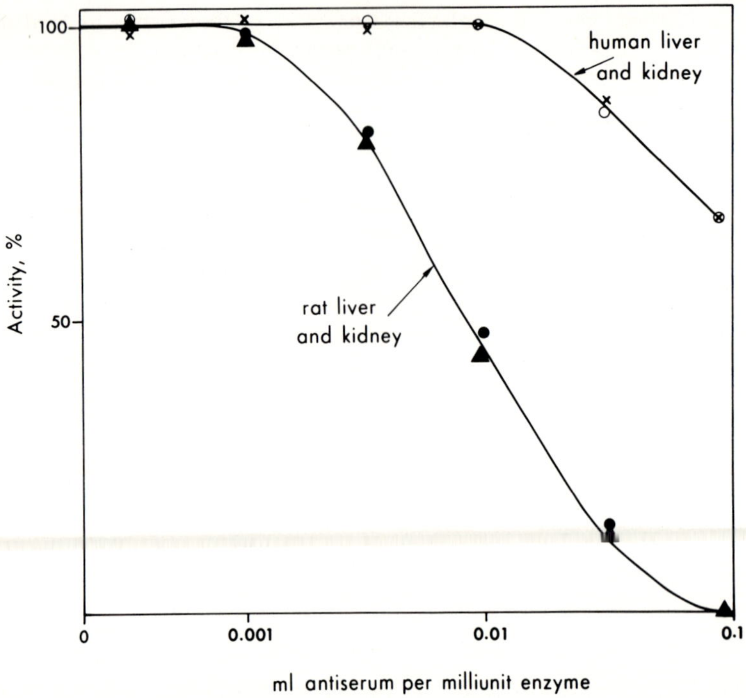

FIGURE 1. Precipitation of phenylalanine hydroxylase from rat liver (▲), rat kidney (●), human liver (×), and human kidney (○), with rat liver phenylalanine hydroxylase antibodies. Enzyme was incubated with varying concentrations of antiserum for 30 minutes at 25°C and 3 hours at 0°C. Enzyme–antibody complex was then precipitated by 33% saturation with ammonium sulfate, and the enzyme activity remaining in the supernatant was assayed after precipitation with 50% ammonium sulfate. Each point on the graph is the average of four measurements.

ase is in the kidney, it is possible that when the liver enzyme is defective the kidney enzyme may be more active. If there are forms of phenylketonuria in which the kidney enzyme remains active, activation or induction of this enzyme might provide a means of treatment.

ACKNOWLEDGMENT

This work was supported in part by USPHS Grant Nos. HD-05061 and HD-04612.

REFERENCES

1. Ayling, J. E., Boehm, G. R., Textor, S. C., and Pirson, R. A. Kinetics of phenylalanine hydroxylase with analogs of tetrahydrobiopterin. *Biochemistry*, 1973, **12:** 2045–2051.

2. Ayling, J. E., and Helfand, G. D. Active sites of phenylalanine hydroxylase. *Fed. Proc., Fed. Am. Soc. Exp. Biol.*, 1974, **33:** 1243.
3. Ayling, J. E., Helfand, G. D., and Pirson, W. D. Phenylalanine hydroxylase from human kidney. *Enzyme*, 1975, **20:** 6–19.
4. Ayling, J. E., Pirson, W. D., Al-Janabi, J. M., and Helfand, G. D. Kidney phenylalanine hydroxylase from man and rat: Comparison with the liver enzyme. *Biochemistry*, 1974, **13:** 78–85.
5. Berry, H. K., Cripps, R., Nichols, K., McCandless, D., and Harper, C. Development of phenylalanine hydroxylase activity in guinea pig liver. *Biochim. Biophys. Acta*, 1972, **261:** 315–320.
6. Dixon, M., and Webb, E. C. *Enzymes*. New York: Academic Press, 1964.
7. Grimm, U., Knapp, A., and Teichmann, W. Phenylalaninhydroxylase-Aktivitatsbestimmungen in Leberhomogenat gesunder probanden. *Acta Biol. Med. Ger.*, 1971, **27:** 443–446.
8. Grimm, U., Knapp, A., Tischer, W., and Schlenzka, K. Phenylalanine hydroxylase activity in hyperphenylalaninemia and classical phenylketonuria. *Acta Biol. Med. Ger.*, 1972, **28:** 549–552.
9. Justice, P., O'Flynn, M. E., and Hsia, D. Y. Phenylalanine hydroxylase activity in hyperphenylalaninemia. *Lancet*, 1967, **1:** 928–929.
10. Kaufman, S. Phenylalanine hydroxylating cofactor in phenylketonuria. *Science*, 1958, **128:** 1506–1508.
11. Kaufman, S. Hepatic phenylalanine hydroxylase and phenylketonuria. This volume, Chapter 16.
12. Kaufman, S., and Max, E. Studies on the phenylalanine hydroxylating system in human liver and their relationship to pathogenesis of PKU and hyperphenylalaninemia. In: *Phenylketonuria.* (H. Bickel, F. P. Hudson, and L. I. Woolf, Eds.). Thieme, Stuttgart, 1971: 13–19.
13. La Du, B. N., and Zannoni, V. G. Inhibition of phenylalanine hydroxylase in liver. In: *Phenylketonuria and Allied Metabolic Diseases.* (J. A. Anderson, and K. F. Swaiman, Eds.). US Govt. Printing Office, Washington, D. C., 1967: 193–202.
14. McGee, M. M., Greengard, O., and Knox, W. E. The quantitative determination of phenylalanine hydroxylase in rat tissues. *Biochem. J.*, 1972, **127:** 669–672.
15. Raiha, N. C. R. Phenylalanine hydroxylase in human liver during development. *Pediat. Res.*, 1973, **7:** 1–4.
16. Tourian, A. Activiation of phenylalanine hydroxylase by phenylalanine. *Biochem. Biophys. Acta*, 1971, **242:** 345–354.
17. Tourian, A., Goddard, J., and Puck, T. T. Phenylalanine hydroxylase activity in mammalian cells. *J. Cell. Physiol.*, 1969, **13:** 159–170.
18. Wallace, H. W., Moldave, K., and Meister, A. Studies on conversion of phenylalanine to tyrosine in phenylpyruvic oligophrenia. *Proc. Soc. Exp. Biol. Med.*, 1957, **94:** 632–633.

17

Studies on the Molecular Defect in Galactosemia

THOMAS A. TEDESCO*

Department of Human Genetics, University of Pennsylvania School of Medicine, Philadelphia, Pennsylvania

INTRODUCTION

Galactosemia is an inborn error in metabolism first described as a clinical abnormality by von Reuss in 1908 (19). Since this observation numerous investigators have contributed to our understanding of the enzymology, genetics, and pathology associated with mutants of galactose metabolism in man (6). We have advanced considerably in our understanding of the galactose metabolic pathway and have developed sophisticated quantitative and qualitative techniques for identifying mutant genes as well as some of their physiological effects in various cell types. Although it is now well recognized that classic galactosemia is a consequence of a deficiency of galactose-1-phosphate uridyltransferase activity, little is known about the type or number of different mutations that can produce this disease, or what the different molecular defects are that can cause catalytic malfunction of this enzyme. The research to be presented here is primarily concerned with answering two questions about galactose-1-phosphate uridyltransferase deficiency in man: (a) is there genetic heterogeneity among transferase deficiency galactosemics and (b) does the mechanism of action of normal human transferase suggest that we can distinguish at a molecular level the basis of defective catalytic function in mutant enzymes?

* Present address: Department of Pediatrics, University of South Florida, College of Medicine, Tampa, Florida.

THE GALACTOSE PATHWAY

There are two enzymes in the galactose metabolic pathway, galactokinase (kinase) and galactose-1-P uridyltransferase (transferase), that are deficient in two distinct forms of galactosemia, both of which are autosomal recessive diseases in man. Kinase deficiency results in the inability to convert galactose (gal) to gal-1-P. This enzyme deficiency first described by Gitzelmann (4) produces galactosemia (i.e., elevated blood galactose), and cataracts appear to be its principle clinical consequence. Transferase deficiency results in the classic form of galactosemia. Since the conversion of gal-1-P to glu-1-P does not occur normally, both gal-1-P and gal accumulate in the tissues of these patients (6). The clinical abnormalities associated with transferase deficiency include failure to thrive, often manifest within the first few weeks of life, cataracts, and liver and neurological dysfunction, the last frequently leading to mental retardation.

Figure 1 shows the galactose metabolic pathway and its relationship to several areas of metabolism. There is good evidence that the conversion of galactose to galactitol by aldose reductase in lens tissue produces osmotic effects which lead to cataract formation (6) common in both kinase and transferase

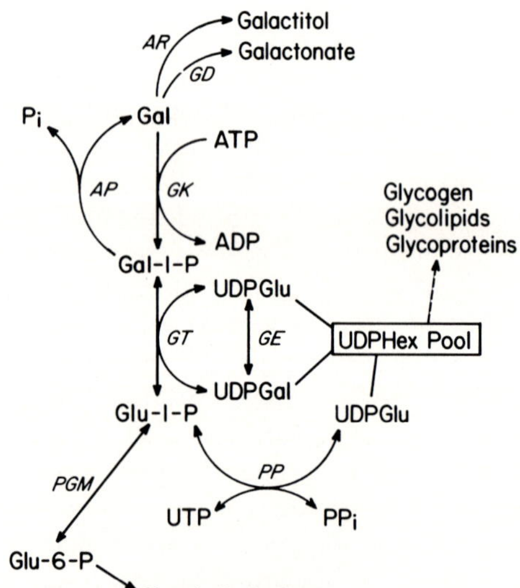

FIGURE 1. The galactose metabolic pathway and its relationship to several areas of metabolism. *AR*, aldose reductase; *GD*, galactose dehydrogenase; *AP*, nonspecific phosphatase; *GK*, galactokinase; *GT*, galactose-1-P uridyltransferase; *GE*, UDPgalactose-4-epimerase; *PGM*, phosphoglucomutase; and *PP*, UDPglucose pyrophosphorylase.

deficiency, and more recent evidence describes a specific inhibitor of aldose reductase that prevents this effect (3).

The obvious clinical and biochemical differences between kinase and transferase deficiency suggest that the accumulation of intracellular gal-1-P is related to the more severe clinical consequences found in transferase deficiency. Gal-1-P has been reported to accumulate in red blood cells (2) and skin fibroblast cell cultures derived from galactosemic patients (10). The toxic effects of gal-1-P as a metabolic inhibitor have been suspected, yet no good evidence has been produced along these lines. Several enzymes have been tested and found to be unaffected by gal-1-P (15). With concentrations up to 2 m*M* we have found that gal-1-P has little or no effect on the activity of UDPgal-4-epimerase or UDPglu pyrophosphorylase under standard assay conditions. Phosphoglucomutase (PGM), an important link in galactose, glucose, and glycogen metabolism, has been reported to be inhibited by gal-1-P, but only in the absence of the coenzyme glu-1,6-diP (15). We have confirmed this finding with PGM extracted from human diploid fibroblast cell cultures. There was no detectable inhibition when glu-1,6-diP was added to the reaction mixture and only about 50% inhibition with a gal-1-P/glu-1-P ratio of 100/1 when glu-1,6-diP was deleted from the reaction. The levels of PGM found in extracts of human fibroblasts are 4 to 5 fold higher when cells are cultured in glucose medium than when grown in galactose medium. This difference, however, may be due to decreased levels of the coenzyme glu-1,6-diP in the galactose-grown cells similar to the finding of decreased levels of this metabolite in the tissues of galactose-fed rats (15).

A vicious cycle of phosphorylation–dephosphorylation has been postulated by some investigators as a toxic mechanism in galactosemia (7,8,10). The action of nonspecific phosphatases on gal-1-P would cause repeated phosphorylation of galactose at the expense of ATP. However, in the livers of rats fed a 50% galactose diet, AMP levels decreased, ADP levels were unchanged or only slightly increased, and ATP levels increased (15) suggesting stimulation of ATP-generating systems rather than exhaustion of ATP by cyclic phosphorylation of galactose. Since no true animal model exists for transferase deficiency galactosemia, it is difficult to compare the data from studies in which normal animals are fed diets of 20 to 50% galactose with those obtained from galactosemic patients or cultured cells derived from them. Our preliminary data show that transferase deficient cells in culture accumulate gal-1-P when grown in galactose medium to levels severalfold that found when these cells are grown in glucose medium; and under the same conditions, normal cells contain barely detectable levels of gal-1-P. These results agree with those recently reported by Mayes and Miller (10) who demonstrated that gal-1-P accumulates in galactosemic cells. In cells derived from heterozygotes for transferase deficiency they found gal-1-P accumulations intermediate between those found in normal and galactosemic fibroblasts. These results correlate well with the relative activities of transferase and kinase activity described by us in normal, heterozygote, and galactosemic fibroblasts (17). Normal cell extracts contain ratios of transferase/kinase greater than 1.0 and heterozygous cells have ratios less than 1.0. Galactokinase appears to be rate limiting in normal cells, but when transferase activity is decreased or absent as in heterozygous and galactosemic cells, transferase becomes rate limiting as reflected in the accumulation of gal-1-P. If the accumulation of intracellular gal-1-P leads to the pathology of galactosemia, studies with fibroblast cells in culture that are truly deficient in transferase activity should elucidate its mechanism, both in cellular and molecular terms.

THE GENETIC NATURE OF THE DEFECT

One first approach toward determining what kind of mutation produces transferase deficiency galactosemia was to prepare a rabbit antiserum to transferase purified to electrophoretic homogeneity from human liver (16). By double immunodiffusion techniques it was found that red blood cell extracts from galactosemic patients contained a cross-reacting material (CRM) immunologically indistinguishable from the transferase found in normal red blood cells (18). Transferase CRM has now been identified in 16 different galactosemic families; we have not yet found a transferase-deficient patient who lacks CRM, suggesting that this disease is due to a structural gene mutation. Proof that the antibody we were using reacted specifically with galactosemia CRM was demonstrated by quantitative immunoprecipitation techniques. Normal transferase was titrated with antiserum to determine the amount needed to neutralize an aliquot of normal enzyme activity. This volume of antiserum was then absorbed with different amounts of partially purified red blood cell extract from transferase'deficient patients, and the amount of transferase-specific antibody remaining was measured. The results clearly showed that these galactosemic red cells contained an antigen that reacted with transferase antibody, and the amounts of antigen were similar to those found in normal red blood cells (18). The lack of transferase activity in galactosemia thus appears to be due to a mutant protein present in apparently normal quantities in the red cell that is defective in its catalytic function. Normal transferase and galactosemic CRM are also similar in molecular size as determined by a standardized Sephadex G-200 gel filtration column. The elution volume of normal transferase determined by specific enzyme activity was identical to that of galactosemic CRM, identified by its immunoreactivity in double immunodiffusion against transferase-specific antiserum (16). These data indicate that the transferase CRM found in galactosemia has the same molecular size and antigenic determinants as the normal enzyme.

GENETIC HETEROGENEITY AMONG GALACTOSEMICS (1)

Although there is a transferase CRM in 16 different galactosemic families, immunologically indistinguishable from normal transferase, we have considered whether there is molecular heterogeneity within this group. Nadler *et al.* (12) showed that complementing hybrids with transferase activity could be produced by fusing certain pairs of galactosemic fibroblast cell culture lines. From this result, the predictions that can be reasonably made are (a) there are functionless proteins in the parental cells, (b) transferase is composed of subunits, and (c) there is heterogeneity among various galactosemic mutations. The presence of CRM in galactosemia where molecular size is similar to normal transferase has already been discussed and thus the first prediction is satisfied. Human transferase purified from liver as well as red blood cells when electrophoresed on SDS polyacrylamide gels, yields a single species with an apparent molecular weight of 30,000 (16). These data satisfy the second prediction since the normal enzyme and galactosemic CRM have an apparent molecular weight in the range of 90,000. The third prediction was satisfied by obtaining evidence for molecular heterogeneity among galactosemics by quantitative and qualitative immunochemical techniques. The content of CRM in red blood cell extracts from different galactosemic patients were analyzed by electroimmunodiffusion in an agarose layer containing human transferase-specific antiserum (9).

Results for five different patients are listed in Table I. On each plate a dilution series was run for each galactosemic sample along with an identically treated normal control. Immunoprecipitin peaks of similar size were chosen from each dilution series and the protein content of that particular sample calculated. On each plate the peak height in millimeters/microgram protein was determined for the control and each galactosemic sample. The amount of CRM in each galactosemic sample is expressed as the ratio of CRM/control. As seen in Table I, two samples have a ratio of 0.96 indicating that these two patients have CRM levels in their red cells similar to the controls. One patient

Table I Quantitative Variation of Human Transferase CRM from the Red Blood Cells of Different Galactosemic Patients[a]

Galactosemic Patient	*Peak Height (mm)*	*CRM*		*Control*	
		Protein (μg)	*Peak Height/Protein*	*Peak Height/Protein*	*CRM/Control*
DT	16.5	11.36	1.450	1.51	0.96
LW	12.5	7.20	1.740	1.81	0.96
FR	15.0	7.45	2.010	1.63	1.23
CW	12.5	16.04	0.779	1.81	0.43
AM	10.0	16.25	0.615	1.92	0.32

[a] Based on electroimmunodiffusion in agar containing antibody to human transferase.

Table II Variation in Electrophoretic Mobility of Transferase CRM in Red Blood Cells from Different Galactosemic Patients Identified by Electroimmunodiffusion

Galactosemic Patient	Electrophoretic Mobility		CRM/Control
	CRM R_f (mm)	Control R_f (mm)	
DT	43	43	1.00
MW	52	54	0.96
WW	55	54	1.01
FR	56	52	1.07
AM	37	43	0.86
LL	44	52	0.84

has 20% more CRM than normal (FR), and two have only 32 and 43% of the control sample (AM and CW, respectively). This quantitative variation in red cell content of galactosemic CRM may indicate that different mutant transferases have different stabilities or that the structural alterations in these proteins affect their rates of synthesis or degradation. Variation in electrophoretic mobility was also found for galactosemic CRM extracted from red cells of different patients. By employing a two-dimensional system in which the samples are separated by electrophoresis in the first dimension, followed by electroimmunodiffusion in the second dimension (11), into an agarose gel containing transferase-specific antiserum, the electrophoretic mobility of CRM can be determined. The results obtained from six different galactosemic patients are listed in Table II. Normal and mutant transferases were run on the same plate, and the electrophoretic migration (R_f) of each galactosemic CRM is expressed as a ratio of CRM R_f/control R_f. Four patients have transferase CRM with the same electrophoretic mobility as the control sample. Patients MW and WW are brothers with transferase deficiency. Two other patients from different families have transferase CRM which migrates at a significantly slower rate than normal (AM and LL).

THE MECHANISM OF ACTION OF HUMAN TRANSFERASE (20)

To understand the structural basis of defective catalytic function in mutant enzymes, the mechanism of action of the normal enzyme needs to be thoroughly characterized. We have analyzed the kinetics of normal human red cell transferase purified to electrophoretic homogeneity; initial velocities as a function of substrate concentration, in both forward and reverse directions, have been determined. From these studies we have concluded that human transferase functions by the Ping-Pong mechanism for a two-substrate enzyme

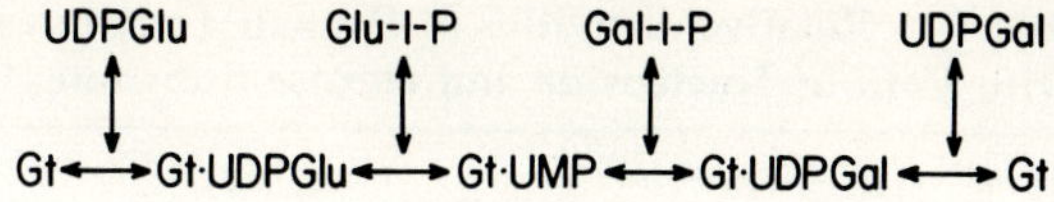

FIGURE 2. Scheme showing the Ping-Pong mechanism of action for human galactose-1-P uridyltransferase.

(18). Such a mechanism implies that both substrates are not simultaneously complexed with the enzyme. The enzyme recognizes the first substrate and proceeds through a half-reaction to produce the first product and a reactive intermediate. The reactive intermediate then complexes with the second substrate and proceeds through the second half of the reaction to yield the final product and free enzyme.

The reaction sequence suggested for the transferase enzyme is illustrated in Figure 2 with an enzyme-UMP complex as the reactive intermediate. Product inhibition patterns for both forward and reverse reactions reveal that glu-1-P and gal-1-P compete with each other as do UDPglu and UDPgal, but UDP-hexose and hexose-1-P (either glu or gal) do not compete with one another. Therefore this enzyme must have separate binding sites for UDPhexose and hexose-1-P. The enzyme shows no apparent preferential affinity for glu or gal as the hexose in these substrates in either the forward or reverse direction. This can be supported by isotope exchange reactions with either glu or gal as illustrated in Figure 3. The ability of human transferase to exchange isotope between UDPgal and gal-1-P was previously described by Segal *et al.* (14). The nonspecificity of human transferase for either glu or gal raises a general question of substrate specificity. We found that human transferase is highly specific for uridine as the nucleotide substrate in the isotope exchange reaction with ^{14}C-glu-1-P (Table III) and for glu-1-P and gal-1-P as the hexose-1-P substrate. Several other hexoses, including glu-1,6-diP, were found to be unreactive in the isotope exchange reaction with UDPglu-^{14}C (Table III). Transferase therefore is a molecule that is highly specific for uridine diphosphate hexose, and for hexose-1-P, but glu and gal readily substitute for one another as the hexose in these substrates.

Although a reactive intermediate has not been isolated, the Ping-Pong mechanism predicts a transferase-UMP complex. This has been supported by experiments in which increasing concentrations of glu-1-P were found to compete with gal-1-P for the reactive intermediate, and by demonstrating that

$$\text{Glu-1-P} + \text{UDPGlu}(^{14}\text{C}) \longleftrightarrow \text{Glu-1-P}(^{14}\text{C}) + \text{UDPGlu}$$

$$\text{Gal-1-P} + \text{UDPGal}(^{14}\text{C}) \longleftrightarrow \text{Gal-1-P}(^{14}\text{C}) + \text{UDPGal}$$

FIGURE 3. Isotope exchange reactions catalyzed by human galactose-1-P uridyltransferase with glucose and galactose substrates.

Table III Relative Activities of Human Transferase with Various Nucleoside and Hexose Substrates[a]

Nucleoside-DPglu	*% Activity*	*Hexose*	*% Activity*
UDPglu	100	Glucose-1-P	100
TDPglu	5.9	Mannose-1-P	0
CDPglu	2.9	Glucose-6-P	0
ADPglu	1.9	Glucose-1,6-diP	0
GDPglu	1.9	Glucose	0

[a] The reaction mixture for testing various nucleoside diphosphate glucose substrates contained in a final volume of 75 μl; 0.06 μmoles of the substrate to be tested; 20 μmoles Tris, pH 8.5; 0.52 μmoles dithiothreitol; 0.2 mg of partially purified red cell transferase protein (specific activity, 0.03 units/mg); and 0.16 ^{14}C-glu-1-P (specific activity, 0.6 μCi/μmole). The same reaction mixture was used to test the various hexose substrates except that 0.03 μmoles UDPglu-^{14}C (specific activity, 3.3 μCi/μmole) replaced ^{14}C-glu-1-P. After 1 hour incubation at 37°C an aliquot of the reaction mixture was chromatographed on DEAE-cellulose paper with 0.05 *M* NaCl to separate hexose-1-P from UDP-hexose which were then counted in a liquid scintillation spectrometer.

glu-1-^{32}P reacts with transferase to produce U-P-^{32}Pglu. A scheme for the hexose-1-P competition experiments is illustrated in Figure 4. Increasing concentrations of glu-1-P were added to the isotope exchange reaction mixture containing UDPgal and ^{14}C-gal-1-P. UDPgal-^{14}C formation was measured by scintillation spectrometry after separating UDPhexose from the reaction mixture with DEAE-cellulose paper chromatography (13). The formation of UDPglu in the reaction mixture was measured with UDPglu dehydrogenase. The results plotted in Figure 5 clearly show that UDPglu formation increases as a function of glu-1-P concentration, and that UDPgal-^{14}C formation decreases proportionately as UDPglu increases. When glu-1-^{32}P is used as a substrate in this reaction the label is transferred to U-P-^{32}Pglu, further evidence that an enzyme–UMP complex is the reactive intermediate in addition to indicating which ester bond is involved in the reaction. Obviously one of the

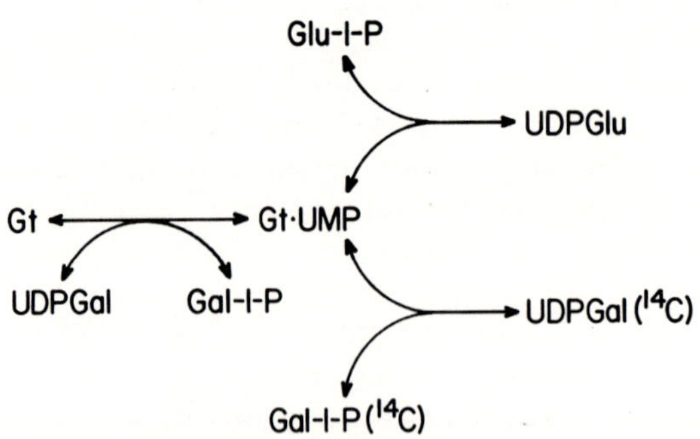

FIGURE 4. Scheme describing the hexose-1-P competition for the reactive intermediate in the transferase reaction.

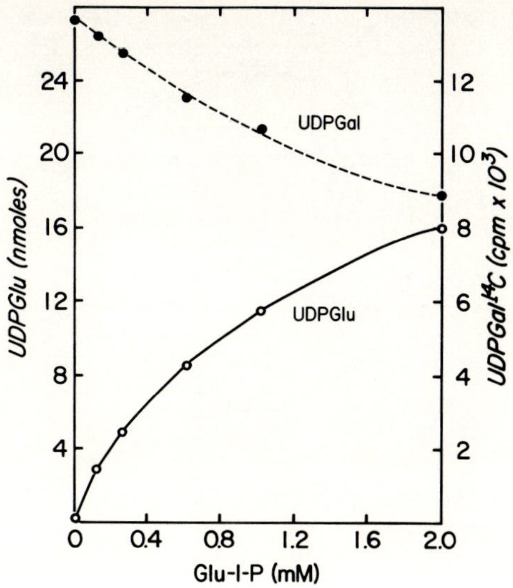

FIGURE 5. The results of hexose-1-P competition for the reactive intermediate in the transferase reaction, as illustrated in Figure 4. Increasing concentrations of glucose-1-P were incubated in a reaction mixture which contained in a final volume of 85 μl; 10 μmoles Tris, pH 8.5; 0.52 μmoles dithiothreitol; 2 mg of partially purified red cell transferase protein (specific activity, 0.03 units/mg); 0.19 μmoles UDPgalactose; and 0.14 μmoles ^{14}C-galactose-1-P. (Specific activity, 0.7 μCi/per μmole.) UDPgal-^{14}C was measured by liquid scintillation spectrometry after separation from the reaction mixture by DEAE-cellulose paper chromatography (13). UDPglucose was measured with UDPglucose dehydrogenase.

bonds in the ester linkage between the two phosphates in the UDPhexose substrate is being broken and reformed in the course of this reaction. Appropriate experiments with specifically labeled ^{18}O-UDPhexose (U-P-^{18}O-Pglu) should now indicate exactly which covalent bond is involved.

The interpretation of these data is summarized in Figure 6 which illustrates the activity of human transferase broken down into six individual steps, each of which is reversible. We are now attempting to detect half-reactions by measuring hexose-1-P formation from UDPhexose in the absence of a hexose-1-P substrate, as well as other individual parts of this sequential reaction. Artificial substrates may provide some of this capability. For example, UMP-*p*-nitrophenol complex, an assay for the first step in the reaction (Figure 6) will not react with the enzyme to produce enzyme-UMP and free *p*-nitrophenol. If we can successfully separate and quantitatively measure the enzyme-UMP-*p*-nitrophenol complex, an assay for the first step in the reaction (Figure 6) will be available for testing mutant transferases to determine if they can perform this part of the reaction. With the use of additional artificial substrates we would ultimately hope to develop the ability to assay each of the individual steps in the total reaction. This would allow the determination of the specific

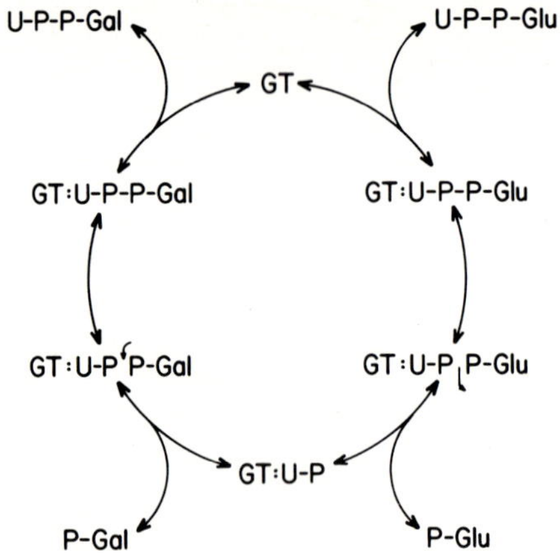

FIGURE 6. The reaction sequence proposed for human galactose-1-P uridyltransferase. Activity moving clockwise represents the forward reaction.

catalytic defect in different galactosemic transferases. Presumably those nonfunctional parental enzymes that are complementary in cell hybridization experiments will have different types of functional defects.

SUMMARY

The galactose metabolic pathway and some of the consequences of deficient galactokinase or gal-1-P uridyltransferase activity have been discussed. The existence of CRM in transferase deficiency galactosemia is presented as evidence that this disease is the result of a structural gene mutation. The finding of both quantitative and qualitative variation in transferase CRM among different galactosemic patients argues that genetic heterogeneity exists within this group. Data supporting a Ping-Pong mechanism of action for human transferase have been presented, and a sequence of six individual steps in the transferase reaction is proposed.

ACKNOWLEDGMENTS

I gratefully acknowledge Dr. William J. Mellman, Chairman, Department of Human Genetics, University of Pennsylvania School of Medicine, for his critical evaluation and direction throughout the course of this work; Dr. Roland G. Kallen, Associate Professor of Biochemistry, for consultation and advice in the studies on the mechanism of action of human transferase; Karen Miller, Jr. Research Specialist, for her work on all phases of this project; Dr. Joseph W-T Wu, Post Doctoral Fellow, for his work on the molecular studies; Francie Boches, graduate student in biochemistry, for her work on genetic heterogeneity of transferase CRM; and last but not least, Barbara Needleman and Constance Page for their cell culture work.

This work was supported by NIH Grant Nos. HD-00588 and HD-04861.

REFERENCES

1. Boches, F., Tedesco, T. A., Miller, K., and Mellman, W. J. Unpublished observations.
2. Donnell, G. N., Koch, R., and Bergren, W. R. Observations on results of management of galactosemic patients. In: *Galactosemia.* (D. Y. Y. Hsia, Ed.). Chapter 31. Thomas, Springfield, Illinois, 1969: 247–268.
3. Dvornik, D., Simard-Duquesne, N., Krami, M., Sestauj, K., Gabbay, K. H., Kinoshita, J. H., Varma, D. S., and Merola, L. O. Polyol accumulation in galactosemic and diabetic rats: Control by an aldose reductase inhibitor. *Science,* 1973, **182:** 1146–1148.
4. Gitzelman, R. Hereditary galactokinase deficiency, a newly recognized cause of juvenile cataracts. *Pediat. Res.,* 1967, **1:** 14–23.
5. Hersh, L. B., and Jencks, W. P. Coenzyme A transferase; kinetics and exchange reactions. *J. Biol. Chem.,* 1967, **242:** 3468–3480.
6. Kalckar, H. M., Kinoshita, J. H., and Donnell, G. N. Galactosemia: Biochemistry, genetics, pathophysiology, and developmental aspects. In: *Biology of Brain Dysfunction.* (G. E. Gaull, Ed.). Chapter 2. Plenum, New York, 1973: 31–88.
7. Kozak, L. P., and Wells, W. W. Effect of galactose on energy and phospholipid metabolism in the chick brain. *Arch. Biochem. Biophys.,* 1969, **135:** 371–377.
8. Kozak, L. P., and Wells, W. W. Studies on the metabolic determinants of D-galactose induced neurotoxicity in the chick. *J. Neurochem.,* 1971, **18:** 2217–2228.
9. Laurell, C. B. Quantitative estimation of proteins by electrophoresis in agarose gels containing antibodies. *Anal. Biochem.,* 1966, **15:** 45–52.
10. Mayes, J. S., and Miller, L. R. The metabolism of galactose by galactosemic fibroblasts *in vitro. Biochim. Biophys. Acta,* 1973, **313:** 9–16.
11. Minchin Clark, H. G., and Freeman, T. Quantitative immunoelectrophoresis of human serum proteins. *Clin. Sci.,* 1968, **35:** 403–413.
12. Nadler, H. L., Chacko, C. M., and Rachmeler, M. Interallelic complementation in hybrid cells derived from human diploid strains deficient in galactose-1-phosphate uridyltransferase activity. *Proc. Natl. Acad. Sci. USA,* 1970, **67:** 967–982.
13. Ng, W. G., Bergren, W. R., and Donnell, G. N. Assay of hemolysate gal-1-P uridyltransferase activity by radioactivity. In: *Galactosemia.* (D. Y. Y. Hsia, Ed.). Chapter 13. Thomas, Springfield, Illinois, 1969: 98–104.
14. Segal, S., Rogers, S., and Holtzapple, P. G. Liver galactose-1-phosphate uridyltransferase: activity in normal and galactosemic subjects. *J. Clin. Invest.,* 1971, **50:** 500–506.
15. Sidbury, J. B., Jr. Investigations and speculations on the pathogenesis of galactosemia. In: *Galactosemia.* (D. Y. Y. Hsia, Ed.). Chapter 2. Thomas, Springfield, Illinois, 1969: 13–29.
16. Tedesco, T. A. Human galactose-1-phosphate uridyltransferase: Purification, antibody production, and comparison of the wild type, Duarte variant, and galactosemic gene products. *J. Biol. Chem.,* 1972, **247:** 6631–6636.
17. Tedesco, T. A., and Mellman, W. J. Galatose-1-phosphate uridyltransferase and galactokinase activity in cultured human diploid fibroblasts and peripheral blood leukocytes. *J. Clin. Invest.,* 1969, **48:** 2390–2397.
18. Tedesco, T. A., and Mellman, W. J. Galactosemia; evidence for a structural gene mutation. *Science,* 1971, **172:** 727–728.
19. von Reuss, A. Zuckerauwscheidung in Sauglinsalter. *Wien. Med. Wochenschr.,* 1908, **58:** 799.
20. Wu, J., Tedesco, T. A., and Kallen, R. G. Human galactose-1-phosphate uridyltransferase; kinetic mechanism, substrate specificity, and exchange reactions. (Submitted to *J. Biol. Chem.*)

18

The Enzymology of Tay-Sachs Disease and Its Variant Forms

JOHN F. TALLMAN
Developmental and Metabolic Neurology Branch,
National Institutes of Health,
Bethesda, Maryland

A. INTRODUCTION: THE CATABOLISM OF GANGLIOSIDES

The study of certain progressively degenerative neurological disorders known as the lipidoses (1–3) has necessitated an intensive investigation of reactions involved in the catabolism of gangliosides and related neutral glycosphingolipids. These compounds which are derivatives of sphingosine, $CH_3(CH_2)_{12}—CH=CH—CH(OH)—CH(NH_2)—CH_2OH$, contain a long chain fatty acid bound in an amide linkage to the nitrogen atom on C-2. This *N*-acylsphingosine complex is called ceramide. Additional constituents, such as mono- or oligosaccharides, may be linked through the primary hydroxyl group of sphingosine to yield the glycosphingolipids. The gangliosides are glycosphingolipids which are characterized by the presence of one or more molecules of sialic acid (*N*-acetyl or *N*-glycolylneuraminic acid) (Figure 1).

It is presently believed that the catabolism of a ganglioside proceeds stepwise from the nonreducing terminus of the carbohydrate portion of the molecule toward the ceramide moiety (Figure 2) (35). The enzymes catalyzing these reactions are located in the lysosomes and exhibit properties characteristic of such enzymes. Of the numerous enzymes involved in ganglioside breakdown, clinical disorders have been associated with deficiencies in each of the reactions (with the exception of the neuraminidase). A discussion of these disorders is available (1–3,36,40). This review will be concerned with Tay-Sachs disease and its variants (known collectively as the G_{M2}-gangliosidoses).

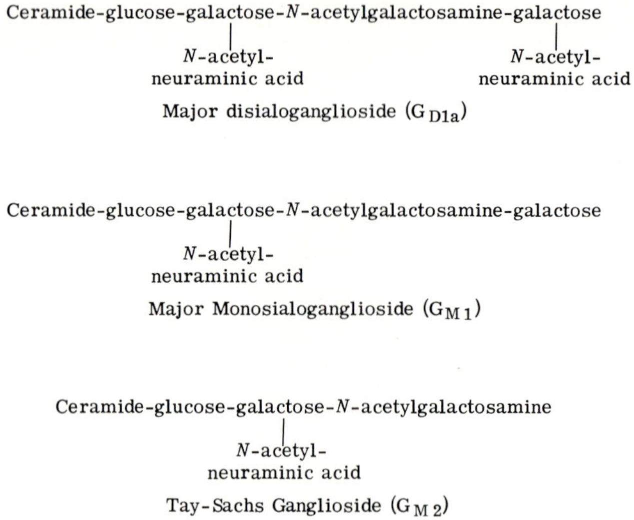

FIGURE 1. The structure of important gangliosides.

B. TYPE I G_{M2}-GANGLIOSIDOSIS (TAY-SACHS DISEASE)

1. Clinical Signs

The original descriptions of this disorder date from the last century and were made separately by Warren Tay (41) and Bernard Sachs (24) in children of Ashkenazic Jewish descent. Since these primary descriptions, numerous cases have been reported. It is this form of G_{M2}-gangliosidosis which is rightly called Tay-Sachs disease. Motor weakness is an early sign and is usually manifest between the third and sixth postnatal month. This weakness progresses and after 1 year of age, increasing mental retardation becomes apparent. The patient declines with the further appearance of blindness, deafness, and convulsions. Affected children commonly die between age 3 and 4.

2. Pathology

Patients with Tay-Sachs disease are characterized by the presence of a cherry-red spot in the macular region of the eye (41). Macrocephaly occurs after 1 year but there are no visceral changes such as hepatosplenomegaly or bony changes in Tay-Sachs patients.

Microscopic signs of an acute lipid storage disease are found in neuronal cells in various organs. The cytoplasm of these cells is distended and contains numerous granules which on electron microscopic examination appear as spiral laminated structures with a cross section of 50 Å (25) (Figure 3). Through

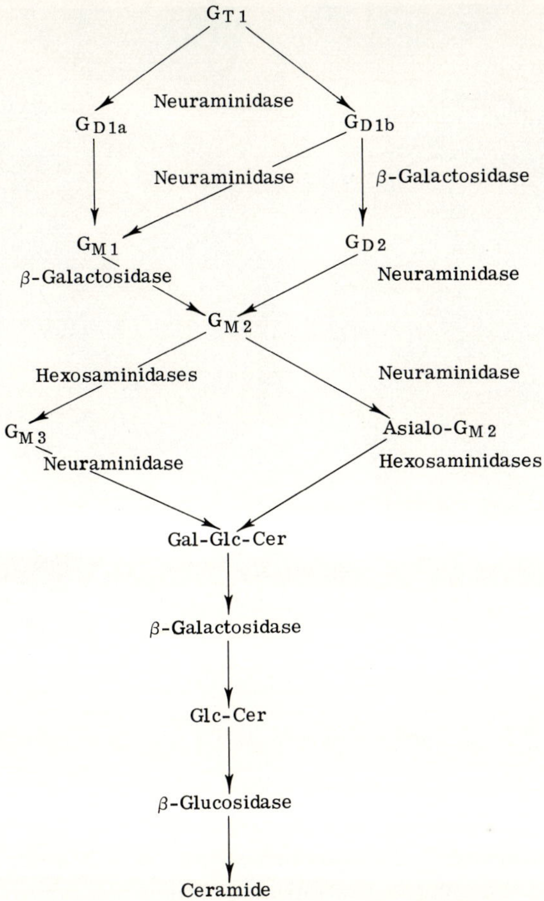

FIGURE 2. Enzymatic hydrolysis of gangliosides.

the use of both continuous and discontinuous sucrose gradient centrifugation, it has been possible to isolate these bodies and show that they contain a large quantity of the ganglioside G_{M2} (Figure 1) (25). Enzymatic analysis indicates that these isolated membranous cytoplasmic bodies contain high levels of various enzymes which are characteristic of the lysosome; this finding points out their probable lysosomal origin (38). Degeneration of the axons, followed by demyelination, may also occur in Tay-Sachs patients (42).

3. Chemistry of the Storage Material

An alteration in the chemical composition of the brain of patients with Tay-Sachs disease was first detected by Klenk (11) who showed an increase in the

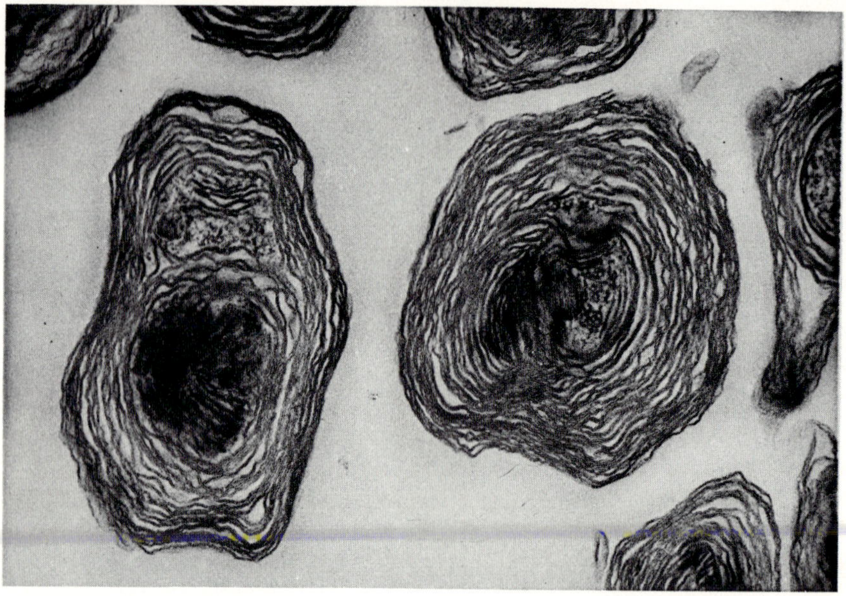

FIGURE 3. Typical isolated MCB from a patient with Tay-Sachs disease magnification ×34,000. Courtesy Dr. Suzuki.

acidic glycosphingolipid (ganglioside) content of such patients. Confirmation of this report followed and the particular ganglioside present in elevated quantities was identified as G_{M2} by Svennerholm (33). Its structure was later determined (16) and this compound came to be called Tay-Sachs ganglioside (Figure 1). The total ganglioside content of Tay-Sachs brain is elevated to 4 to 5 times normal and the greatest proportion of this is G_{M2} (about 80%). The asialo derivative of G_{M2}, *N*-acetylgalactosaminylgalactosylglucosylceramide(G_{A2}) is also present in the brains of these patients (about 1 mole G_{A2}/8 moles G_{M2}) and is elevated approximately 20 to 50 times normal (29).

4. Nature of the Metabolic Defect

Based on previous studies concerning the nature of enzymatic defects in related lipidoses, such as Gaucher's disease and Niemann-Pick's disease (1), a logical site for a defect in Tay-Sachs disease was in the catabolism of the accumulating ganglioside (G_{M2}) and asialo derivative (G_{A2}). Since G_{M2} is branched at its nonreducing terminus, catabolism of G_{M2} could conceivably proceed either through the removal of *N*-acetylneuraminic acid (neuraminidase) to yield G_{A2} or *N*-acetylgalactosamine (hexosaminidase) to yield G_{M3} (Figure 2). Using artificial chromogenic substrates, initial studies on human hexosaminidases indicated that there was a higher total hexosaminidase activ-

Table I Subcellular Distribution of Cortical G_{M2}-Hydrolases[a]

Fraction	*G_{M2}-Sialidase (pmoles/mg protein/hr)*	*G_{M2}-Hexosaminidase (pmoles/mg protein/hr)*
Homogenate	62	31
Myelin-rich	0	0
Nerve endings, mitochondria, and some lysosomes	79	56
Lysosome-rich[b]	198	140
Cytosol	26	10

[a] Data from Tallman and Brady (34).
[b] 64% of total G_{M2}-sialidase activity; 81% of total G_{M2}-hexosaminidase activity.

ity in brain tissue from patients with Tay-Sachs disease than in controls (28). The possibility had to be considered that a G_{M2}-neuraminidase deficiency was responsible for the ganglioside accumulation and that the storage of the asialo compound was secondary to G_{M2} accumulation. To investigate this alternative, G_{M2} was biosynthetically labeled in the *N*-acetylneuraminosyl portion of the molecule from a specific sialic acid precursor, *N*-acetylmannosamine (13). A neuraminidase which possessed activity toward ^{3}H-Acneu-G_{M2} was demonstrated in mammalian tissue (15,34) and possessed a lysosomal subcellular distribution (Table I). The activity of this neuraminidase was determined in skeletal muscle (14) and brain tissue (39) from normal and Tay-Sachs patients. The specific activity of this neuraminidase was similar in tissue specimens from normal humans and patients with Tay-Sachs disease (Table II).

Table II Ganglioside Catabolism by Human Brain Lysosomes[a]

Source of Tissue	*Enzyme Activities*		
	Hexosaminidase		*Neuraminidase,*
	G_{M2}-^{14}C-Ganglioside[b]	*Artificial Substrate[c]*	*G_{M2}-^{3}H-Ganglioside[b]*
Control series ($n = 7$)	140 ± 53	134 ± 11	219 ± 33
G_{M2}-Gangliosidosis patients			
1. V.D. (Type I)	0	513	225
2. J.K. (Type I)	0	1416	Not determined
3. D.T. (Type II)	6	3	232
Mixed experiment			
Control + D.T.	138 (Theory = 98)	Not determined	210 (Theory = 224)

[a] Data from Tallman *et al.* (39).
[b] Picomoles G_{M2} hydrolyzed/mg protein/hour.
[c] Nanomoles 4-methylumbelliferyl-*N*-acetyl-D-glucosaminide hydrolyzed/mg protein/hour.

Resolution of the discrepancy between these results and the existence of G_{M2} storage (and Tay-Sachs disease) depended on a number of observations. Two hexosaminidase isozymes (A and B) had been demonstrated in human tissues (23). Using both heat denaturation (activity of hexosaminidase A is labile to heating at 50°C for 4 hours at pH 4.4) and electrophoretic techniques (A is a more acidic protein), Okada and O'Brien (20) were able to show a deficiency in hexosaminidase A in tissues from patients with Tay-Sachs disease. At that time, the activity of the hexosaminidases with regard to their ability to break down G_{M2} had not been thoroughly investigated. The release of *N*-acetylgalactosamine from doubly labeled G_{M2} was diminished in skeletal muscle preparations from patients with Tay-Sachs disease (14); however, the possibility of a two-step reaction in which *N*-acetylneuraminic acid was first removed could not be ruled out. Using G_{M2}, specifically labeled in the *N*-acetylgalactosaminyl portion of the molecule (22), it was possible to show that direct hydrolysis of *N*-acetylgalactosamine from G_{M2} occurred in brain lysosomes (Table I), that the enzyme involved in this process (a hexosaminidase) possessed many properties different from the neuraminidase [e.g., different pH optimum (Figure 4)] and, most importantly, that this G_{M2}-hexosaminidase activity was missing in the brain tissue of patients with Tay-Sachs disease (Table II). It is critical to mention at this point that in these studies (14,34,39) no attempt was made to separate hexosaminidase A from B and that these results indicated that a deficiency in G_{M2} hydrolysis was the underlying cause of Tay-Sachs disease. It seemed likely at the time by the correlation of our findings with those of Okada and O'Brien (20) that hexosaminidase A alone possessed hydrolytic activity toward G_{M2}; subsequent experiments with purified enzymes have shown this to be false. (See E for a further discussion of this topic.)

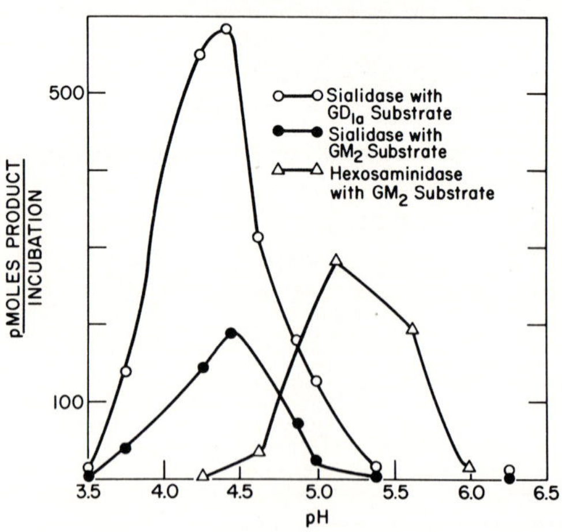

FIGURE 4. Effect of varying pH on brain lysosomal hydrolases. Data from Tallman and Brady (34).

In order to obtain a full understanding of the pathological biochemistry of Tay-Sachs disease, several additional considerations must be taken into account. A hexosaminidase B-like protein, which is present in the tissues of patients with G_{M2}-gangliosidosis Types I and III, can catalyze the hydrolysis of G_{A2} produced by G_{M2}-neuraminidase which is still active in these patients. Since the specific activity of this B-like enzyme is elevated (29), why does G_{M2} accumulate at all?

The question may be partly resolved by the fact that in Type II G_{M2}-gangliosidosis (Section C) in which patients lack both hexosaminidase A and B isozymes, the absolute quantity of G_{A2} accumulating in brain is higher and the ratio of G_{A2} to G_{M2} is larger (⅓) than in Tay-Sachs patients (Type I) (29). This finding suggests that the alternate pathway does participate in G_{M2} breakdown but is insufficient to handle the load of G_{M2} caused by rapid ganglioside turnover in early life. The insufficiency of this pathway may be due to a number of factors including: nonoptional spatial arrangement of the Tay-Sachs patient's hexosaminidase B-like enzyme to the neuraminidase, inhibition of G_{A2} hydrolysis in later stages of the disease by G_{M2} (26), inhibition of the neuraminidase activity against G_{M2} by the di- and trisialogangliosides since the same enzyme works on all these substrates (35), or nonoptimal pH conditions for one or both of the alternate enzymes (pH 3.8 optimum for G_{A2} hydrolysis and see Figure 4). The existence of this alternate pathway may also account for the relatively insignificant accumulation of G_{M2} outside the central nervous system.

5. Prenatal Diagnosis and Treatment

Screening for carriers of Type I G_{M2}-gangliosidosis has been successfully undertaken utilizing the heat denaturation method on serum hexosaminidases. Large-scale testing programs for high risk populations are currently being implemented (6,10) and successful intrauterine diagnosis of Tay-Sachs disease has been made directly on amniotic fluid samples (30) and cultured amniotic cells (19). There is no current therapy for Tay-Sachs disease and the success of enzyme replacement trials seems slight because of the barrier (9) to enzyme entrance into the brain.

C. TYPE II G_{M2}-GANGLIOSIDOSIS (SANDHOFF'S DISEASE)

1. Clinical and Pathological Aspects

These patients have neurological signs similar to those of patients with Type I G_{M2}-gangliosidosis. Additionally, there are changes in visceral organs attendant on the accumulation of neutral glycosphingolipid called globoside: *N*-acetylgalactosaminylgalactosylgalactosylglucosylceramide in both liver and spleen

(28). The progression of this disease is similar to Type I. There is no predilection to Jewish ancestry in these patients.

Microscopically, there is little difference between the neuronal inclusions in Type I and II G_{M2}-gangliosidosis. The predominant difference is the presence of numerous membranous cytoplasmic bodies in the liver cells of Type II patients. On electron microscopic examination these bodies appear quite similar to those described in the brains of patients with Type I disease.

2. Chemistry of the Storage Material

Patients with Type II G_{M2}-gangliosidosis are also characterized by the accumulation of G_{M2} and its asialo derivative in neuronal cells. It is interesting to note that the amount of G_{A2} accumulation relative to G_{M2} is greater than in Type I (about 1 mole G_{A2}/3 moles G_{M2}). This may be related to the nature of the enzymatic defect and alternate pathway discussed in Section B, 4. In Type II patients, there is also a significantly higher accumulation of G_{M2} in liver compared to Tay-Sachs patients where G_{M2} accumulation is minimal (12).

3. Metabolic Defect, Diagnosis and Treatment

Patients with Type II G_{M2}-gangliosidosis are characterized by a total lack of hexosaminidase activity when measured with artificial substrates (29). These patients also lack the ability to degrade G_{M2} (Table II) (39) and neutral glycosphingolipids containing a terminal molecule of *N*-acetylgalactosamine (12,29). Detection of heterozygotes for Type II G_{M2}-gangliosidosis is possible and prenatal detection of this disease has been carried out (12).

Treatment of patients with Type II G_{M2}-gangliosidosis has been attempted by the intravenous injection of highly purified hexosaminidase A (9). Although some lowering of the serum globoside levels was obtained, there was no increase in hexosaminidase activity in the brain. Thus, this therapeutic effort must be regarded as unsuccessful.

D. OTHER VARIANT FORMS

4. Type III G_{M2}-Gangliosidosis

A patient with Type III G_{M2}-gangliosidosis has been described who appeared clinically as a Type I patient and did not show any visceral changes. The amount of both G_{M2} and G_{A2} accumulated in the brain of this patient were higher than in Type I patients, although the relative proportions are close to those of Type I patients (29).

When artificial substrates are used to monitor activity, both hexosaminidases A and B appeared to be present although the ability of this patient to break down G_{M2} is diminished (29). These results are interpreted and discussed in Section F.

2. Hexosaminidase A-Deficient Adults

Very recently, normal adults have been described who are totally lacking in hexosaminidase A and yet do not exhibit any of the signs of Tay-Sachs disease (18,44). In these cases, prenatal diagnosis is impossible using current methods. A possible explanation of this seeming paradox is presented in Section F.

E. PROBLEMS IN G_{M2} HYDROLYSIS

The problems in establishing G_{M2} hydrolysis were almost insurmountable. It was impossible to show directly by colorimetric methods the reaction products from either G_{M2}-hexosaminidase or G_{M2}-neuraminidase. For this reason, the use of G_{M2} specifically labeled either in the *N*-acetylgalactosaminyl and *N*-acetylneuraminosyl portion of the molecule was initiated. When the labeled substrates are used, it is possible to show the low levels of activity reported in Tables I and II. Both enzymes have specific activities that are much lower than the other enzymes of the ganglioside catabolic pathway [e.g., glucocerebrosidase is 100 times more active in the same system (37)] and make it likely that hydrolysis of G_{M2} is the rate-limiting step in ganglioside turnover.

The brain was chosen for study because the predominent effects in Tay-Sachs disease are manifest in this organ. To mimic as closely as possible the physiological state, a crude lysosomal system was prepared and great care was taken to avoid rupture of the lysosomes. Many attempts were made to optimize the incubation conditions. Detergents and various cations had no significant stimulatory effect and in many cases were inhibitory. Fresh tissue (never frozen) was used in all these studies because freezing inactivated the hexosaminidase with G_{M2} as substrate. Sonic disruption of the intact lysosomes which possessed hexosaminidase activity toward G_{M2} resulted in preparations which no longer possessed G_{M2} cleaving activity; activity toward the artificial substrate, 4-methylumbelliferyl-*N*-acetyl-β-D-glucosaminide, was unaffected by this treatment and G_{M1}-β-galactosidase activity was also unaffected. Multistep hydrolysis of GalNAc-^{14}C-G_{M1} with the release of GalNAc-^{14}C (22), which we were able to demonstrate in this system was also lost. It is fatuous to disregard the amount of activity reported in these studies by blithely declaring that optimal conditions have not been achieved. Indeed, it is likely that effective G_{M2} hydrolysis may depend on a membrane-bound hexosaminidase or the association of this enzyme with a critical lipid or protein

Table III Activity of Normal Lysosomes after the Addition of Various Purified Enzymes[a]

Addition	*Activity (pmoles GalNAc/incubation/hr)*
Lysosomal extract	49
Urinary hexosaminidase A	0
Urinary hexosaminidase B	0
Lysosomal extract ($\frac{1}{2}$) + U. Hex A + U. Hex B	23

[a] Data from Tallman *et al.* (39).

inside the lysosomal membrane as was obtained in intact lysosomes. Disruption of this system or ultrastructure leads to drastic loss in G_{M2} hydrolysis by the hexosaminidase. If this is true, it would also explain our inability to bring about stimulation of the G_{M2}-cleaving ability of exogenous hexosaminidase added to the lysosomal system (39) (Table III).

Very recently, we (37) have been able to purify hexosaminidase A and B extensively from fresh human placenta. Using these purified enzymes we found that both normal human placental hexosaminidases A and B possess activity toward GalNAc-^{14}C-G_{M2} (Table IV). Hydrolysis of this substrate was obtained only in the presence of the detergent sodium taurocholate. This dependence is in contrast to the studies in crude brain lysosomes where no detergent was required for G_{M2} hydrolysis. Again, in studies in crude tissue preparations no attempt was made to separate the activities of hexosaminidase A and B. A higher ratio of natural to artificial substrate hydrolysis was also obtained in crude preparations (1:1000 versus 1:10^6 for the purified enzyme). The lysosomal preparations also showed a more basic pH optimum than the highly purified enzymes (compare Figures 4 and 5) and a classical kinetic situation (compare Figures 6 and 7). With the use of either purified enzyme, a complex response of the enzyme to increasing substrate concentration was noted and an optimal detergent to substrate ratio could be established. However, the low levels of activity obtained in these experiments with the purified hexosaminidases cannot be considered physiologically significant.

Table IV Ratio of G_{M2} Cleaving to Artificial Substrate Activity of Purified Hexodaminidases[a]

Enzyme	*Artificial Activity (μmoles/hr)*	*G_{M2} Activity (pmoles/hr)*	*Ratio Natural/Artificial (pmole/μmole)*
Hexosaminidase A	2.4	121	50.4
Hexosaminidase B	0.6	35	57.5

[a] Data from Tallman *et al.* (39).

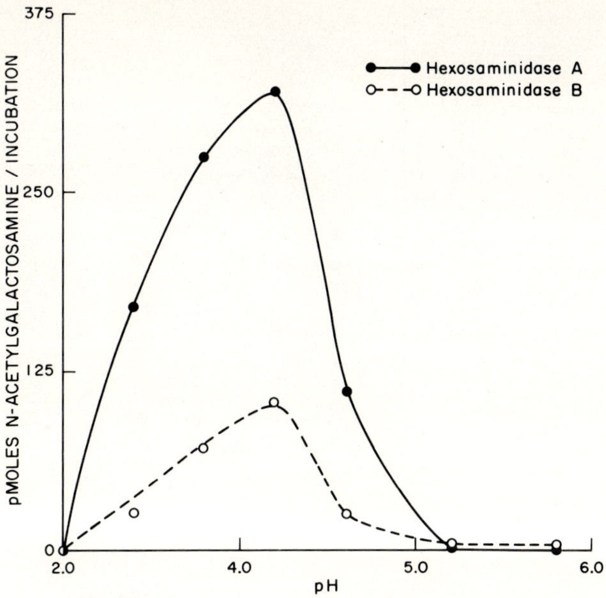

FIGURE 5. Effect of varying pH on G_{M2} hydrolysis by purified hexosaminidase A or B. Data from Tallman *et al.* (37).

Similar experiments (27) using a purified preparation of hexosaminidases from human liver demonstrated the hydrolysis of $^3H-G_{M2}$ (reductively tritiated in the sphingosine moiety) using long-term incubations (24 hours) in the presence of sodium taurocholate. Only hexosaminidase A was capable of this hydrolysis. Purified B had no activity. However, because of the small

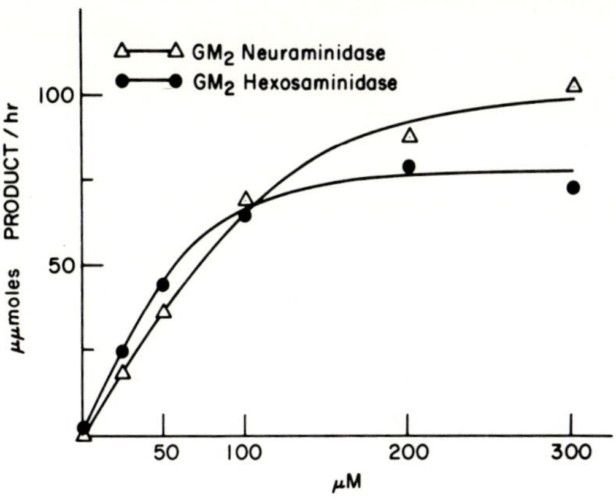

FIGURE 6. Effect of varying substrate concentration on G_{M2} hydrolysis by brain lysosomal hydrolases. Data from Tallman and Brady (34).

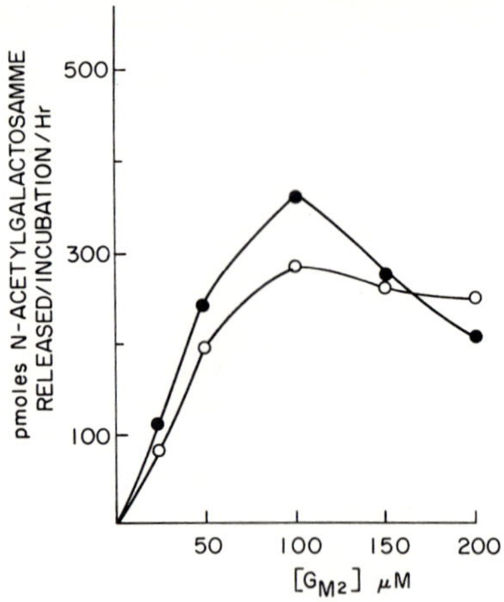

FIGURE 7. Effect of varying substrate concentration on G_{M2} hydrolysis by purified hexosaminidases A or B. Dark circles, hexosaminidase A. Open circles, hexosaminidase B. Data from Tallman *et al.* (37).

amount of product (G_{M3}) (~5%) formed and the complicated assay procedure necessitated by the nature of the labeling, a significant decrease in the activity of hexosaminidase B during the course of the incubation would make it difficult to detect activity present only in the initial stages of the reaction (i.e., a smaller amount of product). Such a decrease in activity was noted in our experiments (Figure 8) and might account for the inability to demonstrate activity with B.

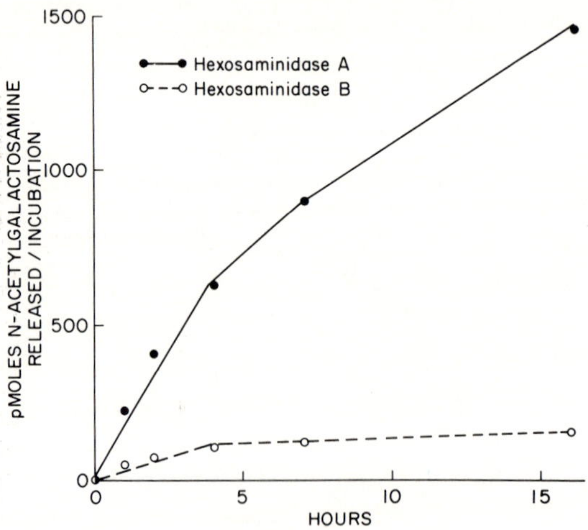

FIGURE 8. Linearity of G_{M2} hydrolysis with time by purified hexosaminidase A or B. Data from Tallman *et al.* (37).

The use of frozen tissue as the purification source may account for the difficulties of another group (45) in demonstrating any G_{M2} hydrolysis. Since I have been emphasizing the necessity of fresh tissue to study adequately the ganglioside catabolic enzymes in light of our experience, their inability to demonstrate activity is not surprising. However, in their experiments, the addition of a bacterial neuraminidase led to a significant conversion of G_{M2} to lactosylceramide. The pH of this incubation was 3.8, the optimum for the hydrolysis of G_{A2} and far from the optimum of the bacterial neuraminidase. It is not clear from their data whether this is a two-step process involving G_{M2} hydrolysis to G_{A2} followed by the hydrolysis of this compound to lactosylceramide or an abstruse mechanism using a "neuraminidase–hexosaminidase" complex. Our attempts to reconstruct this experiment with our optimal substrate/detergent ratio were unsuccessful. We showed a slight inhibition of our active hexosaminidase A at pH 3.8 by the addition of neuraminidase (Sigma, Type VI). At pH 5.0 in our hands, either stabilization of the hexosaminidase or some conversion of G_{M2} to G_{A2} followed by release of *N*-acetylgalactosamine from this compound is obtained. Based on this evidence and our previous negative results (Table III) in which we studied possible synergistic effects after the addition of purified mammalian neuraminidase to both crude lysosomal preparations from human brain and purified human hexosaminidases, we feel that the postulation of a "complex of neuraminidase and hexosaminidase" is premature and clouds the mechanism of an otherwise "simple" hydrolase. It is also possible that a contaminant in their neuraminidase, such as a lipid, led to stimulation of their hexosaminidase in the same way as the detergent, sodium taurocholate.

Very recently, Li and co-workers (17) have reported the presence of a heat-stable factor from liver supernatant which, when added to partly purified hexosaminidases in the absence of other detergents, stimulated the A form but not B. Although a provocative finding, and perhaps of physiological significance, their fully stimulated hexosaminidase was only one-tenth as active as our purified A or B was with sodium taurocholate. Thus, their heat-stable factor merely stimulates their enzymes of no activity into low activity. They do not approach a physiologically significant level by several orders of magnitude and further work is required to assess the significance of this finding.

F. PHYSICAL PROPERTIES AND POSSIBLE RELATIONSHIP OF HEXOAMINIDASES

The apparent molecular weight is identical for both hexosaminidase A and B as determined by gel filtration on Sephadex G-200. Our value of 127,000 daltons is in agreement with that reported earlier (29) for human liver and slightly lower than the reported weights of the beef spleen enzymes (43).

When the molecular weights of hexosaminidases A and B were determined using gel electrophoresis in the presence of urea, sodium dodecylsulfate, and reducing agent at high pH, a uniform subunit with a mass of 33,000 daltons is obtained. Subunits of masses of 33,000 and 66,000 daltons were seen after preincubation in the presence of these agents near neutrality. These results are in the range of subunit weights obtained with the beef spleen enzymes (43) and the presence of only a single band on the high pH gels when hexosaminidases A and B are run simultaneously indicates that the subunits of each enzyme are of identical mass. In separate experiments, when both enzymes were added to the same gel, no differences could be detected. An interesting difference was noted when urea and reducing agents were not included in the preincubation. In this case, only trace amounts of the 33,000 molecular weight unit were seen. Hexosaminidase A had a dark band at the 65,000-dalton level and trace amounts of a set of higher (~120,000–140,000) molecular weight proteins. In contrast, hexosaminidase B was rather resistant to breakdown into its subunits and displayed a pattern of proteins of molecular weight ranging from 120,000 to 140,000 daltons (Figure 9). This pattern was qualita-

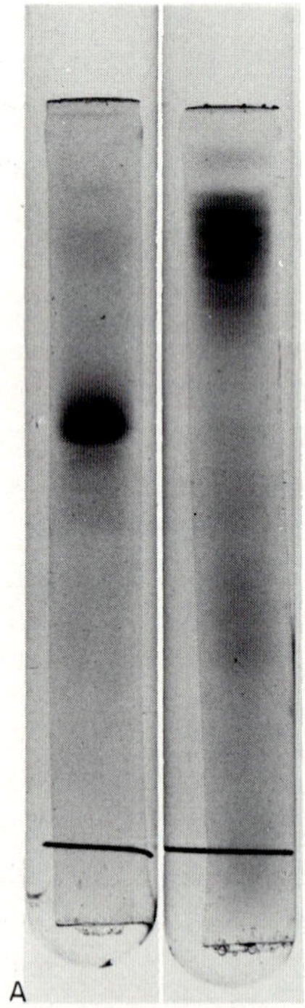

FIGURE 9A. Polyacrylamide gel electrophoresis of purified hexosaminidases A (left gel) and B (right gel) after preincubation in the presence of 0.1% SDS at pH 7.2. Tallman *et al.* (37).

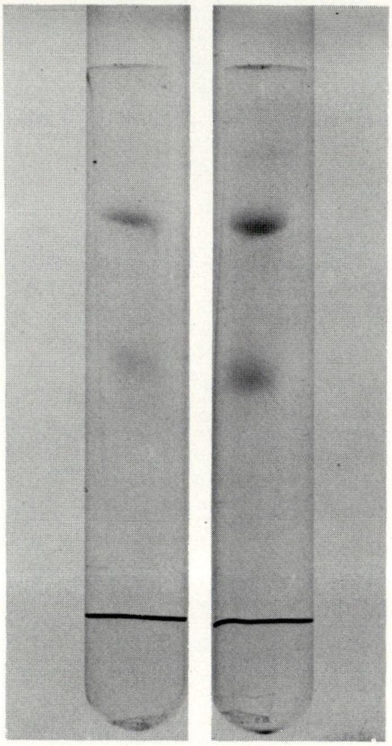

B

FIGURE 9B. Polyacrylamide gel electrophoresis of purified hexosaminidases A (left gel) and B (right gel) after preincubation in the presence of 0.1% SDS, 10% mercaptoethanol, 3 *M* urea, and 0.5% dithiothreitol at pH 7.2. Tallman *et al.* (37).

tively like the trace amounts of high molecular weight A. From these data it would seem that disulfide bonds play an important part of the association of the two 65,000 units in B forming the tetramer. In hexosaminidase A, this type of band does not yet exist or is labile under the conditions employed; indeed, it is likely that the units are hydrophobically associated but not covalently linked. The heterogeneity of both enzymes on SDS gels at the high molecular weight range is interesting because it may represent the association of varying amounts of SDS with the enzyme. Presumably, the enzymes are quite close to their native state and may contain varying amounts of carbohydrate (43); such side chains change the interaction of SDS with proteins (31).

It is possible to convert hexosaminidase A into B by heating at various temperatures in dilute pH 6.0 buffer (Figure 10), and this conversion approaches 100% at 50°C. A mechanism in which the complementary–SH groups are in close apposition after heating and form one or more disulfide bridges seems to be implied by this experiment. This may be due to an initial change in the hydrophobic interactions of the subunits. The inability to convert B back into A to a degree greater than the error in the monitoring of each form is also

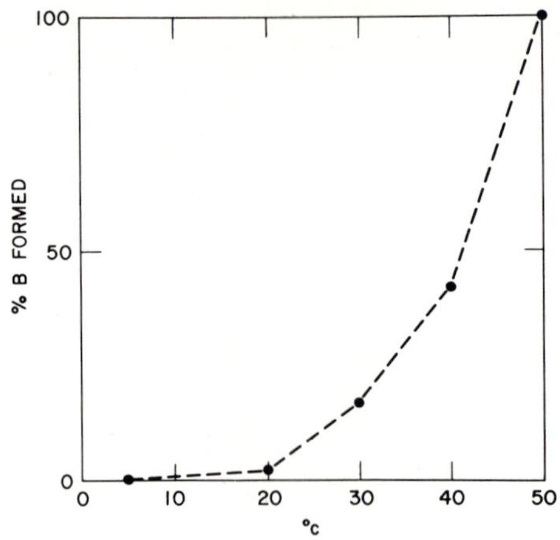

FIGURE 10. The conversion of hexosaminidase A to B. Purified hexosaminidase A was heated in pH 6.0 buffer for 2 hours at the temperatures indicated. Percentage B was determined as described in Tallman *et al.* (37).

explained by the presence of this new disulfide bond. Inherently, B would then appear to be the more stable protein and differences in the charge properties of the two enzymes may exist because of the conformational changes of the protein either preceding or accompanying the formation of the new disulfide bond(s). In dilute solution, where chain–chain interactions are of great importance, similar thermostability profiles for both hexosaminidases are observed (Figure 11). An intermediate in the denaturation of A in such solutions might be a "B-like" species. In serum and crude tissues, one might not expect conversion of A to B, but rather unfolding of the A protein on heating under acidic conditions and interaction of the critical sulfhydryl groups of A with other components of the protein-rich mixture leading to loss of enzymatic activity. Hexosaminidase B might not be expected to show this denaturation in serum.

Other evidence supports this concept of the close relationship of the hexosaminidases. In human placenta, the amino acid content of both enzymes was quite similar, and the only differences between the two species was in their sialic acid and neutral carbohydrate content. Immunological evidence (described below) also supports this close relationship.

I would like to submit a working model for the interrelationship of hexosaminidases which is based on our evidence and that published by other investigators. It is fully realized that the concept may have to be modified or even rejected as a consequence of further studies, but for now it represents to us the clearest explanation for the data obtained for normal enzymes and the enzymes from the various clinical forms of Tay-Sachs disease.

Hexosaminidases A and B represent different conformational states of the

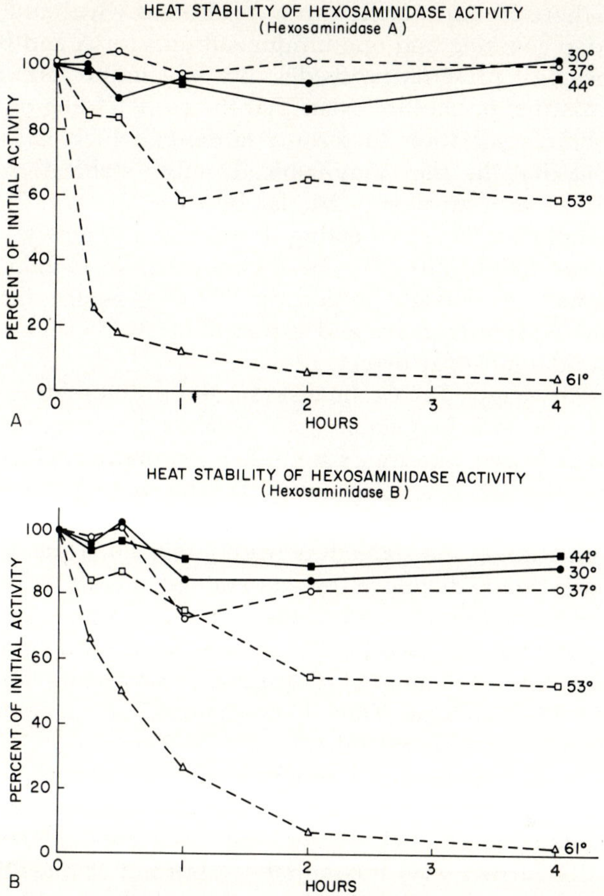

FIGURE 11. A and B. Thermostability of purified hexosaminidase A and B in pH 6.0 buffer. From Tallman *et al.* (37).

same enzyme. Evidence for this theory is based on the almost identical kinetic patterns obtained when the catalytic activity with various substrates is investigated, on identical thermal denaturation curves in dilute solution near neutrality, on identical number of subunits per holoenzyme and identical molecular weights of these units, on essentially identical amino acid composition of purified placental enzymes, and on immunological evidence (5,32) which indicates that A and B cross react extensively. Adsorption of anti-A by hexosaminidase B has been said to lead to the production of specific anti-A antiserum (32), although the other groups (5) have disputed this finding. The specific antiserum A may result from an antigen characteristic of the hexosaminidase without the disulfide bond. Reduction of such bonds has been shown to change the antigenic properties of other proteins (4). It is significant, however, that there are no specific anti-B antibodies which might be expected if there were one common and one unique subunit for A and B.

Since synthesis of proteins proceeds from the amino terminal end of the molecule, the distinct possibility exists that the early folding of the subunits is followed by their association to form a tetramer which is a metastable A, despite the fact that the thermodynamically more stable form may be hexosaminidase B. In fact, an energy barrier between the two forms may exist, and this barrier is overcome by heating. If extrusion of newly synthesized enzyme after glycosylation into the extracellular medium is followed by uptake to form lysosomes (8), a high proportion of the A isoenzyme might be expected in tissue culture medium and extracellular fluids such as fresh plasma where A is found almost exclusively (21).

In patients with classic Tay-Sachs disease, the initial folding of the enzyme in the A conformation is less stable than usual or the energy barrier between the two forms is lower because of a missense mutation which results in an amino acid substitution at a point critical for the folding of the subunits and their association (hydrophobic region). In this case, the disulfide bond necessary for the formation of the stable B is readily formed. Thus, hexosaminidase B is formed almost immediately at the moderate temperatures of the body. The increased instability of the A form of the enzyme accounts for the missing A in Tay-Sachs patients and their lack of the A-specific antigen (32). These patients do have a very small amount of residual (newly synthesized?) A activity and elevated "B-like" enzyme. They do not have a full complement of inactive A protein. It is interesting to note that the "B-like" enzyme which is formed in these patients is not the normal B which would be necessary if the common and unique subunit theory held, but an enzyme which moves more slowly toward the anode in neutral pH electrophoretic schemes; the residual A moves similarly (5). Concurrent with this mutation, but not as a result of the loss of the A conformation above, there is a loss of the ability of either form (A or B) to catalyze the breakdown of G_{M2}. This loss of G_{M2}-cleaving ability is the real deficit in the G_{M2}-gangliosidoses.

In the "O" variant (Sandhoff's disease) both hexosaminidase A and B cross-reacting proteins are said to be present (32), although this has not been totally established (5). The mutation, different from that in classic Tay-Sachs disease, would be at a site which is important in the actual mechanism of hydrolysis of *N*-acetylhexosamine from any of the substrates. Thus, a mechanistically important amino acid is implicated in this disease and not necessarily an amino acid involved in conformational aspects.

In the "AB" variant where both isozymes are present, G_{M2} degradation is decreased. Here we have a mutation which involves G_{M2} hydrolysis but does not affect the conformational stability of the A form; accordingly, A is present.

One might predict, on theoretical grounds, that since both A and B have activity against G_{M2}, there may exist a benign condition in which patients might lack the A isozyme yet their B may retain G_{M2}-hydrolyzing ability. These patients would present no clinical signs and would only be noticed as a result of the mass-screening programs presently based on differential heat denaturation of hexosaminidase A. Recently, such patients have been described by Navon (18) and Vidgoff (44).

REFERENCES

1. Brady, R. O. The Sphingolipidoses. *N. Engl. J. Med.*, 1966, **275:** 312.
2. Brady, R. O. Lipidoses. *Biochimie*, 1972, **54:** 723.
3. Brady, R. O. Hereditary diseases—causes, cures, and problems. *Angew Chem.* [*Engl.*], 1973, **12:** 1.
4. Brown, R. Studies on the antigenic structure of ribonuclease. *J. Biol. Chem.*, 1962, **237:** 1162.
5. Carroll, M., and Robinson, D. Immunological properties of *N*-acetyl-β-D-glucosaminidase of normal human liver and of G_{M2}-gangliosidosis liver. *Biochem. J.*, 1973, **131:** 91.
6. Graves, R., Manunes, P., and Bakerman, S. Screening for Tay-Sachs disease carriers. *Fed. Proc.*, 1973, **32:** 866.
7. Handa, S., and Yamakama, T. Biochemical studies in cat and human gangliosidosis. *J. Neurochem.*, 1971, **18:** 1275.
8. Hickman, S., and Neufeld, E. A hypothesis for I-cell disease: Defective hydrolases that do not enter lysosomes. *Biochem. Biophys. Res. Commun.*, 1972, **49:** 992.
9. Johnson, W. G., *et al.* Intravenous injection of purified hexosaminidase into a patient with Tay-Sachs disease. *Birth Defects, Orig. Art. Ser.*, 1973, **9:** 120–125.
10. Kaback, M. M., and Zeiger, R. Heterozygote detection in Tay-Sachs disease: A prototype community screening program for the prevention of recessive genetic disorders. In: *Sphingolipids, Sphingolipidoses and Allied Diseases.* (B. Volk, and S. Aronson, Eds.). Plenum, New York, 1972: 613–632.
11. Klenk, E. Uber die ganglioside des gehirns bei der infantlen amaurotischen Idiotie von Typus Tay-Sachs. *Ber. Deut. Chem. Ges.*, 1942, **75:** 1632.
12. Kolodny, E. H. Sandhoff's disease: Studies on the enzyme defect in homozygotes and detection of heterozygotes. In: *Sphingolipids, Sphingolipidoses and Allied Diseases.* (B. Volk and S. Aronson, Eds.). Plenum, New York, 1972: 221–341.
13. Kolodny, E. H., Brady, R. O., Quirk, J. M., and Kanfer, J. N. Preparation of radioactive Tay-Sachs ganglioside labeled in the sialic acid moiety. *J. Lipid Res.*, 1970, **11:** 144.
14. Kolodny, E. H., Brady, R. O., and Volk, B. W. Demonstration of an alteration of ganglioside metabolism in Tay-Sachs disease. *Biochem. Biophys. Res. Commun.*, 1969, **37:** 526.
15. Kolodny, E. H., Kanfer, J. N., Quirk, J. M., and Brady, R. O. Properties of a particle-bound enzyme from rat intestine that cleaves sialic acid from Tay-Sachs ganglioside. *J. Biol. Chem.*, 1971, **246:** 1426.
16. Ledeen, R., and Salsman, K. Structure of the Tay-Sachs ganglioside. *Biochemistry*, 1965, **4:** 2225.
17. Li, Y. T., Mazzotta, M., Wan, C., Orth, R., and Li, S. C. Hydrolysis of Tay-Sachs ganglioside by β-hexosaminidase A of human liver and urine. *J. Biol. Chem.*, 1973, **248:** 7512.
18. Navon, R., Padeh, B., and Adam, A. Apparent deficiency of hexosaminidase A in healthy members of a family with Tay-Sachs disease. *Am. J. Hum. Genet.*, 1973, **25:** 287.
19. O'Brien, J. S., Okada, S., Fillerup, D. L., Veath, M. L., Adornato, B., Brenner, P., and Leroy, J. Tay-Sachs disease—prenatal diagnosis. *Science*, 1971, **172:** 61.

20. Okada, S., and O'Brien, J. S. Tay-Sachs disease: Generalized absence of a β-D-*N*-acetylhexosaminidase component. *Science*, 1969, **165:** 698.
21. Price, R., and Dance, N. The demonstration of multiple heat stable forms of *N*-acetyl-β-glucosaminidase in normal human serum. *Biochim. Biophys. Acta*, 1972, **271:** 145.
22. Quirk, J. M., Tallman, J. F., and Brady, R. O. Preparation of trihexosyl- and tetrahexosyl-gangliosides specifically labelled in the *N*-acetylgalactosamine moiety. *J. Label. Compounds*, 1972, **8:** 484.
23. Robinson, D., and Stirling, J. L. *N*-Acetyl-β-gulcosaminidases in human spleen. *Biochem. J.*, 1968, **107:** 321.
24. Sachs, B. On arrested cerebral development with special references to its cortical pathology. *J. Nerv. Ment. Dis.*, 1887, **14:** 541.
25. Samuels, S., Korey, S., Gonatas, J., Terry, R., and Weiss, M. Studies on Tay-Sachs disease. IV. Membranous cytoplasmic bodies. *J. Neuropathol. Exp. Neurol.*, 1963, **22:** 81.
26. Sandhoff, K. Auftrennung der Sanger *N*-Acetyl-β-Hexosaminidase in multiple formen durch elektrofokussierung. *Hoppe-Seyler's Z. Physiol. Chem.*, 1968, **349:** 1095.
27. Sandhoff, K. The hydrolysis of Tay-Sachs ganglioside by hexosaminidase A. *FEBS Lett.*, 1970, **11:** 342.
28. Sandhoff, K., Andrea, U., and Jatzkewitz, H. Deficient hexosaminidase activity in an exceptional use of Tay-Sachs disease with additional storage in three variants of Tay-Sachs disease. *J. Neurochem.*, 1968, **18:** 2469.
29. Sandhoff, K., and Wassle, W. Anreicherung and Charakterisierung zweier Formen der Menschlichen *N*-acetyl-β-hexosaminidase. *Hoppe-Seyler's Z. Physiol. Chem.*, 1971, **352:** 1119.
30. Schneck, L., Adachi, M., and Volk, B. Chemical pathology of Tay-Sachs disease in the fetus. In: *Sphingolipids, Sphingolipidoses and Allied Diseases.* (B. Volk, and S. Aronson, Eds.). Plenum, New York, 1972: 385–394.
31. Segrest, J., and Jackson, R. Molecular weight determination of glycoproteins by polyacrylamine gel electrophoresis in sodium dodecyl sulfate. In: *Methods in Enzymology*. Vol. 28, Part B. (V. Ginsberg, Ed.). Academic Press, New York, 1973: 54.
32. Srivastava, S., and Beutler, E. Hexosaminidase A and Hexosaminidase B Tay-Sachs and Sandhoff's disease. *Nature* (*Lond.*), 1973, **241:** 463.
33. Svennerholm, L. The chemical structure of normal human brain and Tay-Sachs gangliosides. *Biochem. Biophys. Res. Commun.*, 1962, **9:** 436.
34. Tallman, J. F., and Brady, R. O. The catabolism of Tay-Sachs ganglioside in rat brain lysosomes. *J. Biol. Chem.*, 1972, **247:** 7570.
35. Tallman, J. F., and Brady, R. O. The purification and properties of a mammalian neuroaminidase (sialidase). *Biochim. Biophys. Acta*, 1973, **293:** 434.
36. Tallman, J. F., and Brady, R. O. Disorders of ganglioside catabolism. In: *The Sialic Acids.* (C. Schelgrund and A. Rosenberg, Eds.). 1975: in press.
37. Tallman, J. F., Brady, R. O., Quirk, J. M., Villalba, M., and Gal, A. E. Isolation and relationship of human hexosaminidases. *J. Biol. Chem.*. 1974, **249:** 3489.
38. Tallman, J. F., Brady, R. O. and Suzuki, K. Enzymatic activities associated with membranous cytoplasmic bodies and isolated brain lysosomes. *J. Neurochem.*, 1971, **18:** 1775.
39. Tallman, J. F., Johnson, W. G., and Brady, R. O. The metabolism of Tay-Sachs ganglioside: Catabolic studies with lysosomal enzymes from normal and Tay-Sachs brain tissue. *J. Clin. Invest.*, 1972, **51:** 2339.
40. Tallman, J. F., Pentchev, P. G., and Brady, R. O. An enzymological approach to the lipidoses. *Enzymes*, 1974, **18:** 136.
41. Tay, W. Symmetrical changes in the region of the yellow spot in each eye of an infant. *J. Ophthalmol. Soc. U. K.*, 1881, **1:** 55.
42. Terry, R. D., and Weiss, R. Studies in Tay-Sachs disease. II. Ultrastructure of the cerebrum. *J. Neuropathol. Exp. Neurol.*, 1963, **22:** 18.

43. Verpoorte, J. Purification of two β-*N*-acetyl-D-glucosaminidases. *J. Biol. Chem.*, 1972, **247:** 4787.
44. Vidgoff, J., Buist, N., and O'Brien, J. S. Absence of the β-*N*-acetyl-D-hexosaminidase A activity in a healthy woman. *Am. J. Hum. Genet.*, 1973, **25:** 372.
45. Wenger, D., Okada, S., and O'Brien, J. Studies on the substrate specificity of hexosaminidase A and B from liver. *Arch. Biochem. Biophys.*, 1972, **153:** 116.

18A

Discussion: Metachromatic Leukodystrophy, An Unusual Case with a Subtle Cerebroside Sulfatase Defect

HAYATO KIHARA

The Neuropsychiatric Institute, Pacific State Hospital, Research Group, Pomona, California

Metachromatic leukodystrophy (MLD) is one of the genetically determined sphingolipidoses in which there is a deficiency of the lysosomal enzyme arylsulfatase A. As a consequence, cerebroside sulfates (sulfatides) accumulate in tissues, particularly in the central and peripheral nervous systems. There are demyelination and progressive neurological degeneration (4).

MLD has been arbitrarily divided into three forms, late infantile, juvenile, and adult, based on the age of onset of clinical symptoms. Each of the forms appears to be an independent autosomal recessive disorder with only one form occurring in any kinship.

In several other lipidoses, the degree of enzyme deficiency has been decidedly less severe in variants with delayed age of onset than in the infantile type (5), for example, an enzyme level of 10 to 20% of normal compared to less than 5% of normal in the infantile type. In contrast, arylsulfatase A activity in urine, leukocytes, or cultured fibroblasts from all forms of MLD is uniformly present at a level less than 5% of that found in normal samples. It has been difficult, therefore, to rationalize how some patients reach adulthood without clinical symptoms.

Cultured fibroblasts derived from patients with MLD are deficient in arylsulfatase A, but under normal conditions they do not have metachromatic inclusions. They can, however, be induced to become metachromatic when sulfatides are provided in the culture medium (7). This deposition of the sphingolipid can be quantified by the use of ^{35}S-labeled sulfatides. Control fibroblasts also incorporate exogenous sulfatides, but their normal complement of arylsulfatase A enables them to degrade the ingested sulfolipid and release radioactive inorganic sulfate into the growth medium.

This intact cell cerebroside sulfate sulfohydrolase system has provided the first indication that latent forms of MLD do possess attenuated but finite levels of cerebroside sulfatase while the infantile form does not appear to have any functional enzyme (Figure 1) (2,8). There is a direct correlation between age of onset of clinical symptoms and intact cell enzyme activity. Adult MLD fibroblasts appeared to dispose of the intracellularly accumulated sulfatides about one-half as rapidly as normal cells under this test condition, yet the arylsulfatase A level in extracts of these cells was below our limits of reliable quantification (less than 5% of normal). Various approaches failed to provide extracts with reliably assayable levels of enzyme, so 100 times the usual number of cells were cultured, extracts prepared, and fractionated with ammonium sulfate. In this way we were able to show hydrolysis of an experimentally significant proportion of the sulfatide in the assay mixture, eliminating any uncertainty about its validity. This represented 1% of the sulfatidase activity in control fibroblasts. Titration with anti-arylsulfatase A serum showed that adult MLD fibroblasts contained about one-tenth as much antibody reacting material as normal cells (2). Thus, the mutant arylsulfatase A in adult MLD fibroblasts appeared to be catalytically less efficient as well as present in diminished quantity. We have presumed that the latter was due to increased

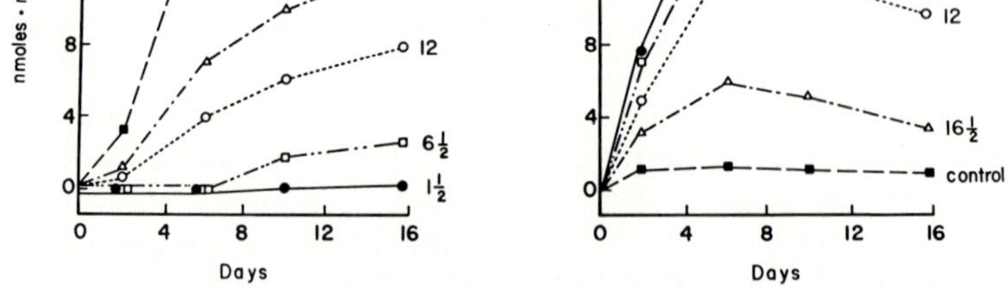

FIGURE 1. Correlation of intracellular cerebroside sulfate sulfohydrolase activities with age of onset of clinical symptoms. Petri dishes (60 mm) were plated with fibroblasts (300,000/dish) in 3 ml medium containing ^{35}S-cerebroside sulfate (23 nmoles/ml; 3.6 × 10^3 cpm/nmole). On the days indicated each cell strain was analyzed for intracellular ^{35}S-sulfatide and extracellular ^{35}S-sulfate. The MLD cells were derived from patients whose age of onset of clinical symptoms are indicated by the numbers opposite the plots. From Kihara *et al.* (2,p.22).

Table I Leukocyte and Urinary Arylsulfatase A Activities

Subject	Specific Activity (nmole/hr/mg)	
	Leukocyte	Urine
Proband	5	30
MLD patients	7	0
Control	208 ± 97	558 ± 97

lability of the mutant enzyme. While we were interested in characterizing the defect in the adult MLD mutant enzyme, its extremely low catalytic activity has served as a deterrent.

We have discovered what appears to be a new variant of MLD. A mentally retarded patient with neuropathy of undetermined etiology showed a deficiency of arylsulfatase A in leukocytes typical of MLD (Table I). Urinary enzyme level was also greatly depressed and the urine contained metachromatic granules which yielded lipids cochromatographing with cerebroside sulfate. The patient presented with the biochemical benchmarks of sulfatide lipidosis, although there were clinical inconsistencies. Neuropathy and myopathy had been evident from infancy. Development was slow and childhood years were stormy because of emotional disturbances. However, she has remained unchanged neurologically for many years and there has been no evidence of progressive degeneration.

A fibroblast culture was initiated from a skin biopsy. Surprisingly, fibroblasts contained about 10% of normal arylsulfatase A activity by the assay with the synthetic substrate, 4-nitrocatechol sulfate (Table II). However, no enzyme activity could be demonstrated toward the physiological substrate, cerebroside sulfate. Fibroblasts cultured in the presence of exogenous sulfatides failed to exhibit metachromasia, suggesting the presence of functional cerebroside sulfatase activity in intact cells. The ^{35}S-sulfatide loading technique was applied, and the results indicated that these cells were able to dispose of sulfatides at a level intermediate between adult MLD and normal cells (Figure 2).

A large batch of these cells was cultured and processed in the same manner as the adult MLD cells. Again, ample activity toward the synthetic substrate

Table II Fibroblast Arylsulfatase A Activity

Subject	Specific Activity (nmole/hr/mg)
Proband	131
MLD patients	72
Control	1335 ± 652

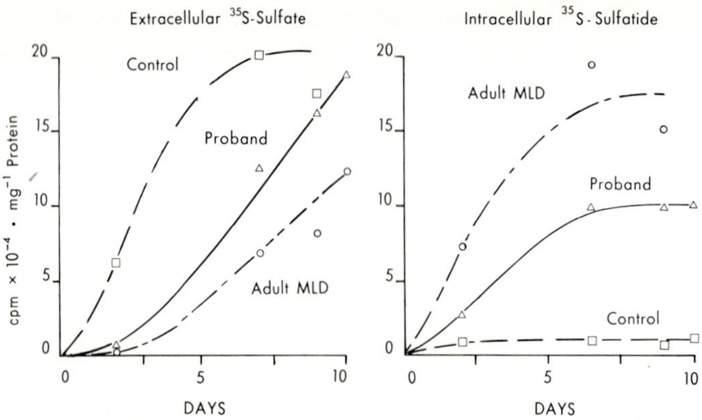

FIGURE 2. Subnormal intracellular cerebroside sulfate sulfohydrolase activity of fibroblasts from the proband. Conditions were similar to those described for Figure 1.

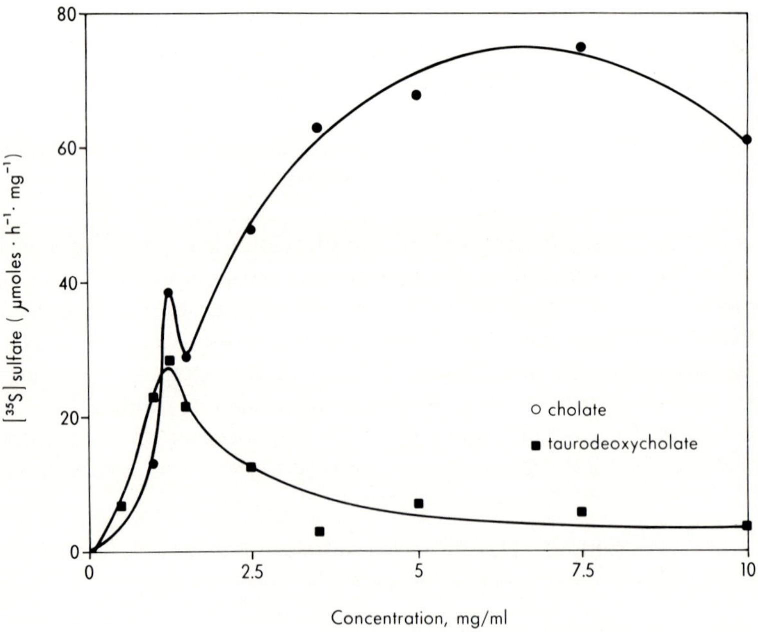

FIGURE 3. The effect of varying concentrations of sodium taurodeoxycholate or sodium cholate on cerebroside sulfate sulfohydrolase activity. Assay conditions were as described previously (6) with bile salt as indicated. The enzyme was human urinary arylsulfatase purified to a specific activity of 2400 μmoles of 4-nitrocatechol sulfate hydrolyzed per hour per milligram of protein.

Table III Cerebroside Sulfate Sulfohydrolase Activities

Subject	*Sodium Cholate (mg/ml)*	*Activity (nmole/hr/ml)*
Proband	1.25	0
	2.50	0
	5.00	189
Control	1.25	2850
	2.50	770
	5.00	4730

was present, but we could not demonstrate any activity toward the physiological substrate. Fractionation procedures, including ammonium sulfate precipitation and DEAE-cellulose chromatography, showed that synthetic substrate activity fractionated like enzyme from control fibroblasts. A comparison of the variant and normal enzyme by such parameters as migration properties on polyacrylamide gel electrophoresis, precipitin reaction with antibodies, rate of heat inactivation, and inhibition by Ag^+ failed to reveal any difference between the enzyme from both sources.

The *in vitro* cerebroside sulfate sulfohydrolase reaction has an obligatory bile salt requirement which can be met by either sodium taurodeoxycholate or sodium cholate (3,6). We normally use taurodeoxycholate because results have been more reproducible than with cholate. On the other hand, we have found that the cholate system provides a greater degree of activation in an unusual bimodal pattern (Figure 3). Thus, when the fractionated variant enzyme was examined in the taurodeoxycholate system and cerebroside sulfatase activity still could not be demonstrated, we reexamined the enzyme in the cholate-activated system. In this way, we were finally able to observe measurable cerebroside sulfatase activity in the extract from the proband (Table III). Quantitative comparisons have been difficult because of the poor reproducibility, but it did appear that the cerebroside sulfatase activity was less than what would be expected from the 4-nitrocatechol sulfate assay.

The arylsulfatase A of this variant form of MLD represents the first mutant enzyme of this disorder amenable for studies of the defect at the molecular level. Such studies would be facilitated by an understanding of the action of cholate on the normal enzyme. There is evidence that taurodeoxycholate acts by dispersing cerebroside sulfate micelles (1). Cholate may also act in this capacity at its lower activity peak, which is coincident with that of taurodeoxycholate. At higher cholate concentrations, precipitated cholic acid appears to play a dominant role. This unusual second, broader activity peak probably results from surface adsorption of the enzyme, substrate, or both. Systematic studies of this phenomenon have been difficult because we have not yet been able to achieve cholate activation in a reliably reproducible manner.

ACKNOWLEDGMENT

This investigation was supported in part by Grant Nos. NS-8839, NS-9479, and HD-4612 from the National Institutes of Health.

REFERENCES

1. Jerfy, A., and Roy, A. B. The sulphatase of ox liver. XVI. A comparison of the arylsulphatase and cerebroside activities of sulphatase A. *Biochim. Biophys. Acta,* 1973, **293:** 178–190.
2. Kihara, H., Porter, M. T., and Fluharty, A. L. Enzyme replacement in cultured fibroblasts from metachromatic leukodystrophy. *Birth Defects, Orig. Art Ser.,* 1973, **9:** 19–26.
3. Percy, A. K., Farrell, D. F., and Kaback, M. M. Cerebroside sulphate (sulphatide) sulphohydrolase: An improved assay method. *J. Neurochem.,* 1972, **19:** 233–236.
4. Moser, H. W. Sulfatide lipidosis: Metachromatic leukodystrophy. In: *The Metabolic Basis of Inherited Diseases.* (3rd ed.) (J. B. Stanbury, J. B. Wyngaarden, and D. S. Fredrickson, Eds.). McGraw-Hill, New York, 1972: pp. 688–729.
5. Okada, S., Veath, M. L., and O'Brien, J. S. Juvenile GM_2 gangliosidoses: Partial deficiency of hexosaminidase. *J. Pediat.,* 1970, **77:** 1063–1065.
6. Porter, M. T., Fluharty, A. L., de la Flor, S. D., and Kihara, H. Cerebroside sulfatase determinations in cultured human fibroblasts. *Biochim. Biophys. Acta,* 1972, **258:** 769–778.
7. Porter, M. T., Fluharty, A. L., Harris, S. E., and Kihara, H. The accumulation of cerebroside sulfates by fibroblasts in culture from patients with late infantile metachromatic leukodystrophy. *Arch. Biochem. Biophys.,* 1970, **138:** 646–652.
8. Porter, M. T., Fluharty, A. L., Trammell, J., and Kihara, H. A correlation of intracellular cerebroside sulfatase activity in fibroblasts with latency in metachromatic leukodystrophy. *Biochem. Biophys. Res. Commun.,* 1971, **44:** 660–666.

19

Role of Biochemistry in Research on Mental Retardation

GEORGE POPJÁK

Mental Retardation Research Center and Department of Biochemistry, University of California Los Angeles, Los Angeles, California

A few years ago I attended a clinical session on psychosomatic medicine. Two cases were presented: one was that of a woman in her late thirties with the signs and symptoms of gross thyrotoxicosis, goiter, exophthalmos, cardiac involvement, and all the rest; the second case was that of a boy, about age 12, with the classic signs and symptoms of Hirschprung's disease, including the X-ray evidence. It was proposed during that session that these two patients should be given psychoanalytical treatment to rid them of their thyrotoxicosis and "encaprosis." Obviously not everybody shares the biochemists's Credo, that expressions of functions are manifestations of carefully controlled body chemistry integrated with cellular structure, and particularly not when the psyche or mental faculties may be involved—nor, apparently, even the movements of the bowel.

Thus mental retardation might share in the disbelief that it has anything to do with a biochemical abnormality. What I am going to say necessarily must be simplistic because I cannot possibly roll into 45 minutes all of biochemistry and one-half of Stanbury, Wyngaarden, and Fredrickson's textbook (10). Certainly, up to 1934 no one knew, and could not even suspect, that at least some of the mental retardations, or oligophrenias as I learned them, were associated with an abnormality of metabolism. As everyone knows, and as you have heard it reaffirmed by Dr. Kaufman this morning, it was in 1934 that Følling reported the presence of phenylpyruvic acid in the urine of 10 imbeciles and established the first correlation between a metabolic abnormality and mental retardation. The title of Følling's paper deserves to be remembered: "Über Ausscheidung von Phenylbrenztraubensäure in den Harn als Stofwechselanomalie in Verbindung mit Imbezillität," i.e., "About the excretion of phenylpyruvic acid in the urine as a metabolic anomaly associated with imbecility" (3).

Of course, it was Garrod (4), before Følling, at the turn of the century, who first recognized the genetic basis of metabolic disorders, which he called "inborn errors of metabolism." From his studies on alkaptonuria, cystinuria, albinism, and pentosuria, Garrod developed the concept that certain diseases can arise because an enzyme, controlling a single metabolic step, is either missing or is severely impaired in its function. He appreciated quite correctly, e.g., that homogentistic acid was a normal intermediate in the metabolism of tyrosine and that its accumulation in the body in alcaptonuria must have been the result of the absence of the enzyme oxidizing this acid. Garrod's prediction was proved correct 50 years later by La Du and his associates (8). In the case of phenylketonuria—again, as related by Dr. Kaufman—it was not until 1953 that Jervis (6) established that absence of phenylalanine hydroxylase was responsible for the metabolic abnormality. But we have also heard from Dr. Kaufman how extraordinarily difficult it was even in subsequent years to pinpoint precisely the abnormality. The biochemist has much difficulty when working with human beings or on human problems.

The last 40 years of biochemical research resulted in the description of probably all the major metabolic pathways. In the early 1940's Beadle and Tatum established experimentally the concept of "one gene, one enzyme" (1). Then came the identification of the structure of DNA by Crick and Watson (13). There followed the identification of the genetic code and of the functional unit—the cistron—of the DNA controlling the structure of a single polypeptide chain. Thus the concept of "one gene, one enzyme" was translated into the concept of "one cistron, one polypeptide." Study of bacterial genetics produced evidence implicating the participation of two other genes in the transcription of the structural gene into enzyme protein. These are the regulator and operator genes. The function of the regulator gene is to produce repressors which interact with a locus on DNA adjacent to the structural gene. This latter locus is known as the operator gene and, when combined with an active repressor, does not permit the transcription of the structural gene.

There was much speculation about the origin of human metabolic disorders resulting from the absence or deficiency of an enzyme. In the second edition of our "bible," "The Metabolic Basis of Inherited Disease," it was postulated that probably all the abnormalities of amino acid metabolism and the storage diseases associated with mental retardation resulted from regulator or operator gene mutations such as those that prevented the transcription of a structural gene coding for a specific enzyme. From what you have heard from previous speakers it is unlikely that regulator or operator gene mutations are responsible for defects associated with the absence or impairment of a single enzyme. The defects in all closely examined instances are now attributable to structural gene mutations. Even the evidence provided by the study of bacterial systems makes it unlikely that an abnormality arising from the silence or low activity of an enzyme would result from mutations in regulator or operator genes. Experiments with mutants of *E. coli* containing the gene for the inducible enzyme, β-galactosidase, have shown that mutations in the regulator or operator gene loci (excepting the deletion of the operator gene in O^- mutants of *E. coli*) resulted not in the repression of the inducibility of the enzyme—on the contrary, such mutations resulted in the derepression of β-galactosidase and the appearance of the enzyme as a constitutive protein in the bacteria. By analogy I would expect a regulatory or operator gene mutation in man, excepting again the less likely total deletion, to manifest itself not by repression of enzyme synthesis but by abnormally high levels of certain enzymes. Mammalian systems and particularly human cellular systems have been much neglected during the past 10–15 years at the expense of *E. coli*. However, there is plenty of evidence that amends will be made during the years to come. The recognition that fibroblasts in culture and leukocytes can express the metabolic pattern—normal or abnormal—of a phenotype is now being exploited vigorously in many laboratories. Study of fibroblasts and leukocytes taken from individuals afflicted by a metabolic disease should answer many questions of enzyme regulation in mammalian systems and decide conclusively whether regulator and operator genes exist in mammalian cells, and, if they exist, what might be the consequences of mutations in these. Gordon Tomkins' experiments with tyrosine aminotransferase (12), and Don Haggerty's, in our laboratory, on phenylalanine hydroxylase in cultures of hepatoma cells strongly suggest the existence of operator genes even in mammalian cells. Certainly, that assumption is the simplest one that can be invoked to explain the "induction" of these enzymes by corticosteroid hormones.* An even stronger evidence as to the existence of an operator gene in mammalian cells came to light only during the last few months from the study of leukocytes and fibroblasts taken from heterozygous and homozygous individuals afflicted by familial hypercholesterolemia. Alan Fogelman found in our laboratory that the leukocytes of such heterozygotes responded to incubation in a lipid-free serum with a far greater induction of hydroxymethylglutaryl-CoA reductase than the leukocytes of normal individuals. Similar findings with fibroblasts were reported by Goldstein and Brown in the October issue of the *Proceedings of the National Academy of Science* (5). Goldstein and Brown have had an opportunity to examine also fibroblasts of homozygous individuals and found that in these the HMG-CoA reductase was permanently elevated and furthermore that the levels of

* Tomkins and his associates have interpreted their observations as indicating a "posttranscriptional" control of enzyme induction by steroid hormones. This interpretation has been challenged repeatedly (2,7). The data of Tomkins and of others are more readily understood on the assumption that the role of steroid hormones in enzyme induction is the derepression of an operator gene thus facilitating the synthesis of specific mRNA.

the enzyme could not be repressed in the homozygous cells, as they can in normal cells, by low density lipoprotein. The inference from these experiments is that in familial hypercholesterolemia a mutation of the operator gene results in the inability of the operator to bind the repressor and hence lead to elevated levels of the enzyme. This is the precise analogy of the derepression of β-galactosidase, or its appearance as a constitutive enzyme in noninduced *E. coli* with mutated regulator or operator genes. Of course, familial hypercholesterolemia has nothing to do with mental retardation, but the problems of genetic mutations are most pertinent.

Although it is dangerous to extrapolate from the singular to the general, I suggest that probably all single enzyme deficiencies are the result of structural gene mutations. I am excluding from this prognostication the major chromosome abnormalities, such as the trisomies in which affairs are probably far more complex, and I doubt if amenable to biochemical analysis at present.

I ventured into these historical reflections because they represent, to me at least, the role of biochemists in seeking an understanding of the living world, an explanation of life in terms of comprehensible chemistry.

Believing as I do that manifestations of abnormal function result from abnormal metabolism, my concept of the role of biochemists in the study of mental retardation is the same as they fulfilled historically in the understanding of the living world. This role was great; nevertheless biochemists engaging, or planning to engage, in the study of the vast problems of mental retardation in man, are severely handicapped: first, because a large number of mental retardations, those resulting, e.g., from birth injuries, intrauterine infections, and major chromosomal aberrations, are not amenable to biochemical analysis by our current techniques. The second handicap most present-day professional biochemists have is that they cannot plan any rational exploration of mental retardation until after clinical colleagues have identified a syndrome or disease entity, and specifically a disease entity which, by the study of the patient's pedigree, is inheritable. Once a genetic background is established, the biochemist is on fairly firm ground. Even so, the study of a metabolic disorder in man, be that a synthetic or catabolic step, is beset with much difficulty, as humane and ethical considerations limit the number and nature of samples a biochemist can take. One is largely restricted to urine, blood, CSF, and occasional biopsies from limited sites.

You have heard Dr. Kaufman's difficult decision on how to make the best use of 20 mg of a liver biopsy. In spite of these limitations such specimens are sufficient for the analysis of chemical composition and hence recognition of a major metabolic error. In this respect we can be guided by past experience which showed that in all metabolic errors of genetic origin there were no abnormal metabolites in the body and body fluids, only normal metabolites in abnormal amounts. From the knowledge of metabolic pathways one can predict, of course, that accumulation or absence of a metabolite must be the result of a block in a chain of reactions. Such a block may have a variety of consequences. Let us assume three reactions in which substance A is transformed into B, which goes to C which is the immediate precursor of D. If the enzyme converting C into D is not functioning, metabolite C may accumulate if the reaction C→D is the only pathway of its metabolism. However, if the preceding steps A→B→C are freely reversible, the precursors farther away from the metabolite whose reaction is blocked may accumulate. A good example of such a case is the accumulation of methionine in the blood of patients with cystathioninuria, although the metabolic block is several steps away from methionine.

The metabolic block between C and D may result in the exaggeration of a perhaps minor alternative pathway of compound C and lead to the accumulation of other metabolites. The classic example is, of course, phenylketonuria, in which not only phenylalanine, but also its secondary metabolites, phenylpyruvic and phenyllactic and phenylacetic acids, accumulate in the body and lead to their excretion in the urine in abnormal amounts.

A failure to form product D may have several consequences if D itself is a vital metabolite or a precursor of a vital metabolite. Thus, as you have heard from Dr. Kaufman this morning, tyrosine, which is not an essential amino acid in normal individuals, becomes an essential amino acid in phenylketonurics. Or a failure to iodinate tyrosine leads to failure of the production of triiodotyronine and thyroxine and results in goitrous cretinism.

If substance D has the role of a feedback regulator in a metabolic cycle or chain, its absence may lead to the overproduction of a precursor which it controls. Thus in orotic aciduria the overproduction of orotic acid may be ascribed partly to deprivation of the body of pyrimidine nucleotides, which act, at least cytidine triphosphate, as feedback inhibitors of carbamyl-phosphate synthetase and aspartate transcarbamylase.

Although examination of metabolic patterns leads ultimately to the identification of a defective, absent, or silent enzyme, this tells us nothing about the origins of mental retardations associated with metabolic errors. If the abnormal metabolic patterns have a message, we are unfortunately unable to read that message. We are totally ignorant of the fundamental causes of the failure of the maturation of the central nervous system or the failure of the development of the high cognitive powers in any of the inborn errors of metabolsim. It was the fond hope of many investigators that a study of phenylketonuria might provide an answer to this fundamental question, yet we are as ignorant on this point after some 30 years of research as we were of the metabolic abnormality itself before Følling dropped ferric chloride into the urine of some imbeciles.

Our ignorance on this question stems primarily, I believe, from our ignorance of the biochemical mechanisms underlying the normal developmental and maturation processes in the central nervous system, i.e., the processes of differentiation. Many of the presentations we heard at this conference went a long way in providing much new information on this question. We may argue whether it is of any material interest what is the mechanism of mental retardation resulting from an inborn error of metabolism. My stand on this point is that it is of paramount importance, not just for an understanding of mental retardation, but also for an understanding of the normal processes of mentation that earned us the self-styled rank of *Homo sapiens*. Inborn errors of metabolism are nature's experiments, which, although exacting a heavy price from those afflicted, have taught us volumes about human biochemistry. Besides, recognition of the nature of a metabolic error led at least in a few instances to rational therapy (PKU, galactosemia, orotic aciduria, methylmalonic aciduria, goitrous cretinism).

I feel therefore that one of the important contributions biochemists can make in the study of mental retardations is the study of metabolic abnormalities and a search for such abnormalities among mentally retarded, and particularly among those whose disease is of unknown etiology and is suspected of being of genetic origin.

There are at present about 150 known inborn errors of metabolism. One cannot help suspecting that there are many more as yet undiscovered. I would like to recall that in 1950 there were known only seven abnormalities of amino acid metabolism. By 1970 there were 50. Our recognition of metabolic errors has grown logarithmically since the 1950's. Apart from the suspicion that there may be many more as yet undiscovered metabolic errors, there is the fact of spontaneous mutation. The spontaneous mutation rate in germ cells is estimated to be about one allele in 10^5 loci per generation. This means in practical terms that in each generation one new mutation is added for every 40 preexisting ones, or a load of 2.5%. Of course, these mutations need not necessarily result in mental retardation, but some undoubtedly will.

The mere establishment of a metabolic error is insufficient to characterize the disease fully. Thus it is not enough to know that someone is excreting excessive amounts of orotic acid. It is the biochemist's duty to establish the cause of such excessive excretion, i.e., the identification of the defective enzymes and the nature of the enzymatic defect. The identification of the defective enzyme seems to me most important as this may well suggest an appropriate treatment. In the example of orotic aciduria, I quoted, recognition that two enzymes are blocked (at least in one form of the disease)—orotidylic pyrophosphorylase and decarboxylase—led to the realization that patients suffering from this disease were really suffering from pyrimidine deprivation. They are well treatable by the oral administration of uridine and cytidine. There are already several examples of successful treatments of disease by the supply of a missing protein among which the latest is the treatment of Fabry's disease with normal human plasma, which contains α-glucosidase, the enzyme which is inactive in Fabry's disease and to which Dr. Tallman had referred earlier.

The final step in the description of an enzyme defect is the identification of the nature of the defect in the enzyme itself. This defect may range from impaired catalytic activity, impaired affinity for coenzyme or substrate, to total loss of catalytic activity. With the great advances that have been made in protein chemistry, the nature of the abnormalities can now be probed. This is not an easy task. First, a reference normal enzyme must be obtained from human sources, from individuals presumed or attested to be or to have been normal. With a few exceptions, a major human organ may be needed for such a purpose, i.e., for the preparation of a reference specimen of an enzyme in a state of homogeneous purity. Although organs are available from postmortems, not many enzymes survive proteolysis after death. Also, physician colleagues will attest that death, excepting those resulting from acute cardiovascular accidents or from violence, inflicted by man or machines, comes slowly to man. During the protracted period of dying many changes occur in organs. Some enzymes, such as phenylalanine hydroxylase, may decay to undetectable levels during the agony of dying.

Then, even if one succeeded in obtaining a quantity of the pure normal enzyme—several milligrams—sufficient for all the needed physical measurements and production of antibodies, one needs an adequate source of the abnormal enzyme also. It is not at all like working with *E. coli,* either the wild type or any of its mutants, which can be obtained, if necessary, in cultures of hundreds of liters and reproduced at will. Apart from the difficulties in obtaining sources of human enzymes, another factor must govern our choice in studying the nature of an enzyme defect. This is, for technical reasons, the molecular weight of the protein, or to be more precise the molecular weight of the subunits of the protein. It would be foolhardy at present to undertake research on the molecular abnormality of a protein, which had a subunit molecular weight of over 60,000 and in which the abnormality may have arisen by the replacement of one or two amino acids.

It is no wonder that the only abnormalities of protein synthesis in man that have been deciphered so far are those of hemoglobin. Hemoglobin is readily available without great sacrifice or discomfort on the part of the donor, and its subunits have molecular weight of only 16,000. The amino acid composition of these subunits and their low molecular weight limits the number of peptides one obtains by tryptic or other proteolytic digestion and allows the identification of the presence of a deviant peptide in the digest. For these reasons, it is my prediction that the nature of an enzymatic abnormality that will be first defined will be that of the transferase deficiency galactosemias. I am predicting this with confidence (a) because of the work of Drs. Tedesco and Mellman on this enzyme (11); (b) because the galactose-1-P uridyl transferase is readily obtainable from erythrocytes; (c) because George Dale in our laboratory obtains now this enzyme in 90–95% purity in high yield with about two days of work; and (d) because it contains two identical subunits of 31,000 molecular weight.

There may be some who might say, "Alright, you have established that a glutamic acid in the hemoglobin molecule was replaced by valine; so what?" My reply is that I learned that this replacement caused specific changes in the solubility properties of the protein causing it to quasicrystallize in the red cell with the consequent sickling and lysis of the cell. From the study of the physical properties of this Hb we also learned that its solubility properties can be restored to nearly normal by its carbamoylation with cyanate. A relatively simple chemical modification of an abnormal protein may now relieve the suffering of many Negroes afflicted by sickle cell anemia. I have given already a sufficient number of examples to show that unraveling the nature of enzyme deficiencies of inborn errors of metabolism may give clues as to treatment.

Before closing I should like to touch briefly on one further topic related to genetic abnormalities and to which biochemistry had already made substantial contribution. This is the prenatal diagnosis of a threatening genetic abnormality. Cytologists can now diagnose, by the culturing and microscopic examination of fetal amniotic cells, chromosomal aberrations associated with major genetic defects. Biochemists can also decide by the study of the enzymatic complement of such cells whether the conceptus is likely to be normal or to carry the genes of some major inborn error; at least a few of such diseases can be diagnosed as early as the fifteenth week of gestation. If one believes in eugenics, then one can assert that no child with Down's syndrome or Tay-Sachs' disease need be born. The further study of the phenotypic expression of genes in amniotic fetal cells by biochemical techniques may extend the scope of prenatal diagnosis of threatening disease beyond our present capability.

At present only a limited number of metabolic abnormalities can be treated even after the full understanding of the nature of the abnormality. All the successful treatments have been, so far, dietary: restrictions (amino acids) and supplementations (hormones and vitamins). We have to await the evaluation of the long-term effects of the treatment of Fabry's disease by the transfusion of normal plasma referred to by Dr. Tallman.

It is unfortunate that most of the metabolic abnormalities known to be associated with enzyme deficiencies and mental retardations are complex reactions involving also cofactors and auxiliary enzymes. If it were not for such a complex situation, it would be possible to "anchor" a missing enzyme onto an insoluble matrix, to enclose such a stabilized enzyme in a dialysing bag, and insert it in a body cavity. Some such treatment, however Utopian an idea this may seem today, might be practicable in years ahead.

I would like to make a last speculation. Perhaps somatic hybridization of genetically incompetent cells with competent cells could or might be, beyond eugenics, an ultimate solution to correcting metabolic abnormalities that lead to mental retardation. You might think this suggestion now to be mere science fiction. Three years ago I was laughed out of court during a site visit when I proposed the culturing of liver cells for the study of factors affecting the phenotypic expression of phenylalanine hydroxylase. We were duly disapproved for trying to do something that no one else had done before.

In less than 1 year afterward the culturing of hepatocytes became a reality and, today, we have two cell culture lines which contain phenylalanine hydroxylase as a constitutive enzyme. We have also about ten cell lines, reputedly of hepatic origin, which contain no detectable levels of this enzyme. Don Haggerty has shown in our laboratory that the phenylalanine hydroxylase in the cultured cells of hepatocytes was also under a hormonal control; glucocorticoids caused at physiological concentration, at about 5×10^{-7} *M*, a 4-fold increase in the levels of the enzyme in 18 hours by the induction of the synthesis of a specific protein. Horse serum, i.e., the serum of an adult animal, contains an as yet unidentified non-steroidal factor or factors which also stimulate the levels of phenylalanine hydroxylase. There is a rather interesting phenomenon in the expression of phenylalanine hydroxylase associated with the growth cycle of the cells. When confluent cultures of fully induced cells are divided for subcultivation, the levels of the enzyme in the sparsely populated new cultures decline in 18 to 24 hours to very low levels and remain so until the cells become confluent. Thereupon within 24 hours there is a sudden rise in phenylalanine hydroxylase and the cells become exceptionally sensitive to the stimulating action of corticoids and adult serum. The phenomenon is not unlike the sudden appearance of phenylalanine hydroxylase in the liver of the newborn rat; whereas 2 days before birth the enzyme is undetectable.

Although we have already learned a little about the regulation of phenylalanine hydroxylase levels in tissue culture cells, we do not understand at all the mechanism of repression and derepression of this enzyme in mammalian cells. What happens in the confluent H-4 cells that triggers off suddenly the synthesis of phenylalanine hydroxylase? Did the RLC and HTC cells of liver origin, which contain no phenylalanine hydroxylase, suffer a deletion of the phenylalanine gene or is the translation of that gene merely repressed? We are hoping to get some answers to these very basic questions by hybridizing the active H-4 cells with the inactive RLC and HTC cells and by examining the properties of the hybrids.

This brings me back to the question of whether it might be feasible one day to correct a metabolic error resulting from genetic defect by somatic hybridization. I must leave the question unanswered and to your imagination. Correction of a genetic abnormality by cell hybridization *in vitro* was already achieved by Nadler's group 3 years ago (9). Dr. Tedesco has reported that Nadler, Chacko, and Rachmeler succeeded in demonstrating galactose-1-phosphate uridyl transferase in hybrid cells made by the fusion of human diploid fibroblasts obtained from different galactosemic patients. The cells contained no detectable enzyme activity before hybridization. Among the seven lines of galactosemic cells studied, three combinations, out of the possible 21, gave enzymically active hybrid cells. In all three instances the fusion of the cells of one particular individual [Gal. $(-)_D$] with the cells of 3 others (A,

C, and E) led to the formation of active enzyme. These very remarkable experiments suggest at least two nonidentical point mutations in transferase deficiency galactosemia and suggest furthermore that if somatic hybridization could be achieved *in vivo,* metabolic abnormalities resulting from simple point mutations might be amenable to correction.

In this sketchy summary of the very large areas pertaining to inborn errors of metabolism and amenable to biochemical analysis I wished to convey the philosophy that guided me and my colleagues in preparing a research program for the biochemistry section of the Mental Retardation Research Center at UCLA for the coming years. They are also the thoughts that parts of this conference have evoked in me. I should also like to leave the message that we are concerned not with mice but with men.

REFERENCES

1. Beadle, G. W., and Tatum, E. L. Genetic control of biochemical reactions in *Neurospora. Proc. Natl. Acad. Sci. USA* 1941, **27:** 499–506.
2. Butcher, F. R., Bushnell, P. E., Becker, J. E., and Potter, V. R. Effect of cordycepin on induction of tyrosine aminotransferase employing hepatoma cells in tissue culture. *Exp. Cell Res.,* 1972, **74:** 115–123.
3. Følling, A. Über Ausscheidung von Phenylbrenztraubensäure in den Harn als Stoffwechselanomalie in Verbindung mit Imbezillität. *Hoppe-Seyler's Z. Physiol. Chem.,* 1934, **227:** 169.
4. Garrod, A. E. "Inborn Errors of Metabolism." (Croonian Lectures). *Lancet,* 1908, **2:** 1, 73, 142 and 214.
5. Goldstein, J. L., and Brown, M. S. Familial hypercholesterolemia: Identification of a defect in the regulation of 3-hydroxy-3-methylglutaryl coenzyme A reductase activity associated with overproduction of cholesterol. *Proc. Natl. Acad. Sci. USA,* 1973, **70:** 2804–2808.
6. Jervis, G. A. Phenylpyruvic oligophrenia: Deficiency of phenylalanine-oxidizing system. *Proc. Soc. Exp. Biol. Med.,* 1953, **82:** 514–515.
7. Kenney, F. T., Lee, K. L., Stiles, C. D., and Fritz, J. E. Further evidence against posttranscriptional control of inducible tyrosine aminotronsferase synthesis in cultured hepatoma cells. *Nature (London),* 1973, **246:** 208–210.
8. La Du, B. N., Zannoni, V. G., Laster, L., and Seegmiller, J. E. The nature of the defect in tyrosine metabolism in alcaptonuria. *J. Biol. Chem.,* 1958, **230:** 251–260.
9. Nadler, H. L., Chacko, C. M., and Rachmeler, M. Interallelic complementation in hybrid cells derived from human diploid strains deficient in galactose-1-phosphate uridyl transferase activity. *Proc. Natl. Acad. Sci. USA,* 1970, **67:** 976–982.
10. Stanbury, J. B., Wyngaarden, J. B., and Fredrickson, D. S., Eds. *The Metabolic Basis of Inherited Disease.* (3rd ed.) McGraw-Hill, New York, 1972.
11. Tedesco, T. A., and Mellman, W. J. Galactosemia: Evidence for a structural gene mutation. *Science,* 1971, **172:** 727–728.
12. Tomkins, G. M., Gelehrter, T. D., Granner, D., Martin, D. M., Samuels, H. H., and Thompson, E. B. Control of specific gene expression in higher organisms. *Science,* 1969, **166:** 1474–1480.
13. Watson, J. D., and Crick, F. H. C. Genetical implications of the structure of deoxyribonucleic acid. *Nature (Lond.),* 1953, **171:** 964–967.

Epilogue

ALBERT DORFMAN
Joseph P. Kennedy, Jr., Mental Retardation Research Center, Department of Pediatrics, Pritzker School of Medicine, The University of Chicago, Chicago, Illinois

In the following remarks I will try to give my impressions of the window into neurobiology as seen first from the point of view of a biochemist and cell biologist and finally from the point of view of a pediatrician concerned with the care of children with mental retardation.

In the recent past, biochemists have become more and more concerned with the integration of metabolic systems. The earliest biochemical studies were concerned with the end results of metabolic systems as evidenced by the analyses of whole organisms, blood, urine, etc. With the developments starting just before World War II and expanding rapidly thereafter, such systems were dissected by the isolation of enzymes and determination of metabolic pathways. While such isolated systems seemed originally distant from physiology, it has now become quite clear that information derived from such studies was necessary for the understanding of physiological systems. Perhaps one of the great milestones of scientific achievement has been the development of the understanding of the mechanism by which genetic information is transmitted from generation to generation as well as the mechanism by which this information controls the expression of cell activity. For the most part, this progress has been made utilizing prokaryotic systems. We are now entering an era of more intensive study of the eukaryotic cell. Research on prokaryotic cells has provided a wealth of information of the basic biochemical and genetic mechanisms characteristic of living matter. We now must utilize this information to determine which mechanisms obtain in eukaryotic cells and which new mechanisms have been evolved to carry out the functions unique to eukaryotic cells.

Two striking differences between the two types of systems are immediately apparent. Prokaryotic cells are self-contained entities which carry out all their functions as individual cells while eukaryotic cells exist in organisms with specialization of function for individual types of cells. Furthermore, the specialized cells of the organized systems are mutually interdependent and appear to send messages to each other, that is they engage in cell talk. At present, a large part of biological research is concerned with this problem. The implications of such communication are profound. Involved is a determination of: (a) the stimulus which results in sending of messages, (b) the nature of the message, (c) the receptor for the message, and (d) the manner in which the receptor converts the message to change the behavior of the receiving cell. The development of all these functions represents the problem of differentiation of eukaryotic cells.

It has become increasingly apparent that the cell membrane is of critical importance in all of these phenomena. Already great progress has been made in dissecting the structure of membranes. Most important has been the recognition of the complex and dynamic structure of such membranes, particularly the realization of the presence of macromolecules which serve to act as receptors for particular messages.

In the case of certain types of cells such as the erythrocyte, a clearer picture of this integrated system is beginning to emerge. It seems likely that an understanding of the structure of membranes of a wide variety of other cells will eventually lead to greater comprehension of the nervous system. If one adopts a developmental and evolutionary point of view, one may regard the nervous system as the ultimate in a system of cells specialized for the purpose of communication. The nervous system probably utilizes the general mechanisms but has additionally evolved new and specialized mechanisms.

The great progress in understanding communication in cells, other than in the nervous system, has occurred largely as a result of improved methods of tissue culture. In the case of the cells of the nervous system this is as yet limited, although progress is being made. The reports of Dr. de Vellis and Dr. Dichter give us an insight into the status of such studies. With the development of tissue culture lines of mouse neuroblastoma and rat glial cells there has been intense activity in many laboratories. Much valuable information regarding the metabolic properties of such cells has been obtained. With use of explants some information regarding integration is beginning to emerge. However, the use of cell or organ culture of the nervous system continues to have severe limitations compared with work on other tissues. The failure of normal differentiated neurons to divide in culture represents a serious stumbling block. The available systems of culture are not yet satisfactory for the study of differentiation of the nervous system.

I would like to digress to point out the kind of studies which are being carried out in culture in other tissues. In our own laboratory we have been primarily concerned with the differentiation of cartilage. We have used this model because of the existence of a considerable background of information regarding the biochemical parameters which constitute the phenotypic expression of this tissue and because differentiation of cartilage may be observed in cell culture. These studies have been recently reviewed (4). When chick limb-bud cells at stage 24 are dissociated and cultured on plastic dishes at usual cell densities, cartilage differentiation does not occur when measured by morphology, formation of metachromatic matrix, or synthesis of large amounts of chondroitin sulfate proteoglycan. If, however, such cells are cultured at very high density or over agar for 48 hours and then subcultured on plastic dishes, differentiation to cartilage is rapid. Apparently during this short period of time some event occurs which activates the machinery for expression of the cartilage phenotype. It has been possible to show that cells cultured over agar or at high density go on to produce large amounts of chondroitin sulfate proteoglycan and cartilage specific collagen.

In recent years a large literature has appeared demonstrating that the thymidine analog, 5′-bromodeoxyuridine (BrdU), inhibits the phenotypic expression of a number of specialized cells. This effect appears to be due to the replacement of thymidine in DNA by BrdU. When limb buds are subjected to BrdU during the early period of culture and subsequently subcultured in the absence of BrdU, differentiation does not subsequently occur even though no detectable BrdU remains in the DNA. In contrast, when differentiated cartilage cells are subjected to BrdU, the suppression of differentiated function is reversible. Similar experiments have now been performed in a number of other systems. These results suggest that in the course of differentiation of eukaryotic cells there is a specific sequence of events which is time ordered. Once this sequence is disturbed, the opportunity may not again occur.

In the case of the nervous system the problem of differentiation appears to be more complex. The studies presented by Drs. Rakic and Altman begin to give some insight into some of the phases of differentiation. It seems likely that the multiplication and initial differentiation of neuroepithelial cells may be more akin to the differentiation of cartilage or muscle. Subsequently, other important events must occur before an integrated nervous system is formed. It is important to note that at least two developmental processes, myelination and migration, require the cooperation of at least two different cell types. The experiments of Dr. Rakic indicate that migration may be guided by glial elements. A most interesting question that has not to my knowledge been addressed is the nature of the milieu through which cells migrate. It might be expected that the matrix between cells plays an important role in migration. The existence of genetic mutants which apparently show disturbances of migration may offer a useful tool for the study of the chemical structure of the glial processes which appear to guide migration as well as the milieu through which such migration occurs.

When one thinks of the many specific cell surface components that have recently been identified, it is unlikely that studies by classic methods of staining will give us answers with respect to developmental deviations in brain development. It also seems unlikely that anatomical studies on patients labeled as mentally retarded will produce meaningful answers until the patients are adequately sorted out from a clinical point of view.

Dr. Popják has already summarized the current state of the art as well as future directions of research concerning metabolic diseases which result in mental retardation. I would like to emphasize the importance of a genetic approach. Whenever we can identify a clinical syndrome for which clearcut Mendelian transmission exists, we have a potent tool for the investigation of etiology. In the case of recessive diseases, it appears safe to assume that the disease stems from an abnormality of a single gene product. No matter how bizarre the combination of clinical manifestations, explanation will be found eventually to have a single biochemical basis which may in turn lead to many complex abnormalities. The self-destructive behavior of patients with the Lesch-Nyhan syndrome is an excellent example of this principle.

In the case of dominant diseases the biochemical basis is less clear. Our own work on Marfan's disease (3,5) suggests an increase of hyaluronic acid synthesis which might involve a regulatory mechanism. The recent studies by Goldstein and Brown (1,2) on Type II hyperlipidemia strongly indicate a regulatory defect in this dominant disease which appears to be due to an absence of a cell receptor. I am emphasizing this point because I believe the road to elucidation of specific syndromes of mental retardation may be the careful clinical description which may in turn lead to appreciation of the genetics and subsequent elucidation of the biochemical defect.

Elucidation of biochemical mechanisms is not confined to genetic diseases. The presentations of Drs. Heller and Tennyson point the way to a new level of understanding of transmission of signals within the nervous system. Whether or not the exact mechanisms postulated turn out to be correct, they represent a step forward in the attempt to fathom the mechanisms by which messages are transmitted.

I would like now to jump ahead to the contributions that we have heard regarding behavior studies. Anyone who has dealt with retarded children realizes the difficulties of classification. Despite great faith in biochemistry and cell biology, we all know that a large part of the problem lies in social, economic, and educational problems. The extent of this is not clear. As is apparent from the presentations, we cannot yet define adequately the mechanisms by which these factors produce retardation. I refer, of course, to importance of *in utero* nutrition or early infant nutrition as compared to the effects of environment on early development. Here, I believe, great progress can be made by psychologists in defining specific characteristics that may be related to etiology. We all now accept that defects in performance may be very specific. The unraveling of these defects may help us define etiology. While we as physicians and scientists cannot control the economic and social environment, whenever we can discover specific etiological factors, the chances of society listening to us are greatly enhanced. Witness the great progress that has been made in the last few years in the control of lead poisoning, an important cause of mental retardation. Although treatment has been of some importance in decreasing the effects of this toxin, most of the progress has been made by control of the environment.

Research in mental retardation is in many ways frustrating because of the very nature of the problem. Since mental retardation involves so many etiologies, each of us has had to confine ourselves to a very limited sphere. In turn, in each sphere progress is dependent on the evolution of fundamental knowledge. In the past few years we have had increasing pressure on research both from limitation of funding and threats of increasing regulation of clinical research. Proposed legislation and administrative regulations would severely hamper work on fetuses which may be of critical importance in studies of development of the brain. Regulation of testing might make further vaccine development virtually impossible. I am not convinced that either the decreased funding or the regulation stems from public outcry, but I think rather from a small group of people who do not understand the issues. I believe it is encumbent on us to attempt to counter these things but not by unrealistic promises or exaggerated claims. Most of all we must be true to ourselves as scientists and physicians and continue to seek the truth for its own sake as well as to alleviate human suffering.

REFERENCES

1. Brown, M. S., Dana, S. E., and Goldstein, J. L. Regulation of 3-hydroxy-3-methylglutaryl coenzyme A reductase activity in cultured human fibroblasts. Comparison of cells from a normal subject and from a patient with homozygous familial hypercholesterolemia. *J. Biol. Chem.*, 1974, **249:** 789–796.
2. Goldstein, J. L., and Brown, M. S. Familial hypercholesterolemia: Identification of a defect in the regulation of 3-hydroxy-3-methylglutaryl coenzyme A reductase activity associated with overproduction of cholesterol. *Proc. Natl. Acad. Sci. U. S.*, 1974, **70:** 2804–2808.
3. Lamberg, S. I., and Dorfman, A. Synthesis and degradation of hyaluronic acid in the cultured fibroblasts of Marfan's disease. *J. Clin. Invest.*, 1973, **52:** 2428–2433.
4. Levitt, D., Ho, P.-L., and Dorfman, A. Differentiation of cartilage. In: *Cell Surface in Development.* (A. A. Moscona, Ed.). Wiley, New York, 1974: Chapter 6, pp. 101–125.
5. Matalon, R., and Dorfman, A. The accumulation of hyaluronic acid in cultured fibroblasts of the Marfan syndrome. *Biochem. Biophys. Res. Commun.*, 1968, **32:** 150–154.

Author Index

Numbers in parentheses are reference numbers and indicate that an author's work is referred to although his name is not cited in the text. Numbers in italics show the page on which the complete reference is listed.

SUBJECT INDEX

A

B

C

A 5
B 6
C 7
D 8
E 9
F 0
G 1
H 2
I 3
J 4